Floral Absolutes

"With deep knowledge, Candice doesn't just describe floral absolutes—she introduces you to them. Each essence becomes a companion on a journey of emotional and energetic healing, turning the reading experience into an intimate, enchanted walk through a soul-lit garden."

JENNIFER JOHNSON, SOMATIC INTUITIVE ADVISOR AND THE FORMER SENIOR DIRECTOR OF CHOPRA GLOBAL MIND-BODY PROGRAMS

"Candice Covington has created a magical journey through the world of floral absolutes. Her descriptive and evocative language guides readers through a dreamscape filled with the wisdom and beauty of these extraordinary oils. This book teaches how to work with the subtle body, craft intentional blends, and infuse scent with story and art. A truly beautiful and inspiring read—a must for anyone passionate about aromatherapy."

AILYNN HALVORSON, CLINICAL AROMATHERAPIST AND AUTHOR OF *The Tarot Apothecary*

"Candice Covington invites you to indulge in a sensual, nature-aligned journey imbued with soul searching and imagination. Within this insightful tome, you will find the unusual alongside the ordinary."

HEATHER DAWN GODFREY, PGCE, B.Sc. (HON), AUTHOR OF *Essential Oils for the Whole Body* AND *Healing with Essential Oils*

"*Floral Absolutes* is a one-of-a-kind treasure for anyone drawn to the beauty and power of scent. Candice Covington goes far beyond the basics, unveiling the soul of each botanical through a stunning blend of science, myth, intuition, and practical wisdom. This book will quickly become your go-to guide for working with the radiance of floral absolutes."

ANITA KALNAY, REGISTERED AROMATHERAPIST RA EOT AND OWNER OF FLYING COLORS NATURAL PERFUMES

"Candice Covington writes with the heart of a mystic and the clarity of a gifted teacher. In *Floral Absolutes*, she offers an extraordinary perspective on plants—seeing them not merely as healing tools but as conscious storytellers and spiritual companions. This book invites a deeper relationship with the natural world."

AMANDA REE, CANINE WELLNESS PRACTITIONER AND OWNER OF SAMA DOG

"More than just a treatise on essential oils or a collection of recipes, *Floral Absolutes* by Candice Covington is an encyclopedic journey into the mysteries of the plant world. Drawing on her profound understanding of floral energetics, Candice weaves together myth, art, story, ritual, and embodied wisdom to create an immersive guide for using scent to heal both body and soul."

LESLIE ZEMENEK, HAND ANALYST, ASTROLOGER, AND LIFE PURPOSE GUIDE

"*Floral Absolutes* is a masterful exploration of floral oils, uniquely enriched by archetypal parallels that bring depth and dimension to Covington's vast knowledge. Her understanding of each plant—alongside the benefits and techniques of working with these oils—is both informative and captivating."

MELISSA CARVER, PH.D., AUTHOR OF *WHO THE HELL TOLD YOU THAT?*

"With the grace of one who walks between worlds, Candice offers us more than a book—this is a soul-born offering, woven with presence and deep devotion. Each page shimmers with timeless wisdom, gently guiding us back to the knowing that lives in our bones. This book is a song to my soul—a gateway to remembrance, reverence, and a tender realignment with the Earth's quiet magic."

KELIE MICHO, FOUNDER OF RUBY ROSE SANCTUARY

"I've read many books and writings on plants, but this one truly stands out. The plants Candice includes—and the stories she shares—feel deeply intentional and refreshingly unique. *Floral Absolutes* is perfect."

CHRISTY SWENSON, FOUNDER OF ALOESWOOD BEAUTY

Floral Absolutes

Aromatic Healing for the Physical, Emotional, and Energy Body

Candice Covington

Healing Arts Press
Rochester, Vermont

Healing Arts Press
One Park Street
Rochester, Vermont 05767
www.HealingArtsPress.com

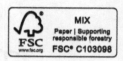

Healing Arts Press is a division of Inner Traditions International

Copyright © 2025 by Candice Covington

All rights reserved. No part of this book may be reproduced or utilized in any form or by any means, electronic or mechanical, including photocopying, recording, or any information storage and retrieval system, without permission in writing from the publisher. No part of this book may be used or reproduced to train artificial intelligence technologies or systems.

Note to the reader: This book is intended to be an informational guide. The remedies, approaches, and techniques described herein are meant to supplement, and not to be a substitute for, professional medical care or treatment. They should not be used to treat a serious ailment without prior consultation with a qualified health care professional.

Cataloging-in-Publication Data for this title is available from the Library of Congress

ISBN 978-1-64411-738-5 (print)
ISBN 978-1-64411-739-2 (ebook)

Printed and bound in the United States by Lake Book Manufacturing, LLC

10 9 8 7 6 5 4 3 2 1

Text design and layout by Kenleigh Manseau
This book was typeset in Garamond Premier Pro with Itangiuh and Rig Sans used as display typefaces.

To send correspondence to the author of this book, mail a first-class letter to the author c/o Inner Traditions, One Park Street, Rochester, VT 05767, and we will forward the communication, or contact the author directly at **DivineArchetypes.org**.

Scan the QR code and save 25% at InnerTraditions.com. Browse over 2,000 titles on spirituality, the occult, ancient mysteries, new science, holistic health, and natural medicine.

*To Mother Nature, our original storyteller and caretaker.
I thank you with all of my heart for all the beauty given.*

Contents

Foreword by Elizabeth Ashley   ix

Acknowledgments   xiii

Introduction
Meeting Nature in Story   1

PART 1
The Profiles
Energetic Signatures of Nature's Gifts

1   Absolutes   8
    Solvent-Extracted Concentrated Plant Extracts

2   Essential Oils   85
    Steam-Distilled or Expressed Plant Extracts

3   Fixed Oils   107
    The Carriers for Blending

4   Other Tantalizing Tidbits   149
    Macerated Oils, Milk Baths, Plant Butters, and Unrefined Salts

PART 2

The Body Ecstatic
Exploring the Body's Energetic Patterns

5   Our Body as Expressed in the Elements   178
    Earth, Water, Fire, Air, Ether

6   The Chakras   205
    The Seven Centers of Spiritual Power

7   Symbolic Anatomy   219
    The Body as Story

PART 3

The Blends
Recipes, Prompts, and Inspiration

8   Alchemical Creations   262
    Blending Story, Art, and Sensations

9   Butter, Scrub, and Oil Recipes   309
    Waking Up Archetypal Stories Within

Appendix Practices for Growth, Heart
Opening, and Deep Purification   336

Resources   349

Notes   352

Bibliography   356

Index   360

About the Author   370

Foreword

Elizabeth Ashley

The current fascination with essential oils is focused on the corporeal aspects of our being. Yet science has increasingly acknowledged that our physical wellness equally depends on our emotional and mental balance, such that today the mind, body, and spirit are equally involved in making a healthy, whole human being. This holistic vision is supported by the emergence in recent years of complementary medicine, a science-based form of medicine that embraces the plant healer's knowledge of natural alternatives. As a result, the internet is flooded with essential oil recipes for pain, depression, anxiety, and many other conditions.

Progress, some might say. In reality, though, most of these recipes are considered mere adjuncts to a doctor's primary recommendations, which nearly always involve taking a pill. Where is the acknowledgement that a person's struggle with environmental factors is what's making their back ache? What about the woman so terrified by her own sensuality that her pelvis screams in agony each month? How does a man, oppressed by his superiors, overcome his workplace strife to slay the dragon, which is the source of his migraine? The true source of a person's pain is rarely addressed by the conventional medical system. To paraphrase Descartes, "I think, therefore I am—in pain!" And it's true—a person's illness can often be explained by some conflict held within the emotional or mental body.

It's the recognition of the union of body-mind-spirit that brings aromatherapy to life. Aromatherapy is no longer considered emergency first aid but instead a holistic journey to self-discovery, an invitation to the Oracle of Delphi's maxim to "Know thyself." Then and only then the perfumery box becomes a wondrous healing tool bursting with safety data and contraindications, but all too frequently lacking "operating instructions" on how to heal the heart.

And it is in the heart where you will find the realm of the mythic, where both flights of fantasy and broken dreams lie dormant, where you will find magic carpets that no longer leave the floor, and hinges too rusty to "open sesame."

For so many of us, the twinkle has been extinguished and the magic has gone out of our lives thanks to age and its concurrent responsibilities. How then can we ever hope to draw forth the magical powers of Excalibur when we don't have the time or even the inclination to create magic? And yet a place of mystery awaits us, where the hero triumphs over demons and everyone lives happily ever after.

I guess the truth is that we all have to start somewhere. The mythologist Joseph Campbell famously said that the hero never begins as a hero. He becomes a hero, and that entails the annihilation of his own unheroic former self through a death and rebirth experience. The hero always undergoes a metamorphosis, from the ordinary to the extraordinary. Like a snake, the hero sheds her skin and takes on a new form.

Ah, but how to train the hero? Now, there's the rub! How do we tempt her away from the computer screen to embark on an odyssey back to herself? What tools are needed for the quest? Most assuredly, a compass to navigate the treacherous journey, a map that points out where the dragons lay and indicates dangerous choppy waters. We need a dark mirror that reflects the soul's shadowy corners and a magical potion consisting of wondrous healing herbs exuding a scent so glorious that nobody can resist it.

But where does one find a twenty-first century sorceress, a guide capable of creating and transmitting knowledge of such a beguiling elixir?

Who better to coach the aromatic apprentice than Candice Covington! Candice is a mistress of myth and a huntress of the most mystical hedgerow bounty who possesses an encyclopedic knowledge of seductive species and unusual herbs. The wonderful stories that Candice has collected for each plant—some of them completely new to me—offer a thousand prescriptions for the challenges we all face day to day.

The glory of a myth is that it is a living, breathing thing. It twists and turns and morphs a tale into a story specifically about us, where we are the hero or heroine, and the gods are close behind. Myths are full of truths and insights about how to progress and where to go next. Archetypical struggles remain as salient and relevant today as they were for the ancient Greeks.

The goddess of abundance and fertility, Demeter, speaks of the harvest but also about the challenges of being a mother and the grief she bears for crimes against her kin, the plant kingdom. We may not have had the good fortune to meet the goddess of love, Aphrodite, on a romantic quest, but her glorious plants stand in her stead, a garden full of species that speak to the trials and tribulations of love. Inexplicably, the stories of these and many more plants unfold in the vapors they exude. And as they speak, they touch aspects of our personality that ordinary conversations simply cannot touch.

I can think of nowhere better to study the lessons of Eden and the medicine of the nose than this treasure map of a book.

Get ready, reader, to embark on a sensory trip like no other, a journey into scentsual myth.

ELIZABETH ASHLEY began using essential oils at the age of eight when she was introduced to them by her mother, who was one of the founding members of the International Federation of Aromatherapists and one of the first aromatherapists in the UK. Since then, Elizabeth has gone on to write over twenty essential oil manuals and several courses, including thirteen Amazon bestsellers. Her most recent book is *Meeting the Melissae: The Ancient Greek Bee Priestesses of Demeter*. She is the co-creator of the *Tongue of the Trees* aromatherapy oracle cards and associated video training packages. Her books track herbal medicines from their first mentions in prehistory right up to the most current scientific research. Elizabeth brings a uniquely balanced approach to the study of aromatherapy, with one foot firmly in the scientific camp and the other drifting dreamily through the land of myth and legend.

Acknowledgments

My heart is so soft as I recently had an extended visit to the valley in Provo, Utah, where I grew up. This has allowed me to reconnect with my parents, Sandra and Harold; my sisters, Andera, Jaime, and Cherilynn; and my childhood best friend, Mary Jane. I have also made new friends, the kind that change one's life, with Lisa and Wendy. Last but not least, I cherish the profound opportunity to once again be hugged by the nature that shaped my early years—the cottonwood, cattails, Russian olives, and pod milkweed!

A heartfelt thank-you to my editors, Jamaica Burns Griffin, whose gentle touch and boundless wisdom help bring the essence of my work to life, and Margaret Jones, whose keen eye and attention to detail ensures everything is as clear as possible. And to Dr. Porter for her timeless inspiration.

Introduction
Meeting Nature in Story

Everything is an expression of spiritual consciousness, which spiritualizes by its inherent life all matter.

ALICE BAILEY

This is not a straightforward, "just the facts" aromatherapy book; instead, it is an invitation to begin the journey of discovering what these plant distillations can awaken, cultivate, or restrain within you—how they can support all levels of your being—body, mind, and spirit. Being human is complex, difficult, and even frightening even in the best of times. We are often faced with worries and uncertainty as we navigate the human experience. So many of my clients have a clear idea of where they want to go and what they want to accomplish, yet they encounter internal and external blocks that stymie them. Past experiences that play out in the mind and emotional body illuminate loss and the road less traveled. All this is held in the vessel of the self as one learns, grows, and hopefully finds contentment and true joy.

Blessed are we, as wisdom traditions from all cultures remind us. The intelligence that organizes the activity of humankind also orchestrates the activity of the universe, as the microcosm that is the human body and the macrocosm that is the entire cosmos are mirror reflections of each other. Understanding this allows for a deeper relationship with nature and shows us how to use her gifts to navigate our own nature.

My hope in writing this book is that when you engage with nature you see her as an extension of yourself and the plants as aspects of you—and you in them. We are intimately and forever intertwined, made from the same raw materials: the same recycled earth, life force, mind, and spirit. The inner intelligence of our bodies is the ultimate and supreme genius of nature and mirrors the wisdom of the universe. I believe nature to be the kindest of teachers, one who is always refining and bringing out the best of us.

Over the years I have been curious about the ways in which nature communicates with us. There are, of course, many ways, but recently I have fallen in love with nature as a storyteller. I once heard Deepak Chopra say that he believed that what pushed human beings forward in their evolution is our ability to value stories and tell stories. *Homo sapiens sapiens* is, as we know, the species to which all modern human beings belong, one of several species grouped into the genus *Homo*, but it is today the only one that is not extinct. This fascinated me, and I started to think about where we got our original stories from. Who shaped what we value? What we fear? What we hold with reverence? What we find beautiful? Why do all cultures share common archetypes? I believe that it was nature who told us our first stories. And if we really listen to her, we discover that nothing is just one thing. It is many things at once.

Paraphrasing Marcel Proust, upon drinking the juice of an orange squeezed into water, it reveals the secret life of its ripening and growth and a hundred mysteries to the senses, but not to the intellect. What mysteries took root in this writer's soul and slowly bloomed into his conscious awareness and in turn shaped his storytelling?

Let's consider the simple act of smelling. A carnation smells like a carnation, although if you ask a perfumer they would say you are smelling clove, green (yes, they use color to explain scent), fresh, wintergreen, fruity, and resinous.

René Magritte (1898–1967), one of my favorite painters, explained his surrealist masterpiece *The Son of Man* as a self-portrait. This famous painting depicts a man in an overcoat and a bowler hat standing in front of a wall, beyond which is the sea and a cloudy sky. The man's face is largely obscured by a large green apple floating in the space in front of him, and his eyes can be seen peeking out from behind the apple. Of the apple, Magritte explains,

> At least it hides the face partly. Well, so you have the apparent face, the apple, hiding the visible but hidden, the face of the person. It's something that happens constantly. Everything we see hides another thing, we always want to see what is hidden by what we see. There is an interest in that which is hidden and which the visible does not show us. This interest can take the form of a quite intense feeling, a sort of conflict, one might say, between the visible that is hidden and the visible that is present."[1]

Magritte featured apples in many of his paintings, and it's fair to say that the ever-complex apple was his constant guide and muse. As a surrealist, Magritte was known for his depictions of familiar objects in unfamiliar, unexpected contexts, which often provoked questions about the nature and boundaries of reality and its representations. His paintings encourage viewers to seek the form behind the form, the story behind the obvious. He once famously remarked that the apple can represent the perpetual tension between the hidden and visible.

The American Buddhist nun and teacher Thubten Chodron believes that nature organizes herself into specific arrangements to teach us that we have the capacity to recognize and understand specific states of being. In her opinion that is why buddhas who can emanate in any configuration choose specific shapes and colors to guide us, expressing themselves in certain ways so that we can understand the qualities being conveyed:

> They need a way to communicate with us to lead us on the path out of suffering to full enlightenment. Since we are embodied beings who relate to color, shape, and other objects of the senses, the compassionate

Buddhas appear in various forms in order to communicate with us ... they appear in different manifestations to emphasize certain characteristics. For example, an artist or a musician has an internal feeling or meaning he wants to express. In order to communicate it, he draws a picture with color and shape ... to express what's going on inside. In a similar way, Buddhas express their realizations in different external forms.[2]

Surely this universal template is based on nature's original design. Nature is the consummate storyteller, possessing an exceptionally rich pallet of colors and hues that shape our deepest places and inform how we think, feel, and grow. Jesus used the mustard seed as a metaphor to teach the principle of faith and patience that is needed to grow from something small into something great. Any metaphor could have been used, but the minuscule mustard seed communicates this concept so well.

English poet John Milton (1608–1674), in Book 5 of his masterpiece *Paradise Lost*, uses plants to shape readers' emotions to create a vivid mental picture that could not be adequately conveyed otherwise:

> *[The archangel Raphael] now is come*
> *Into the blissful field, through Groves of Myrrh,*
> *And flowering Odours, Cassia, Nard and Balm;*
> *A Wilderness of sweets; for Nature here*
> *Wantoned as in her prime, and played at will*
> *Her Virgin Fancies, pouring forth more sweet,*
> *Wild above Rule or Art; enormous bliss.*
> *Him, through the spicy Forest onward come,*
> *Adam discerned, as in the door he sat*
> *Of his cool Bower.*

The great American naturalist and poet Henry David Thoreau (1817–1862), whose soul screamed in ecstasy when it came to nature, expressed these feelings in his writing, which still captivates us today:

Early apples begin to be ripe about the first of August, but I think that none of them are so good to eat as some to smell. One is worth more to scent your handkerchief with than any perfume which they sell in the shops. The fragrance of some fruits is not to be forgotten, along with the flowers. Some gnarly apple which I pick up in the road reminds me by its fragrance all the wealth of Pomona. . . . There is thus about all natural products a certain volatile and ethereal quality which represents their highest value, which cannot be vulgarized.[3]

The stories told by members of the plant kingdom captivate us through their scent and sight, and I believe that through our interdependence with all of nature we are hardwired to resonate with their energies. For example, there is common agreement on what specific colors convey in terms of energy and colors arise from nature. Shapes have long been used to make us feel certain ways, and shapes also arise from nature. There are numerous fascinating studies that have been done on how scent can manipulate the emotions and create mental pictures, and scent arises from nature. Plants are characters in myths, folklore, poetry, art, and contemporary literature; they express states of being and teach us how to navigate the complexity of being human.

For example, blueberries are perfectly round with a five-pointed star shape that is formed at the blossom end of the berry. Their blue skin is the rarest color on earth and is highly evocative. The peach has frequently been used by poets to describe the essence of a woman's moist cleft. The people of ancient Athens, before it was named as such, were given a choice: Athena offered an olive tree while Poseidon offered a horse. The people chose Athena's gift, and she became their patron. Every time you use olive oil it carries the echo of countless stories of those who came before you as well as the story of the goddess Athena, which is embedded in the fruity oil. If you want to know Athena, use olive oil. Myth and folklore are replete with stories of nymphs and humans being turned into plants, children being born of fruit and vegetables, and beautiful women who are really trees.

What I am putting forward is that nature is the more aware side in our conversation with her, and she is highly effective in using language that transcends words. My wish is that this book will help us listen more sensitively to her and really take the time to lean into and decode the wondrous volume of information from those people past and present who are in essence her storytellers.

How to Read This Book

Allow your soul and mind to meet in story. Some of the plant profiles are not exactly "how-to" guides but rather a wonderous and evocative call to dance with the Divine. Allow yourself to be fed, nourished, and grow in ways that you may never have even imagined. Some descriptions are straightforward, where I offer a snapshot of the plant's personality that describes a specific state of being that you can leverage. Some descriptions might leave more questions than answers in your mind. Some might provide the answer to what you have been looking for. Some might be couched in the mythical language of your dreams. A fun aspect of this book is the blending section found in part 3, where we learn how to use plant distillations to express a feeling or a sensation as a way to touch our ephemeral nature.

All the descriptions are in the language of the Divine and as such they offer a way to start a conversation with aspects of yourself that may lie dormant, just waiting for a way to communicate with you, eagerly waiting to help you learn and grow. Hopefully this book will allow you to process mythically, understanding your role on the larger stage that is the universe. This will allow you to view your life with softer eyes and a sense of wonderment. I have found that this makes navigating life, even the hard edges, much more manageable and delightful. Because no matter the situation, nature offers a subtle solution.

PART 1
The Profiles
Energetic Signatures of Nature's Gifts

1

Absolutes

Solvent-Extracted Concentrated Plant Extracts

To see a World in a Grain of Sand
And a Heaven in a Wild Flower
Hold Infinity in the palm of your hand
And Eternity in an hour

WILLIAM BLAKE

An absolute is a plant distillation and one of the most concentrated forms of fragrance, cherished in natural perfumery. It differs from an essential oil in that it contains not only essential oil, but also a higher density of coloring, waxes, and other constituents from the plant. This tells you what an absolute is on the physical level. On a subtle level, these concentrated distillations speak to the rich tapestry of spirit and soul to reveal the subtle and unique aspects of each. We'll turn to His Holiness the Fourteenth Dalai Lama for more insight on spirit and soul:

> I call the light and high aspects of my being *spirit*, and the dark and heavy aspects *soul*. Soul is at home in the deep, shaded valleys. Heavy, torpid flowers saturated with black grow there. The rivers flow like warm syrup.

They empty into huge oceans of soul. Spirit is a land of high white peaks and glittering jewel-like lakes and flowers. Life is sparse and sounds travel great distances. There is soul music, soul food, and soul love. . . . People need to climb the mountain not simply because it is there, but because the soul to find divinity needs to be mated with the spirit.[1]

This chapter is all about absolutes, highly concentrated forms of plant essential oils. The descriptions of the plants speak to aspects of our soul and spirit. By exploring these plant energies in a storytelling form we can access their archetypes, which are also found within us. Reread these profiles from time to time as your deep places morph and change; what stands out for you will match whatever you need. Know that to use a plant distillation is to awaken and energize its living dispositions within you. Its qualities, used with focused intent, move to the forefront of your personality, creating a state of being that allows you to embody the presiding deity or energy and the archetypal traits they radiate.

About Botanical Extractions

A botanical extraction is the process of removing desired chemical components from a plant to separate it from its initial source. For botanicals, many different parts of the plant can be used, such as the stem, root, flower, or fruit. The result is an oil that contains the compounds of interest without the solid plant material.

There are various methods of extraction, some of which go back to ancient Egypt. In this book we are concerned primarily with three methods: solvent extraction, steam distillation, and expression (cold-pressed or expeller-pressed).

Solvent Extraction—Absolutes

An absolute is a highly concentrated extraction used in perfumery and aromatherapy. When steam distillation is not possible due to the delicate nature of many flowers and plants, in which the intense heat of this process would destroy the plant matter and the plant has a relatively low amount of essential oil by volume, then an extraction method that uses an organic solvent is used to "lift" the aromatic plant oils. This method captures far more of the flower's true aroma than is possible with other methods, such as steam distillation, hence absolutes are more potent than steam-distilled essential oils. In addition, because this process does not use heat or water, none of the important water-soluble aromatic compounds are lost as they are in steam distillation. This means a higher yield is obtained from a crop when producing absolutes.

Plant parts (often flower petals) are submerged in an organic solvent such as ethanol or hexane to release their aroma. The solvent mixture dissolves the aromatic compounds of the plant and releases them into the liquid. The solvent is then removed, leaving behind a fragrant, concentrated mixture known as an *absolute*. Absolutes differ from essential oils in that they contain not only essential oil, but also a higher density of coloring, waxes, and other constituents from the plant. These are generally very thick and require a high dilution rate. More and more today you can find absolutes that have been extracted with solvents such as fixed oils and alcohol to coax the aromatic essence out of the plant material, resulting in a bioavailable essence that's been extracted very gently, without added heat, that captures the intricate aroma of the original plant material.

When blending absolutes with a fixed oil (also called *carrier oil* to describe oils such as coconut, olive, and sunflower that can be blended with absolutes and essential oils), I cannot stress this enough: *less is more*! In general absolutes smell better at a 1–2 percent dilution rate with a fixed oil.

Steam Distillation—Essential Oils

Essential oils are located in tiny secretory structures found in various parts of plants such as leaves, berries, grasses, flowering tops, petals, roots, resins, and wood. An essential oil will typically contain more than a hundred different chemical compounds. All essential oils possess antiseptic properties, but many also have antifungal, antiviral, and antibacterial properties as well.

Essential oils are mostly obtained as a result of steam distillation, considered the most commonly used method of extraction. The plant material is placed in a still and then hot steam is passed through it. The intense heat breaks open the essential oil storage chambers within the plant, releasing the volatile oils into the steam. The infused steam rises to the top of the still, where it enters a condenser—essentially a long spiral pipe surrounded by cold water—which condenses the steam back into water form. At the end of the condenser, the water and essential oil are collected in a sequestrator. This specially designed container has two outflows so the essential oil and hydrosol (water byproduct) don't mix. Essential oils are usually lighter than water and so the oil will float above it.

Steam distillation is environmentally friendly, and the equipment is safe and relatively easy to operate. Steam distillation produces pure compounds and reduces impurities better than the other methods. However, steam distillation has several disadvantages. It is slow and requires a long extraction time. The water used in steam distillation must be redistilled to optimize essential oil recovery and to recover dissolved oil components. Redistilling increases utility costs, particularly heating and energy costs.

....

Expression—Heat-Sensitive Essential Oils and Fatty Fixed Oils
Cold expression (or cold-pressed extraction), is the method used primarily in making heat-sensitive citrus peel essential oils as well as seeds, nuts, and certain other fruits. In this method the rinds of fruit (or the seeds or nuts) are squeezed until the oil glands burst, releasing the oil. In the case of citrus, the essential oil is obtained first by abrading or lacerating the citrus peels, which are subsequently centrifuged

to separate the volatile, aromatic molecules from the juice, peel solids, and heavier compounds such as waxes and flavonoids.

This method avoids the application of a direct heat source and operates at low temperatures (typically below 120°F). Cold-pressed extraction controls temperature through several techniques, including reducing screw rotation speed, taking frequent breaks while pressing, and using fans to cool the chamber of the press. Cold-pressed extraction is valued for its simplicity, safety, and its capacity to create premium natural products.

Virtually all fixed oils are expeller pressed. The oil is removed from the plant material—normally from the fatty portions (seeds, nuts, kernels) of foods we eat—by using a screw press or expeller, same as in the cold-pressed method. If the oil has many free-floating particles in it, it is run through an oil filter press. Expeller-pressed oils may have slightly reduced efficacy than cold-pressed oils, as temperatures can sometimes go as high as 200 degrees Fahrenheit during extraction; however, in most cases the difference between this technique and cold pressing is negligible.

❊ Aglaia (*Aglaia odorata*)

Presiding influence: the goddess Aglaia

Key energies: internal radiance, cooperation, reciprocity, state of grace, beauty, refinement, ability to respond in the moment, good luck, the number 6, love, desire, fertility, prosperity, peace, regeneration, sanctification

This small tree commonly known as Chinese perfume tree displays petite, golden-yellow, oval-shaped flowers with six petals that produce a heavenly scent. The number 6 holds the energy of structured dynamism, the ability to spontaneously respond in the moment and allow that feedback to restructure oneself. In Chinese culture, aglaia flowers are auspicious because they look like rice grains and are believed to bring wealth and good luck.

Named after the Greek goddess Aglaia, one of the Three Graces and the daughter of Zeus, she brings the principles of beauty, refinement, peace, and cooperation into everyday life. She is known as one of the goddess Venus's favored companions and a reflection of her traits of love, beauty, desire, fertility, and prosperity. Fifteenth-century Renaissance painter Francesco del Cossa sumptuously depicted Venus, the goddess of love, presiding over the month of April, with Mars (representing the principle of aggression, at least in part) chained at her feet, as doves (representing peace) fly at both sides of her head, with her favorite companion, Aglaia, by her side.

During the Renaissance, the dance of the Three Graces—Aglaia (personifying radiance), Euphrosyne (joy), and Thalia (flowering)—expressed the idea that any deed we do will come back to us. One of the sisters gives, the other receives, and the third returns the benefit. In this way one learns the dance of reciprocity. The Graces are frequently depicted with their hands interwoven in a circle, implying a state of grace that involves becoming whole and suggesting that a spontaneous, unmerited gift of divine favor operates in humankind for regeneration and sanctification.

> **Blending Tip** – Blend equal parts macerated saffron oil (see chapter 4) and fractionated coconut oil (see page 108) with 6 drops of aglaia absolute to cultivate your internal radiance.

❀ Benzoin Resin (*Styrax benzoin*)

Presiding influence: Inanna, Queen of Heaven and Earth; Ereshkigal, Queen of the Underworld

Key energies: being embodied, soul, descent, the underworld, wholeness, ascent, spirit, freedom from, making conscious, shifting awareness, personal struggles, opposing forces, death and rebirth, creative friction, integration, difficult wisdom, soul guide, bat medicine, place out of time, infinite creativity, empty essence

Benzoin resin, derived from the gum benjamin tree native to Indochina, is the essence of descent into and emergence from the underworld, one of the most difficult of all journeys, which is best explored through myth.

Descent into the underworld is about discovery, sitting in uncertainty, and collecting information. It is through descent that things of the mind and heart become embodied—ideas and knowledge become reality, and questions are answered on a meaningful level. Often the underworld is depicted as a fiery hell, a realm ruled by ancient and frightening forces long forgotten. Here lie riches beyond belief—pristine waters, gold, silver, diamonds, rubies, coal, oil, and all that they symbolize. These days, to be a plutocrat is to obtain riches from what lies beneath the earth; Pluto is the Greek god of the underworld, and this can also be read as mining one's psyche, soul, and unconscious for the riches found there.

The soulful aspect of this quest does not involve self-improvement, nor is it task-driven or a way of being released from the pain of being human. It does not explore the proper way to live and does not bestow judgments or reduce things into polarities—these are all the concerns of the upper world. This work touches a different dimension, one not independent from conscious waking life, with its constant problem-solving, but not identical to it either. You care for the soul by honoring its expressions and by creating time to let the soul express itself. You achieve this by living in a way that fosters depth, being (as opposed to doing), curiosity, and inwardness.

Soul is its own reason for being, both a purpose and an end. Here memory is more important than development, artistic expression is more important than reason, and love is more important than organization. Here we form attachments and revel in being alive.

Ascent is celestial in nature; it means climbing out of what makes us human. The goal here is to shed all vices and desires. This journey is *sattvic* in nature according to ayurveda and thus embodies the light-infused energy of purity. *Ascent* is from the Latin *ascendere*, "to climb," and is associated with freedom, emergence, elevation, and sublimation. It can be mythically viewed as taking flight, rising above, or a state of wingedness that suggests a more expansive, bird's-eye perspective. Here is where spirit dwells. Here one has conscious knowledge and moves it into the intellectual realm, assigning value, filtering and sorting, creating a hierarchy of values, and then drawing from earthly principles to arrive at universal concepts.

One of the more challenging aspects of this journey is to recognize the grasping, solipsistic, and very self-centered or selfish aspects of our nature. Then we must prepare to move into a different state of awareness, working with our fears and limitations so we can understand the struggles embedded in our psychic reality that have given rise to these kinds of reactions and behaviors.

Benzoin resin absolute helps give us pause and examine life's opposing forces: feminine and masculine, free will and rules, innocence and burgeoning sexuality, childhood and adulthood, life and death, good and evil, light and darkness, human and the Divine, fear and faith, anger and kindness, consciousness and lack of knowledge, and so on.

Here we get a chance to be reborn, if not physically, then in stages of understanding. This comes from the process of examining the creative friction that arises from a deep examination of opposing forces. This helps dissipate projected fears and distorted ideas so they can be integrated. Integration is the key.

Inanna, Queen of Heaven and Earth, was a most beloved deity of the ancient city of Sumner. The god of knowledge and water, Enki, gifted her with the keys to all positive and negative aspects of civilization and knowledge, known as the *me*. This gave her control over human affairs. Even though she now had the ability to rule both kingdoms, above and below, in perfection, her heart was discontented. She wanted *wholeness*, and so she voluntarily set out to the Great Below.

From the Great Above she opened her ear to the Great Below.
From the Great Above the goddess opened her ear to the Great Below.
From the Great Above Inanna opened her ear to the Great Below.[2]

When Inanna sought entrance to the underworld, she was forced to release the characteristics that constituted her sense of self at each of seven gates, and from there she was required to proceed naked and alone into the darkness of the netherworld. When she hesitated to do so she was told,

> *Quiet, Inanna, the ways of the underworld are perfect.*
> *They may not be questioned.*[3]

Inanna begins her descent into the underworld by abandoning her seven cities and her seven temples. As she descends further, she releases more levels of her projected self—her role as queen, holy priestess, woman, mother, sexual being, and so forth.

Her royal power, her priestly office, her sexual powers, which had helped her in her journey and encounter[s] . . . are of no avail in the underworld. In fact, all that Inanna had achieved on earth weighs against her when she meets the woman [her sister, Ereshkigal] at whose expense Inanna's glories had been attained. The all-seeing judges of the underworld perceive Inanna's hidden, split-off parts and condemn her. Ereshkigal cries out, "Guilty."[4]

Then Ereshkigal condemns her to death:

> *She struck her.*
> *Inanna was turned into a corpse,*
> *A piece of rotting meat,*
> *And was hung from a hook on the wall.*[5]

When three days and three nights had passed and Inanna had not returned, her faithful servant Ninshubur began to ask the gods to intervene for her safe return, as she could not do so herself. After two refusals for help, Enki finally set out to aid her. From under his fingernail he brought forth some dirt and fashioned it into a *kurgarra*, a creature neither male nor female. From under the fingernail of his other hand he produced more dirt and fashioned it into a *galatur*, a creature that was also neither female nor male. Enki gave the water of life to the galatur and the food of life to the kurgarra and told them how to enter the underworld as flies and win the favor of Ereshkigal by showing empathy for the goddess. Ereshkigal was moaning in pain "with the cries of a woman about to give birth," but had no attendants:

> *Ereshkigal, the Queen of the Underworld, is moaning*
> *With the cries of a woman about to give birth.*
> *No linen is spread over her body.*
> *Her breasts are uncovered.*
> *Her hair swirls about her head like leeks.*
> *When she cries, 'Oh! Oh! My inside!'*
> *Cry also, 'Oh! Oh! Your inside!'*
> *When she cries, 'Oh! Oh! My outside!'*
> *Cry also, 'Oh! Oh! Your outside!'*
> *The queen will be pleased.*
> *She will offer you a gift.*
> *Ask her only for the corpse that hangs from the hook on the wall.*
> *One of you will sprinkle the food of life on it.*
> *The other will sprinkle the water of life.*
> *Inanna will arise.*[6]

Ereshkigal is Inanna; she is also you and me. She is the archetype of the dark moon, the third face of the goddess, and wisdom. She is the dark place where difficult wisdom resides. She is the aspect of self from which we hide or shy away, the pieces of the self that have split off due to traumatic life experiences. Hers is also the realm in which one heals and is made whole before rebirth into the next cycle.

Here pure possibility exists—there are no causal laws with which to contend. This is the place of the shaman's death and rebirth, as represented by bat medicine. It is a place out of time and a source of infinite creativity.

There is wisdom in knowing the empty essence, and not merely the qualities that arise in the empty essence. This is an important energy to understand and work with because it is the great Source that exists within all of us, from which all aspects of our being arise, abide, and dissolve. I want you to pause and sit with this. Energy never ceases to be, although in this space you can reorganize any causation patterns—ways of being, thinking, and behaving. Here in the Great Below you can come to understand the lessons and rewards that arise from whatever creative friction you are trying to resolve, and once you have the information required for the next steps in life you can journey back.

A profound example of this sacred journey comes from the Sun Dancers of the Blackfoot Nation, who must fast for three days. During this time the dancer cannot even touch food or water—he or she must abstain from the vibration of food and water completely, and on the fourth day the dancers are revived by the food and water of life (represented by one cup of chicken broth) until they can break their fast the following day. This ritual mirrors the dry void; the three days of the moon's darkness; the hero's journey; and the death of the egoic self as, traversing within, it is stripped of its projections. This journey is the stuff myth is made of and must be undertaken if one desires wholeness.

One of the most fascinating aspects of the myth of Inanna's descent is that she did it with intent. She basically had done everything there was to do on Earth and in the Great Above, so she turned her attention to the last aspect of the self she had not explored and willingly traversed into her depths to reveal what lay in the darkness (which was not very much fun!).

This is unlike Persephone, who took the same trip, but in an unconscious way. Persephone's story starts when Gaia, at the will of Zeus, makes a narcissus bloom, and Persephone reaches down to pluck it and the earth opens, and Hades reaches out to abduct her. Traditionally this story is called "the rape of Persephone," which implies the violence the soul feels when it is not prepared to enter the depths voluntarily and instead waits for circumstances to push it forward on the journey. One aspect of the narcissus bloom (see Narcissus, this chapter) is its identification with the resolution of conflict by going to the center of the problem or fear. Even though Persephone was content to stay on the surface, her growth required a trip into the underworld, ready or not. While waiting for a rescue she eats one pomegranate seed, and from that time forward she spends a third of her time as the Queen of Hades (a role she grows to enjoy, as it is healthy to abide in both our upper and lower worlds). Even though eventually she gets everyone's blessing to return to the land of the living, she is unable to do so on her own without the help of the goddess Hecate, who guides her on her way out.

As we see from these myths, both of these great goddesses, Inanna and Persephone, needed help to leave the underworld once their work there was complete. Similarly, benzoin can act as a soul guide, holding space as you descend to do your inner work, and when that work is completed, helping you ascend.

I cannot emphasize this enough: write down your dreams (and keep a record of them), even if they seem nonsensical. Long before I read the story on Inanna, I had a significant dream that featured leeks, which prepared me for a journey to the underworld. I still do not fully understand the archetypal energy of leeks, but the journey into the depths will take the time it takes until your soul has awakened to what it must know. At this time in my waking life I was preparing to go north for a three-day fast to prepare for the Sundance, and the night before I left I had the following dream:

> *I was sleeping on a high wooden table in a pink mummy bag when a rabid dog that was wobbly and disoriented came up to the table. I was very concerned and frightened. Then a wise woman appeared and told me that during my time fasting I was not to take any flower essences (which*

I was planning on doing) because they managed my internal energy and I needed to do the work without help. I could not introduce an outside template. While in the dream I became aware that the emanation of the dog was an emanation of me. I needed to descend into the three days of darkness with no food, no water, no attendants, and in my case no flower essences. I needed to be alone in the starkness of the void. As I lay there in my dream listening to the wise woman, the dog morphed into a flat leek. This symbol from nature came to me to prepare me for my inner journey, which would repattern me on a deep level.

Many years later, I still cannot completely figure out this dream, and I still await this knowledge to be made conscious. I know I say this a lot and I will say it again—you cannot rush this kind of learning—it simply manifests when it's time.

· ·

Blending Tip – If you want to enter the Great Below but you're not sure how, blend narcissus (see description in this chapter) and benzoin in a pomegranate fixed oil (see chapter 3) to start your journey. Once you arrive, replace narcissus with orris root (see description in this chapter) and combine with benzoin to support your process. Once you're ready to return, use benzoin and labdanum (see description in this chapter) to ascend. I also suggest incorporating leek into your diet in a reverent way, as it helps you determine where you're at in your evolutionary journey.

· ·

❀ Black Currant (*Ribes nigrum*)

Presiding influence: seal

Key energies: twilight, in-between places, oceanic, waters of the womb, night journey, untangling the composite self, curiosity, slow unfolding, paying attention to details, sudden desires, working with the unconscious and dreams, liminal spaces, thresholds, enchantments, uncanny manifestations, magic, ritual, revelations

Day yielding to night reveals twilight. The archway that is the horizon holds within it the final splendor of the sun as it releases itself in a sliver of time, a gap, an in-between place, before mythically embarking on its night journey.

A feeling you could call oceanic arises, an evocation of being in the sea or immersed in the waters of the womb. The sea contains the vast potential of life, but in this aspect you are being asked to surrender some knowledge, thing, or way of being, thereby untangling the composite self and the ethos you have crafted over the years. The night-sea journey is a return to your primordial self and the waters of womb. This return is not to the false self that burns out and falls into judgment, but to your original Self, your higher Self, your greater and deeper being.

When I first started using black currant bud I had this dream:

> I was scuba diving in the pitch-black ocean and couldn't see anything, swimming along the ocean floor feeling with my hands as I swam. At first I was fine, curious and exploring. Suddenly it hit me that I was alone and couldn't see, as I was engulfed in darkness. I panicked and did not want to be there anymore. I swam straight up to the surface. Once I arrived there it was still dark, although the surface of the ocean was dimly lit by the moon and the stars, and it hit me—I was still alone, bobbing in the same body of water—that I was not safer on the surface. I was still exposed to everything that was beneath me, without any sanctuary due to the dim light. I felt helpless as I was pulled by the current, treading water. My scuba suit was not made for this.
>
> While still in my dream I decided to return to the depths to explore. For the longest time I swam along the ocean's floor, pulling myself along on rocks until I found an incline that I knew I needed to climb. It led into a cave, where I was greeted by a seal. I peeled my wetsuit down to my waist and discovered the cave was filled with filing cabinets containing information about all my many questions about my deep self. I was delighted! I immediately started reading. This was not followed by a

sudden download of instant information, but was rather an alert that I would start a cycle of discovery, an intermediate state that was not clearly defined.

During this phase allow yourself to be curious and follow sudden intuitions, such as being drawn to a certain book and flipping open to a specific page to find just the answer you need, or having a strong urge to see a film, play, or art exhibit that explores a question you have. Perhaps you have an inkling to travel to a place that feels luminous, to start a new course of study, to engage in a ritual, to reconnect with old friends from the past or allow new friends in, or to expand your work network. Black currant absolute is powerful for connecting with the collective unconscious and working with your dreams.

Allow the world to inform you. Pay attention to details, and then even smaller details, and then keep going; this helps to reveal the whole and brings understanding.

Seal medicine represents the emergence of unseen knowledge and the life force or new information emerging from the collective unconscious. In my dream, my wetsuit, being half-on and half-off, represents that aspect of myself that is anchored in the night sea and an aspect of myself becoming aware of hidden knowledge and truths—the energy of twilight. I would not have obtained this information if I would have stayed on the surface or in the dark.

The soft, gradual dissolution of sunlight during twilight, which happens simultaneously with the rising of the moon and the evening stars, offers a portal. It opens you to a magical realm where the logical mind must surrender to this liminal space. The word *liminal* comes from the Latin word *limen*, meaning "threshold." To be in a liminal space means to be on the precipice of something new but not quite there yet. You can be in a liminal space physically, emotionally, metaphorically, or energetically. Housed within one's own personal twilight are fantastical, erotic, seductive, melancholy, magical, and ominous possibilities. Being in a liminal space can be uncomfortable—scary and unnerving even—as there is no predictability. Liminal spaces are anything but predictable.

In the energy of twilight, one's perceptions attune themselves differently. Psychic landscapes undergo a blurring and blending of things and ideas, bringing enchantment and uncanny manifestations. It is the place where ritual and magic flourishes and holds great sway, allowing revelations to occur.

> **Blending Tip** – Blend black currant absolute with black currant fixed oil (see chapter 3) to abide in the twilight, in-between realms, where uncanny manifestations, magic, ritual, and revelations unfold.

❀ Brown Boronia (*Boronia megastigma*)

Presiding influence: the embodied self

Key energies: tangible body, having a combative relationship with your body, what makes you unique, loving being embodied, your personal relationship with food, cellular knowledge, tapping into the energies of whole foods, the Annamaya kosha (food body), human incarnation, exploring the world with your five senses, your environment as a sensual paradise, the art of making mistakes, the seed of the Self, the five elements, the kapha dosha (the dosha responsible for the stability, lubrication, substance, and support of our physical body), remembering, evolutionary impulse

This fragrant plant has bell-shaped flowers that are enclosed and point earthward. The flowers are bright yellow inside, while the exterior is a handsome reddish-brown color. In general, bell-shaped flowers explore the concept of embodiment.

Brown boronia offers a fascinating gift: she helps you understand what it means to be embodied and the opportunities this entails. It's tempting to regard the physical body as something we have to transcend, and some people even have a combative relationship with their body such as hating how they look or not valuing the specific gifts they were born with. This flower helps you develop a curiosity about what your specific gift set is, what makes you unique, and what makes you love being in your body.

I frequently teach on vibrational nutrition, about food as our ultimate ally. And no matter how clearly I advertise the course material—food as a means to access the deep self—on average about half of the participants are seeking a means to conquer their body and remake it into the image they have decided on instead of seeking what is stored inside.

Whole food, when treated in a mindful manner, allows us to access the full spectrum of who we are. Brown boronia helps you tap into this innate knowledge and work with the food body—the first layer, or Annamaya kosha—of who you are. This flower's vibration attunes you to the subtle fields of whole foods so you can begin the work of unlocking and accessing the deep self, thereby gaining access to the timeless truths stored in your body.

The Annamaya kosha, or food sheath, consists of flesh, blood, muscles, bones, and internal organs. It is the outermost layer, the tangible physical body, which is nourished and maintained by the food we eat. *Maya* means "veil," implying something that is obscured from view. *Kosha* means "sheath," referring to the layers that make up your being. The body is the vehicle that houses the five elements, a storehouse that holds the energetic imprints of everything we are aware of and not consciously aware of. This includes our senses and our means of understanding and interpreting our body and the world around us. Without a body to house our consciousness we could not execute the profound evolutionary push of existence. All wisdom traditions teach that obtaining a human incarnation is auspicious and rare, as it allows us to learn in an entirely unique way.

There are several myths concerning fallen angels that became jealous of humanity's aspect of free will, which provides opportunities to learn through mistakes and the ability to experience the world through the senses. The ability to taste food, kiss your beloved, bask in the sun, pet a dog, and smell flowers make this life a sensual paradise. This flower helps you to not shut down when you make a "mistake" but rather revel in it as a chance to learn something new. This flower opens you up to drinking in Earth's delights and bask in being alive and experiencing the marvels all around you.

This brings me to the idea of matter as a mediating factor. The physical body acts like a gatekeeper to deeper states of awareness; navigating this can be puzzling. One of the most remarkable aspects of our human design is the act of learning something, then taking it further to true understanding and finally to wisdom in action. The truth of all times and realms is held within our cellular memory. This memory holds the entirety of creation and is held in stasis within the Self. The implication is that it is a dormant potential not yet realized. The question then becomes: How does one harvest this vast knowledge? Let us explore.

We live in juxtaposition. On the one hand we are bound by the material rules of the world. To quote an old pop song lyric, "We are living in a material world, and I am a material girl." We are indeed impacted and formed by the cultures, traditions, families, finances, and inherited physical forms we are born into. We bend to the seasons, compulsions, illnesses, and how much energy we have. We are influenced by vast emotional ranges, cultural conditioning, vacillating thoughts, and a will that feels impotent. We strive for security, thirst for spirituality, and need purpose. These factors are all impacted by our physical bodies, which sometimes feel unchangeable.

On the other hand, our cognitive memory stored within our flesh can be understood as a learning system involving the storage of patterns and data, and it provides access to our vibratory field. According to the Vedas, the memory of all our lives—our own and that of all other organisms—is remembered by the human embryo at the moment it leaves its watery domain in the womb and begins to emerge into the open world. After this passage we gradually lose this understanding. The Vedas teach us how to regain access to our dormant memories. A few starting points involve using the plant kingdom (including absolutes, essential oils, herbs, and fixed or carrier oils), whole foods, yoga, meditation, prayer, and being present and fully feeling what is actually occurring in your life. This flower helps you know what tool to use at any given moment.

At a base level, everything that exists in the material world is formed from the five elements: earth, air, fire, water, and ether/space. This includes the plant kingdom. Although many have forgotten the fundamental understanding of how this works, brown boronia helps us remember. The five elements arise from vibration. These elements are what create the feeling of existing. What we call the *inherent self* is just a label describing emanations of form that help us interpret the self and the environment. For example, what we refer to as *earth* does not mean just "soil" but is to also be understood as a combination of light and vibrational patterns that have collated to act like a specific set of behaviors. So we experience the element of earth as the earth around us, but at the same time it is a set of behaviors that arise internally with us.

To realize we are born with inherent knowledge of the elements is to remember from the beginning to the present. When we consciously start to work with the elements within and all around us, we start down the path of remembrance. And as we deepen our relationship with our inner elements, we can comprehend and work with our deepest underpinnings.

The Bhagavad Gita tells us, "My prakriti [material nature] is of eightfold composition: earth, water, fire, air, ether, mind, intellect, and ego (see entry on narcissus in this chapter for more detailed information on ego). You must understand that behind this, and distinct from it, is the principle of consciousness that is present in all beings and is the source of life. It sustains the universe. Take a minute to sit with this declaration. You are composed of all of the elements, each offering an evolutionary impulse to help you learn specific lessons. You are born with all the tools you need to explore the emanations of form, mind, intellect, and ego. But behind all of this is the ultimate consciousness from which all expressions of form, both subtle and solid, are birthed. Do keep in mind that your body is the means to reach and grow toward the one unified source of life.

The food body consists of earth and water (the kapha dosha in ayurveda), while the cognitive memory is carried in the impulse of everything that has existed through the passage of billions of years, from the beginning of time and space. Food (the plant kingdom), which includes all of the substances in this book, are one of our most tangible forms connecting us to this universal consciousness. Yet paradoxically it is the very density of our physical form that prevents easy access to the subtle and pervasive truths around us! In releasing consciousness from matter using our refined senses, we must see the body as densely packed energy and subtle information, and the five elements as the keys to accessing this information.

Blending Tip.—Try using a blend of brown boronia absolute, Spanish broom absolute, juhi absolute, and borage fixed oil (see chapter 3) to access cellular knowledge and understand both its practical applications and its divine purpose in supporting the wholeness of the self.

❀ Carnation (*Dianthus caryophyllus*)

Presiding influence: the moon

Key energies: moon goddesses, gardening, vegetation, cooking, deepening your relationship with plants, interpenetration, the universal center, caretaking, creativity, deeply nourishing, changeability, the astrological sign Cancer, working with natural rhythms, mistress of dew

The Latin botanical name *Dianthus* comes from the Greek for "heavenly flower." Carnation helps you recognize the divine reality behind the world of things, lives, and minds. It offers a way of being that finds in the soul something similar to or exactly like divine reality. It affords an understanding of the inherent and transcendent ground of all being, the center that is immaterial and universal, and that interpenetrates everything and is interpenetrated by everything. As the poet-prophet William Blake puts it,

The moon like a flower,
In heaven's high bower,
With silent delight,
Sits and smiles on the night.

Carnation helps us explore the interconnectedness of the moon, plants, and ourselves. This flower is sacred to several moon goddesses, including Artemis and Diana (who as huntress rules wild vegetation). It is one of the flowers associated with the astrological sign of Cancer, which is the essence of the moon. The glyph for Cancer displays the male and female seeds; the archetype of Cancer is the cosmic womb, which seeds intuitive creativity, imaginative creativity, and practical creativity and which bursts forth in diverse forms—biological, artistic, and structural. Carnation drives us to explore the primal Mother in her archetypal energy of nurturer and fosters a strong desire in us to take care of small, fragile things such as seeds so we can nurture them to maturity. This flower encourages us to understand and appreciate the divine role of plants as food and how they nourish and caretake us.

Botanist and art historian Marina Heilmeyer says in her book *The Language of Flowers* that carnation has carried many meanings over time. It is associated with Artemis as an apology for flying into a rage and killing a man. Napoleon chose a red carnation as the symbol of the French Legion of Honor. The English upper classes turned their noses up at this flower, declaring it a "workers flower." A symbol of death, Roman Catholics claimed it for the Virgin Mary. During the Middle Ages it came to symbolize love, fertility, and betrothal. It has been associated with vanity and pride. Poets have claimed it as the flower of friendship because it keeps its color to the last. And in 1907 it was declared the official flower of Mother's Day in the United States. Heilmeyer writes, "With so many contradictory meanings and associations, it is little wonder that the carnation was also referred to disparagingly as merely a fashionable flower of no great meaning."[7]

I would argue the mutability and changeability of carnation is, in fact, its gift and strength. The essence of the moon and humankind have the same central impulse—to be ever-changing. And thank goodness we do, or we would be a rather dull lot.

The moon is the celestial body nearest our planet. The moon's kinship with our planet is evident in the protective lunar deities who have watched over us and our food supply: the cow-headed Hathor, whose milk nourishes the world; Nana-Sin, who keeps a watchful eye over shepherds and herds; the black-cloaked Isis, whose misty radiance nurses the happy seeds living in the soil; and Herse, goddess of the dew and a daughter of the moon goddess Selene, whose moisture nourishes the plants in the ground.

Historically it was taught that the moon presides over agricultural cycles of sowing and reaping and over every type of coming into being, and that she is the mistress of moisture, the juice of life. She rules over sap, semen, and menstrual blood (the average menstrual cycle lasts for about twenty-nine days, the same as the lunar cycle), and the nectar in flowers. She governs the moisture that falls as rain or dew, as well as the ebb and flow of every body of water on the earth.

Plant biologist and astronomical researcher Nick Kollerstrom holds that many people today may not believe that the moon holds water, rain, or dew, or that it influences human and animal conception. Yet they still choose to plant their seeds during the waxing and full moon and harvest their crops during the waning cycle. The Persians believed the moon flowed toward pastures to nourish the land, and in Deuteronomy the moon is described as the bearer of all that is precious. Torches of the moon goddess Hekate were carried around the fields after sowing to promote fertility. Until the nineteenth century, many cultures around the world believed that the harvest moon actually ripened the crops by shining through the night.

Growing up, I was taught that tomatoes germinate more quickly during the full moon, so you would start your seeds then. The dark moon was for planting root vegetables, such as radishes. Connecting to Diana and Artemis by working with carnation will help you follow the natural rhythms of vegetation and what makes plants happy, such as planting by the moon. The basic idea behind gardening by the moon is that its cycles affect plant growth. Just as the moon's gravitational pull causes Earth's tides to rise and fall, it also affects the moisture in the soil. So it is believed that seeds will absorb more water during the full moon and the new moon, when more moisture is pulled to the surface of the ground. This causes seeds to swell, resulting in greater germination and well-established plants.

Moon phase gardening considers two periods of the lunar cycle: the time between the new moon and the full moon (the period of the waxing of the moon), and the time between the full moon and the new moon (its waning cycle). It's considered best to plant certain types of plants during the waning moon and other types during the waxing period.

The moon also impacts plant growth through geotropism, which refers to how plants grow in response to gravity. Roots grow downward in the direction of gravity, and stems grow upward to resist gravity. If you plant tomatoes, peppers, cucumbers, or green beans in containers and hang the containers upside-down, the plants, despite being hung upside-down, will respond to geotropism and begin to grow upward.

Planting by the Moon

Plant your annual flowers and fruits and vegetables that grow above ground such as tomatoes, lettuce, melons, and peppers during the full moon. Carnations are an edible flower, so this is also the correct time to plant them (after you harvest them, sprinkle their petals on salads, use in spring rolls, or freeze in ice cubes). During the waxing moon plants are encouraged to grow leaves and stems. Plant flowering bulbs, biennial and perennial flowers, and vegetables that grow below ground such as onions, turnips, carrots, and potatoes during the waning moon. As the moonlight decreases night by night, these plants are encouraged to grow deeper roots, tubers, and bulbs.

Generally in astrology the moon is associated with the food we eat and the act of cooking, such that the more you cook, the more lunar you will become. In their book *Mythic Astrology Applied: Personal Healing through the Planets*, Ariel Guttman and Kenneth Johnson say, "Gardening is also a quintessential lunar activity. If you grow your own food, then cook it yourself: you will be immersed in the Moon's gentle vibration!"[8]

Blending Tip – Using carnation will help you forge a deeper relationship with the plants you cook, eat, and grow.* Try anointing your heart and the palms of your hands with a blend of carnation absolute and a carrier oil such as buriti before cooking or gardening. Your understanding will be magnified, enriched, and expanded. If gardening is not your heart's delight, carnation will encourage a relationship with the wild vegetation that surrounds you.

---

*To explore the magical role of food and how it can powerfully create ways of being, see my book *Vibrational Nutrition: Understanding the Energetic Signatures of Food.*

❀ Cyclamen (*Cyclamen europaeum*)

Presiding influence: butterfly

Key energies: calcified notions, new contexts, transformation, stagnation, perceived reality, seeing clearly, persistence of the past, epiphany, thought processes, interplay between habit and creativity, stages in life activated, intuitive grasp of reality, incubation, loss, birth

The origin of the word *cyclamen* is the Greek word *kyklos*, meaning a circle, a wheel, or a ring, suggesting this flower's petals, which open as elegant, brightly colored butterfly wings floating in tandem and circling the stem. The Chinese artist Zhang Daqian (1899–1983) would make fantastical translations of a flower's scientific name into a Chinese name based on pronunciation. The cyclamen's Chinese name is *xiankelai*, which means "the guest who comes from the fairyland," and indeed the energy of this absolute is ethereal.

Cyclamen gifts the ability to frame things and ideas in new contexts. It is powerfully freeing to see things outside of one's calcified notions. In fact, it is transformative. Cyclamen's other gift is the ability to crystalize this information and anchor it in the material realm to grow.

One of the oddest aspects of being human is how we absorb information. Psychotherapist Barbra Shore addresses this in her fascinating essay "An Absurdist Pantomime." She examines the ways in which our thought processes shape the information that constitutes our perceived reality, including ourselves and our surroundings:

> We have to make room for the possibility that our thought processes do not neutrally report on what is "out there" in an "objective" world. But rather, like the suppositions of theoretical physicist David Bohm, that our thought processes actively participate in forming our perceptions, our sense of meaning, our daily actions. Bohm suggests that "collective thought and knowledge have become so automated that we're in large part controlled by them, with subsequent loss of authenticity, freedom and order." Seen through this hypothesis, thought is not a fresh, direct perception but rather is the past—that which has already been thought—carried forward through memory into the present.[9]

Our growth as a whole requires an interplay between habit and creativity. Without the ability to perceive in a new way, outside of our calcified projections—which is the essence of creativity—no new habits would come into being. Your nature would follow repetitive patterns and behave as if you were governed by devolutionary principles. This is stagnation. On the flip side, without the stabilizing force of habit formation, your new ideas and perceptions could never take root and bear fruit, leading to a turbulent and unproductive life.

This speaks not only to the mysteries of physical metamorphoses, but also to the loveliest transmutations of the soul. This plant helps you know when it's time to anchor down and when it's time to seek change, whether in perception or in one's physical circumstances.

At the most basic level cyclamen helps you perceive where you are in your evolutionary cycle, because aware or not you are always at a certain stage in life. There is always a beginning, and to have a beginning you must have something truly *new*, something that has not existed in your reality before.

For many, a fresh, direct perception is what we call an *epiphany*, a sudden manifestation or perception of the essential nature or meaning of something. It is an intuitive grasp of reality through something such as an event, often simple and striking. The second turn of the wheel is the incubation stage, here lovingly growing your new idea or life circumstance. This is followed by taking your fully formed concept and birthing it into the manifest world; this is where stabilization through habit formation comes into play.

One of the most amazing aspects of this process is what you leave in your wake. Even though you are ready to move on to the next project, idea, or circumstance, what you leave behind might be an ah-ha moment for someone else. In this way we, as one human family, link arms in our evolutionary cycle.

Blending Tip – Blend cyclamen absolute and cranberry fixed oil (see chapter 3) to cultivate the dance between inner discipline, flexibility, restraint, habit, and creativity.

Damask Rose, Pink (*Rosa damascena*)

Presiding influence: Venus, Hera

Key energies: true love rooted in another; deep, passionate, personal love; profound love, romantic love; seeing divinity in your beloved; the desire to pair off and build a life with one special person

There are many types of love. There is *philia*, deep friendship, brotherly or sisterly bonds, and camaraderie. This type of love is the essence of goodwill toward others for a cause or purpose. There is *philautia*, self-love. This can be a narcissistic love of oneself, which is a self-centered approach to life, or it can be the healthy kind of self-love in which we believe in our own worth and worthiness no matter what anyone else thinks or says. And there is *agape*, a transcendent form of love, an altruistic love, a love that mirrors God's love for us and our love for God. This is a selfless love that is extended to all, including strangers and even enemies.

Eros is the essence of physical love and sexual desire—an energy fueled by passion, intimacy, and romance. It is the type of love that ignites the senses and is deeply rooted in longing and connection. Damask rose embodies this energy of true love, but with a special depth: it embodies a love that is not only passionate, but profoundly personal. It is a romantic love that binds two souls together, creating a bond that transcends the physical into something sacred and enduring. This essence speaks to the heart of deeply felt, committed love—a love that is intimate, transformative, and enduring.

Damask rose is the energy of seeing divinity in your beloved, making you want to pair off and build a life with that person. It is the gift of seeing through another's eyes and perceptions and returning that gift wholeheartedly. It is being held in unconditional love and holding the other in the same way. This is the kind of energy that tames, untangles, teaches, and heals. It makes life an adventure that is fun to explore. It helps each person reach their highest potential. It is the kind of love found in the poetry of Rumi:

> *The real beloved is that one who is unique,*
> *who is your beginning and your end.*
> *When you find that one,*
> *you'll no longer expect anything else.*

Damask rose opens you to feeling deeply bonded in a love relationship. This is the kind of love that will bloom within you and allow your relationship to grow over a lifetime. Regular use of damask rose will enhance your relationship with your beloved in so many ways. Consider:

- exploring dreams and life options together, setting goals together, and savoring how this process creates the future you want to bring into reality
- being best friends and playing, laughing, going on adventures together, and enjoying the simple pleasures of traversing the mundane together and keeping a home that is a sanctuary
- taking delight in and celebrating your beloved's accomplishments, showering them with praise and letting them know that not only do you truly see them, you are amazed at what you see
- taking an active interest in your partner's life's work, asking questions, truly listening, and offering support to help them meet their goals
- listening carefully to your beloved's point of view and giving it its due weight when making decisions together
- taking personal responsibility for mistakes that impact your sweetheart and not only clearly communicating what needs to be said, but healing any hurt through right action
- being vulnerable and raw, exposing your true self
- softening your speech and letting your words express your love
- carefully tending the garden of your love, nurturing it until love is all that is
- creating a lifestyle that promotes physical health, including regular exercise, making delicious and healthy meals, and creating a sanctuary for restorative sleep
- exploring spirituality together and finding out what this looks like for you both
- forgiving easily, with a strong desire to move back into equilibrium
- protecting each other

- cultivating mature emotional intelligence and applying that to your daily life
- expressing your love through touch as a form of communication
- making love in a way that expresses your deep connection

Blending Tip – Blend pink damask rose absolute with strawberry fixed oil (see chapter 3) to tenderly care for the garden of your love, nurturing it until love is all that remains.

❀ Elderflower (*Sambucus nigra* ssp. *caerulea*)

Presiding influence: elder mother, the tree herself

Key energies: working with fairies, oracle, guidance, protection, source of strength, shelter from the storm, different points of view, understanding your inner impulses, emphasis on yourself versus an event, cause and effect, clear results, human and nonhuman

The proper and respectful way to approach the spirit of this tree is to understand that she is the physical embodiment of a wise ancient one, holding the energy and memory of the first rooted beings—an oracle and a source of strength and guidance in times of trouble or need.

An oracle is a person or thing that provides wise and insightful counsel or prophetic predictions, including foreknowledge of the future inspired by deities. If done through ritual means it is a form of divination. Elderflowers have a strong connection to the fairies.

I was a professional oracle reader for many years, and quite often people would ask for a prediction, as if the world around them wasn't mutable and in constant flux, not only as a result of their actions but as a result of all the actions of the human and nonhuman collective. Even if you start from a clear vantage point, at any time there can be a swift change of fortune because you cannot control outside factors; you can only react and adjust as needed. This is one of elderflower's special gifts. When life is confusing, this flower helps you look again and see things from a different point of view. Often confusion arises because the wrong questions are being asked, you are operating on incorrect assumptions, or you are being deceptive or deceived either consciously or unconsciously. There will always be variable results if your focus is on controlling your environment or another person.

There is a direct link between asking an oracle for help and not trying to control an outside force, but to understand an internal one. The goal here is not predictability or domination, in fact quite the opposite—the less predictable the person is, the less rigid they are, and as a result spontaneity and creativity increase. The emphasis on the person rather than a specific event switches the energy from something happening to you, to you happening to an event. What skills and knowledge do you want to bring to bear on a situation? This way of working with an oracle emphasizes your potential for creativity and self-actualization and is deemed more important than your limitations, idiosyncrasies, and difficulties with social situations.

Opening yourself up to the vast expanse of your feelings and thoughts, as well as to the range and variety of your experiences, brings freedom. This requires a recognition that you are a process, not a static end product. I want to emphasize that this understanding of freedom does not negate the influence of cause and effect, but rather complements it. One way to understand freedom is through the fulfillment of desire—achieved by intentional actions and a well-ordered life that leads to clear outcomes, while still leaving room for kismet. This creates a sense of spaciousness, free from constraints, allowing you the authentic freedom to be and do as you truly feel—but only after circumstances are nurtured. Cultivating this kind of openness is the long game, yet it is the most reliable way to craft the future you desire. It's a path laid by clear sight and built on a foundation of right action, with enough wiggle room for divine inspiration and serendipity.

Of course, we are not always in a rational frame of mind or have the energetic capability to manage our inner self. Elderflower will come and shelter when you are in need of protection and a soft place to rest. In the past, people were cautioned not to sleep under an elder tree for fear you would transport out of time and place to a fairyland. Sometimes that's what's needed—to be suspended out of time and place, held safe and fast in love and protection until you are strong enough to readdress your problem and have the clarity and energy to work on it.

No matter if you are looking for wisdom and insight to navigate a situation or you need to be held fast in love, ask elderflower for help with respect, love, and reverence, and she will aid you.

Blending Tip – Blend elderflower absolute and borage fixed oil (see chapter 3) to open and soften your inner oracle before using divination tools or seeking wisdom from Elderflower herself.

❀ Frankincense (*Boswellia sacra*)

Presiding influence: the sun
Key energies: bridge between worlds, worship, divinity, regeneration, phoenix energy, spirit, Christ consciousness, transcending, divinity, Tummuz (Sumerian god of fertility and Ishtar's consort)

Frankincense is synonymous with incense (from the Latin *incendere*, "to burn"). The aromatic smoke of incense spiraling upward to the heavens provides a bridge between the worlds, as expressed in Psalm 141: "Let my prayer be set forth before thee as incense, and the lifting up of my hands as the evening sacrifice."

The Bible is replete with references to frankincense. *Boswellia sacra* served as a herald for King Solomon on his wedding day: "What is that coming up from the wilderness like columns of smoke, perfumed with myrrh and frankincense, with all the fragrant powders of a merchant? Behold, it is the litter of Solomon!" (Song of Solomon 3:6–7). It was one of three gifts the Magi presented to the Baby Jesus, emblematic of his divinity. This heavenly scent was key to awakening the Sumerian god of fertility, Tummuz, Ishtar's consort, from his winter slumber, so the Earth would regenerate each spring. The fabled phoenix creates her nest from frankincense and myrrh so that her offspring will be born from its scented ashes and lifted up to the firmament.

The Egyptians used frankincense as an antidote for hemlock poisoning. The Egyptian queen Hatshepsut ground charred frankincense into kohl eyeliner to enhance her beauty and to protect her eyes from the sun and the evil eye. The biblical Jezebel did not enjoy these same benefits and fell from grace after lining her eyes with kohl to impress the rival king Jehu:

> When Jehu came to Jezreel, Jezebel heard of it. And she painted her eyes and adorned her head and looked out of the window. And as Jehu entered the gate, she said, "Is it peace, you Zimri, murderer of your master?" And he lifted up his face to the window and said, "Who is on my side? Who?" Two or three eunuchs looked out at him. He said, "Throw her down." So they threw her down. And some of her blood spattered on the wall and on the horses, and they trampled on her. (2 Kings 9:30–33)

In mythology, Sol (the sun), having an all-seeing eye, told Vulcan, the god of fire, that his wife, Venus, was having an affair with Mars. Venus, not happy with the turn of events, and possessing the power to make any mortal or god fall in love, made Sol fall in love with the fair mortal Leucothoë. Since this was intended as a punishment, Venus made sure Clytie, Leucothoë's sister, found out, and she immediately told their father, who promptly buried her alive.

Unable to awaken his beloved with light, Sol swore to revive the girl and make her rise to the sky. He covered her in the nectar of the Gods. The body of Leucothoë melted away and filled the soil with its fragrance, and out of the earth arose the frankincense tree.[10]

Apollonius, a charismatic teacher and miracle worker from the first century AD, wanting to win the favor of the sun,

> took up a handful of frankincense and said: "O thou Sun, send me as far over the earth as is my pleasure and thine, and may I make the acquaintance of good men, but never hear anything of bad ones, nor they of me." And with these words he threw the frankincense into the fire.[11]

Frankincense is sublime for enhancing meditation or prayer work, stimulating the sixth and seventh chakras, brightening the mind, removing heaviness from the heart, motivating one to altruism, uplifting your spirit, and deepening your connection with the Divine.

Blending Tip — Try blending frankincense with sunflower oil (see chapter 3). Sunflower embodies the essence of the sun, or Sol, while frankincense represents his beloved Leucothoë, lost to him. This blend captures the energy of them reunited. Apply to the solar plexus and heart to cultivate the power of reconciliation.

❀ Gardenia (*Gardenia jasminoides*)

Presiding influence: *natura*, all of nature

Key energies: building an intimate relationship with nature, widening your circle of understanding, plant translator, cosmic body, human body, coevolution, the plants' point of view, natural magic, secrets revealed, listening with your whole body

Gardenia helps you get to know nature in an intimate way and build relationships that are natural and easy, warm, nurturing, full of humor, supportive, loving, community- and family-building, and just flat-out fun.

Albert Einstein writes about us being part of a universal family and asks us to expand our understanding:

A human being is part of the whole called by us "universe," a part limited in time and space. He experiences himself, his thoughts and feelings, as something separated from the rest—a kind of optical delusion of his consciousness. The striving to free oneself from this delusion is the one issue of true religion. Not to nourish it but to try to overcome it is the way to reach the attainable measure of peace of mind.[12]

Wisdom traditions from all cultures teach that the cosmic body and the human body are reflections of each other. The intelligence that organizes the activity of humankind orchestrates the activity of the universe. Knowing this allows us to have a deeper relationship with nature. Gardenia opens you to this understanding. When you engage with nature you see the environment as an extension of yourself and the plants and trees as aspects of you, and you in them. We are intimately and forever intertwined, made from the same raw materials, the same recycled earth, life force, mind, and spirit. The inner intelligence of our bodies is the ultimate and supreme genius of nature, which mirrors the wisdom of the universe. Since we have so much in common, we have the ability to be co-conspirators, friends, and family!

Michael Pollan, in his fascinating book *The Botany of Desire*, describes how he had an epiphany one day while gardening. He was planting potatoes and watching bees pollinating, and it hit him that their role to the plant kingdom was not so different from his own. Previously he had fancied himself more of a lord and master of the garden, choosing what seeds to plant and grow, all his choice. Then he realized that both he and the bees were partners in what is called *coevolution*, when two parties act on each other to advance their individual interests but end up trading favors. Plants that are stationary need another being to help them propagate, and those beings who do the propagating need plants not only to survive, but to create pleasure and enrich life on so many levels.

So the question arose in my mind that day: Did I choose to plant these potatoes, or did the potato make me do it? In fact, both statements are true. I can remember the exact moment that spud seduced me, showing off its knobby charms in the pages of a seed catalog. I think it was the tasty-sounding "buttery yellow flesh" that did it.[13]

This made me laugh out loud! I am always reading seed catalogs and being seduced by various plants' version of Pollan's "knobby charms," and heaven forbid they omit language about the taste of a plant—I swoon and it's all over! I am very susceptible to the plant world's charms, and I am guessing you are too since you're reading this book. As beguiling as Pollan's tale is, I'm not surprised at this description because the energetic role of the potato plant provides a preternatural understanding of something. He was planting a gift from the earth—potatoes—which in my opinion helped facilitate his ah-ha moment. Of course he had a predisposition and most likely a karmic disposition to do so, but I do believe the plant kingdom triggered him and helped him reach his hypothesis.

Pollan goes on to share:

That May afternoon, the garden suddenly appeared before me in a whole new light, the manifold delights it offered to the eye and nose and tongue no longer quite so innocent or passive. All these plants, which I'd always regarded as objects of my desire, were also, I realized, subjects, acting on me, getting me to do things for them they couldn't do for themselves. And that's when I had the idea: What would happen if we looked at the world beyond the garden this way, regarded our place in nature from the same upside-down perspective? ... [This book's] broader subject is the complex reciprocal relationship between the human and the natural world, which I approach from a somewhat unconventional angle: I take seriously the plant's point of view.[14]

Gardenia is a translator; she wants you to connect with the exact plant friend who will help you figure something out or to do anything that is possible in a human incarnation that is linked to understanding how to actually do it. This is the incredible gift of the plant kingdom—for anything you can think of on a subtle level, there is an exact answer for you in the plant kingdom.

This then prompts the question: How can I, outside of memorizing all the properties of plants, really get to know them? How to make the right introductions? Well, look no further than gardenia. Imagine being at a dinner party in the ethers and your astute hostess, gardenia, sees your need and she artfully escorts you to just the right fit. This is a very accurate analogy. Using gardenia in a mindful way, she will help you fill in the gaps in your life by pointing out which plant allies will help you—and we all need help. This book is all about plants that have been taken to their secondary forms as absolutes, essential oils, and fixed oils. But gardenia's gift does not stop here—she would love to introduce you to plants you can eat and grow for pleasure.

I have seen a grown woman cradling a peach like a newborn while gushing about how perfectly soft and fuzzy its skin is—"Look at the coloring" and "Just smell!" Then, of course, she wants to share her joy with you, and now it's my turn to smell and coo about how perfect this peach is! And I too am delighted and rejoice in the wonder of this peach. One doesn't take such personal delight in something that is "other" or alien to you. There could be interest, but not the instant intimacy that signals that we are one with a plant and vice versa.

As always, nature is perfect and finds her familiars. My maternal grandmother's favorite flower was gardenia (and I am sure gardenia nudged her along in her selections and understanding of plants). My grandmother's superpower was her ability to teach using nature and the plant kingdom. Her garden perfectly mirrored her personality, traits, and values. She planted corn and tomatoes in abundance. It was all about the sun ripening tomatoes on the vine until plump and fat, filled with exquisite juice and pulp. I experienced this miracle firsthand as I watched my grandmother tenderly caretake her garden with such love as she watered, weeded, and sang her plants into the fullness of their being. She was also a storyteller—she told us kids endless stories as we helped her weed. I experienced this miracle even further when we gathered as a family to harvest the fruits of our labors and then watch and learn as my grandmother made her famous tomato sauce from scratch. It was her joy to share with us what she had learned from her mother and grandmother. And it was her intention for us to share with the generations to come what she had shared with us. It is nature's design that tomato (see chapter 3, tomato seed fixed oil) teaches love, and my grandmother did not just tend her garden—she was weeding and watering we children in a way, and nature amplified her teachings and profound, perfect love. As I wrote in my book *Vibrational Nutrition*,

> Tomato, first and foremost, teaches togetherness in many forms. Be it a loving family, a robust community, the dance of relationship, a passion, or even courtship, this fruity vegetable is all about the heart. A part of this dynamic is its ability to help you be open to differences and new circumstances and joyfully embrace them.[15]

Corn's vibration (see chapter 3, corn fixed oil) is fertility, understanding the earth, the joys of being a woman, and being in community and family. So my grandma's garden magic was a combination of love plus an understanding of the earth as our community, plus her seemingly endless ability to grow anything. Now *that* is magic!

Another aspect of Grandma's natural magic involved how she heard plants so deeply. We can point to gardenia. This sweet, sweet flower wants you to have an engaged and profound relationship with the plant kingdom. Use gardenia in conjunction with the other oils profiled in this book, and she will reveal their secrets to you. You aren't sure which absolute you need? Meditate with gardenia and see what comes to mind. I always take a bath with whatever new plant distillation I am working with, and I take gardenia to amplify, clarify, and crystalize my thoughts and ideas.

Blending Tip – Blending gardenia absolute with fractionated coconut oil (see page 108) and another oil you want to know better will help you understand the deeper stories of nature; apply to the heart and forehead. Blend gardenia absolute with carnation absolute in fractionated coconut oil before planting a garden or to help you create an intimate relationship with the fruits and vegetables you eat and tend.

❀ Hyacinth (*Hyacinthus orientalis*)

Presiding influence: the element ether

Key energies: the color blue, personal vault of heaven, akasha, fifth chakra; spiritual gifts such as clairvoyance, clairaudience, and being a clear channel; all information beyond the rational mind; good communication skills

Low-growing hyacinth is extremely fragrant and bears many small, star-shaped flowers, often purple or "blue as birds' eggs," according to Homer. Blue is one of the rarest colors to be found in nature. Blue flowers are idyllic fragments of the sky blooming right here on the earth, uplifting and spiritualizing human consciousness and at the same time enfolding the soul in a mantle of soothing reassurance, nurturance, and calm.

According to Alice Bailey (1880–1949), who wrote prolifically on Theosophy and is credited for coining the term *New Age*,

> It is known esoterically that the vegetable kingdom is the transmitter and the transformer of the vital pranic fluid to the other forms of life on our planet. That is its divine and unique function. This pranic fluid, in its form of the astral light, is the reflector of the divine akasha. . . . Those who seek to read the akashic records, or who endeavour to work upon the astral plane with impunity, and there to study the reflection of events in the astral light correctly, have perforce and without

exception to be strict vegetarians. It is this ancient Atlantean lore which lies behind the vegetarian's insistence upon the necessity for a vegetarian diet, and which gives force and truth to this injunction.... Only those who have been for ten years strict vegetarians can work thus in what might be called the "record aspect of the astral light."[16]

Akasha is the Sanskrit term for ether, which is often translated as "space." The element of ether produces the fifth chakra, *vishuddha*, which is located at the throat and whose color is a brilliant blue.

Before we go any further, let's dig in and attempt to sort out what the Akashic field is.

The vibration of this element, ether, is said to be so subtle that it cannot be perceived by the external senses—our senses are simply not tuned to its frequency. Therefore, as long as we function through the five senses we cannot experience the subtle vibration of akasha, or ether.

Akasha is expansion, diffusion, timelessness, and the convergence of past, present, and future. It is limitlessness, the void, an absence of light described as black or transparent, and within this blackness all the colors of creation exist. It is the space of consciousness or inner space that is located in front of the closed eyes, known to yogis as *chidakasha*. Ether is everything and nothing—the All in One. At the level of the mind, ether is said to control the emotions and passions in humankind (*control*, not *generate*) to turn one away from strictly sensorial experiences. It is auspicious for spiritual work and contraindicated for material gain. Without any kind of conscious cultivation, ether is active or dominant in the average person for only five minutes every hour.

Working with akasha opens you to spiritual gifts such as clairvoyance, clairaudience, and channeling—all information sources that exist beyond the rational mind. Akasha teaches and promotes the highest expression of the Self, understanding truth and expressing that understanding as a lifestyle. Ether fosters true creativity and grants an understanding of the gestalt (the organized whole that is perceived as more than the sum of its parts), as well as providing insights into symbolism, myth, and subtle information. It encourages good communication skills, expressing clearly what you mean and feel, along with the ability to really hear what others say, including what is left unsaid.

Since this element is housed in the physical body and is a manifestation of form born from the unified whole, it is subject to dualism. The aforementioned qualities are the gift aspect of ether; the following are its shadow aspects:

Having too little ether in your makeup gives rise to the sensation of feeling contracted and immutable, lacking spiritual connection and the ability to transcend the physical world. You'll have difficulty recognizing and expressing your own truth and difficulty with communication—not hearing what others are saying or not saying what you mean. Having too much unregulated ether in your makeup gives rise to feeling spaced-out and disoriented, afraid of being alone or lost and disinterested in participating in earthly activities that cultivate well-being, safety, and structure.

Hyacinth teaches you how to accesses the information that resides in your personal Akashic records, housed in your throat chakra. A dynamic first step in accessing akasha involves working with this absolute with focused intent.

Blending Tip – If you want to literally feel the sensation of deep blue, blend hyacinth absolute with blueberry fixed oil (see chapter 3) to invoke the energy of saturated blue and to explore your personal vault of heaven.

❀ Juhi (*Jasminum auriculatum*)

Presiding influence: Sri Krishna

Key energies: meditation, asking questions (Who am I?), peering into the navel of creation, deep listening, form behind forms, original impulse, in the beginning, the eternal made manifest, the field, eternal knowledge

Come my love and drink deeply from the well of eternal knowledge. You can call the body "the field" because you sow the seeds of action in it and reap their fruits. A wise person claims the knower is he who watches what takes place within the body. Juhi—otherwise known as jasmine—enables you to discriminate between the field and the knower. Questions arise: What is humankind? Are we *prakriti*, pure form, material in nature? Or are we *purusha*, that which is eternal and beyond perception? What are you? Are you the cosmos? Are you the intellect, the ego? Are you earth, water, and ether, air and fire? Are your organs filled with knowledge? Are you the knowledge and doings of your mind? Are you more than your five senses? Are you hatred and desire? Pain and pleasure? Are you pure consciousness in material form?

It is true, all these blend in the body, with all its limitations and changes. If you seek stability, seek that which is eternal. It is easy to be misled and have what you know to be true clouded over and hidden. It is easy to mistake one thing for another. The acceptance of the unreal as real constitutes a state of bondage. The seed of the Self is indivisible and eternal—the eternal made manifest by the power of its own knowledge. We are born with a veil that hides our true self, just as an eclipse hides the rays of the sun. When the pure rays of divine knowledge are concealed, it is easy to identify with the body and only the body. True, this is a most important root, but juhi helps you meditate and find what lies beyond physical forms.

Now let's explore that which has to be explored on the spiritual path: beginningless, transcendence, and the eternal. What is it to be in this world but not of this world? It is being of your senses but not defined by them. You are all of your experiences but free of them. You are within and without. You understand the subtle, the undivided that seems to divide into objects and experiences, as a way to teach and expand your personal knowledge. The all-encompassing, the eternal, is the root source. Our sense of individuality is a divine gift from which we can explore and learn. From this taproot, all opposites exist to teach us through their friction as we puzzle life's questions. You recognize the pure impulse that is ultimately who you really are, and you work toward that, even as you recognize all the crazy-making and beautiful aspects of yourself that are not eternal and merely temporary expressions of your personality. We are a combination of the material and the eternal. We are all made perfect as we understand the role of the body and that which is timeless and eternal, made one in our holy nature.

Juhi is a lesser-known species of jasmine with remarkable spiritual qualities that differ from the more common varieties, *Jasminum grandiflorum* and *Jasminum sambac*. This delicate flower at present is seldom used in western aromatherapy and perfumery. It offers a unique energy and scent profile that is different from other types of jasmine. Its fragrance is more reminiscent of gardenia—it has a grassy green aspect with top notes of olibanum, tropical fruit, and a rich balsamic undertone. It has traditionally been used as a devotional flower for religious ceremonies and to make garlands for the hair.

Blending Tip – Try blending juhi and brown boronia (this chapter) with goji berry fixed oil (chapter 3) and apply when asking deep questions.

❀ Labdanum (*Cistus ladaniferus*)

Presiding influence: your internal fire

Key energies: inner sun, third chakra (*manipura*), assigning value, "I" consciousness, personal lens, archetypal masculine, protect or destroy, being consumed, intellect, perfectionism, structure, repeatable process, becoming conscious

Labdanum, commonly known as rock rose, has a luminous yellow center with five blazing white petals and a fiery red dot at its base. Labdanum is harvested from the long, sticky stems of a scented gum resin shrub. It is a sun-loving plant that thrives in Mediterranean conditions, and this special relationship with the sun provides the plant with what it needs to produce its fragrance. To use labdanum is to awaken to and understand your inner essence in relation to the sun, an idea beautifully expressed by Pulitzer Prize–winning American poet Theodore Roethke:

> *To have the whole air! —*
> *The light, the full sun*
> *Coming down on the flowerheads,*
> *The tendrils turning slowly,*
> *A slow snail-lifting, liquescent*

Sun (light), spirit, and matter, the transparency of consciousness and the crystallization of light as form . . . The Vedas tell us that we each have a personal sun that resides in our navel. It is called *manipura*, meaning "abode of glittering gems," and it is from here that personal awareness arises. From this vital energy center we start to look at the unified whole as parts and pieces and give each a name and assign a value. From here we gain a sense of "I" consciousness and explore the world through a very personal, subjective lens—I like this, I do not like this—and we apply this to our environment and to other people.

The Vedic science of ayurveda teaches that it is the inner fire that rules physical sight. The Dalai Lama says, "I call the high and light aspects of my being spirit and the dark and heavy aspects soul." Said another way, spirit is the sun and soul is the moon. The sun is the animating force that coaxes dormant yin forces into being. It purifies and wants to transcend.

Most traditions teach that the sun is an archetypal masculine energy, and as all things in our dualistic world have two sides, the sun is often depicted as having the ability to protect or to destroy. It can provide warmth, nurturing, and healing, or be a consuming, devouring force that can be unstable and destructive. In the tale of King Midas we are reminded that all that glitters is not gold, the moral of the story being to not to allow yourself to be consumed by worldly ambitions to the point where your inner life is obliterated. The familiar Greek myth of Icarus and Phaethon is also instructive: to fly too near to the sun is to be consumed by one's own hubris. The Vedas say the solar plexus chakra (our inner sun) is where the personal ego is housed, and if you're not vigilant it's easy to get scorched by this energy.

This energy center, manipura, teaches the earthly lessons of

- **a balanced inner sun:** personal power, the intellect, opinion, logic, will, direction, joy, leadership, action, authority, integrity, radiance, courage, self-worth, consciousness, refinement
- **a distorted inner sun:** anger, pettiness, rage, hatred, ego issues (inflated or deflated), abuse of power (domination, misguided force, using fear to control), feeling superior, "my way or the highway," perfectionism, rigidity, violence, weakness, having no expression of personal choice.

Our inner sun can also be understood as a catalyst for change, growth, evolution, and increase. Attachment arises from here—what do you want to caretake? Foster into fruition? From here also arises the ability to be in a committed, long-term relationship.

The sun is the quintessential protector of those who cannot help themselves. As the heavenly warrior, the sun's blazing light turns back the darkness of primeval chaos; as the hunter, his arrowlike rays unerringly hit their target. He is the majestic solar vitality embodied in the ram, the dragon, the lion, the eagle, and the phoenix. He is the omniscient, all-seeing eye, the exacting guardian of universal order.

J. R. R. Tolkien's wizard character Gandalf, whose "hair was white as snow in the sunshine; and gleaming white was his robe; the eyes under his deep brows were bright, piercing as the rays of the sun,"[17] radiated the protective light of the sun, pushing back the threats that loomed in the darkness to keep the travelers under his protection safe until the true dawn came.

Eastern philosophy teaches that this is the energy center that produces the mind and intellect, which determines how we process and synthesize. The alchemists associated the sun with the act of becoming conscious. Generally speaking, we can only know that which already exists within our realm of awareness, and we must use this small opening to scan the vast ocean of knowledge and information to begin the process of becoming more aware. I believe most creation stories are metaphors for this very process of becoming awake or aware, which is the path of enlightenment.

The ability to derive rich information from the fertile darkness and break it into usable bits and synthesize it until it is a fully formed concept that moves civilization forward is behind all great discoveries that require structure and repeatable processes. Art, music, literature, philosophy, spirituality—all are, to a degree, lunar in that they are not subject to hard and fast rules. In contrast, engineering, architecture, biology, chemistry, aeronautics, surgery, dentistry, and so forth all benefit from a structured body of information. The sun gives rise to being analytical, organized, and methodical.

Blending Tip — Try blending labdanum absolute with Himalayan pink salt and cow's milk in a bath (see chapter 4). This supports learning new concepts—and not just in memorizing facts but in being able to understand how they relate to what we already know. It's crucial to see the connections, because this enables us to apply the knowledge in real-world situations, adapt to new circumstances, and make informed decisions based on a broad understanding of the subject. This deeper level of thinking involves recognizing patterns, anticipating outcomes, and using the knowledge to influence change.

❀ Lilac (*Syringa vulgaris*)

Presiding influence: Pan
Key energies: mythic language, instinctual self, nature spirits, playfulness, sexual intoxication, being capricious, re-wilding, ecstasy as a gateway

to the Divine, high tantra, divine inner marriage, wind instruments, plants as emissaries, counteracts dourness, beyond the mundane

Lilacs have a deep history originating in ancient Greek mythology. It was said that Pan, the god of forests and fields, was desperately in love with a nymph named Syringa. As he relentlessly pursued her, she became so overwhelmed by his advances that she prayed for divine intervention. To Pan's dismay, Syringa was transformed into the delicate lilac plant right in front of his eyes. In despair he removed one of her branches and kissed it, and his breath through the hollow branch produced a melodic, haunting sound. He then cut more branches and created the first pan pipe. Note that the botanical name for lilac, *Syringa vulgaris*, is derived from the Greek word *syrinks*, meaning "pipe."

As you may have noticed, in mythology nymphs are always turning into plants to avoid some god or another. This should not be read as violence; mythic language is complex. This is more along the lines that we as mortals often do not fare well in the raw energy of the Divine, and these plants are their emissaries who allow us to touch an aspect of divinity without getting overwhelmed.

Pan's archetype represents body wisdom, play, and being grounded in oneself and in nature. Magenta-colored lilac is a resonance gateway to this energy. Pan is the primordial god of the earth, the wilds, and sexuality. In antiquity he never had a temple dedicated to him: instead, grottoes, clear lakes, meadows, woods, and caves are his places of worship. His gift is to help us remember the body's wisdom so that we can get out of our heads and back into our instinctual nature.

When you feel overwhelmed by life and yearn for simplicity, nature, quiet, and solitude, call on Pan. His consorts are nymphs (nature spirits), and this dynamic brings playfulness and the kind of sexual intoxication that loosens us from the bonds of the ordinary and sets us free in spiritual ecstasy so that we can let go completely and experience oneness. An invocation of Pan in the form of lilac is truly a supplication of our divine nature.

The different colors of lilac express in part the vibrational action of this flower:

White lilac: purity, innocence, freshness, and simplicity. This bloom resets energy, allowing a blank slate to inscribe a new story on, a new beginning, a fresh start. Use when you cannot forgive and are holding on to energies that hinder your ability to love, grow, and move forward.

Violet lilac: This gentle flower brings the vibration of the breath of love, spring, youthful vigor, and joy. It returns you to the basics, back to your core self. It resets and renews energy for relationships that lack softness and ushers in more sweetness.

Magenta lilac: love and passion. This blossom connects you to your raw, natural self, deeply melding you with nature and activating profound bliss, divine play, true surrender, beingness, and sensuality as an ecstatic gateway to the Divine.

If you are feeling ashamed about any natural impulse—frustrated, bored, agitated, restless, or if you have an unsatisfying physical life that does not feed your soul—these are all signs you are cut off from your deep, natural self. Magenta lilac will help you remember, replenish, and make whole what you have lost.

In the throes of intimacy (with the right partner), you lose your worldly identity and open the gateway to truly letting yourself go completely. A sense of oneness is experienced. This concept is explored in tomes like the Karma Sutra and systems such as high tantra. The Eastern practice of tantra is likened to tending the flames of your sacred energy centers or chakras, burning out any negativity and in the process purifying your body and soul. In so doing you discover the supreme Self hidden deep within your heart. This ancient practice is capable of moving you beyond duality into alignment with the Divine, as in the alchemical concept of the divine marriage, which can be understood as symbolic of the balanced energies combining the divine male and the divine female. Supreme consciousness is the masculine principle that pervades all things; it is the sustainer. This is the ultimate, out of which mind and matter proceed. Nature is the feminine principle and forms this information; she is responsible for procreation, for birthing earthly existence. They are two sides of the same coin. This is the basis of all creation, the power of evolution. It is Shiva-Shakti, yab-yum, yin-yang, Father Sky and Mother Earth—in essence, it is male and female energy combined and giving rise to experience.

Western culture bases so much of life around what we *do*. We define ourselves through our work and judge our worth based on outer accomplishments. Magenta lilac is about *being* rather than *doing*; it is about total surrender to a bliss that is beyond the mundane that we so often strive for.

Blending Tip – Try blending lilac absolute with macerated orchid oil (see chapter 4) to amplify the energy of re-wilding and merge with the archetype of Pan.

❁ Lily (*Lilium candidum*)

Presiding influence: Hera, Mother Mary
Key energies: matrimony, harmony, and unity; the Milky Way; mother's milk, purity, mercy, innocence, chastity, mythic container, psychic integrity, incorruptible and eternal

In China, the lily is celebrated for its regal white blossoms and for what is hidden from sight. Both the fragrant flower and the bulb have the same meaning, and these are frequently depicted in art as wedding symbols. The lily flower and bulb represent harmony and unity. This plant is fittingly named "hundred together" for the many overlapping scales on its bulb. Terese Tse Bartholomew, curator of San Francisco's Asian Art Museum and one of the leading authorities on Chinese iconography, states: "The lily (*baihe*) is thus a pun for 'hundred' (*bai*), as well as for 'togetherness' or 'union' (*he*)."[18]

At the Palace of Knossos on the Greek island of Crete, Lilies grace a replica of a reconstructed Minoan fresco called the "Prince of the Lilies." Fragments of the original were excavated at the site in 1901. Looking at this fresco you can feel the strength of the lily's bulb as it pushes up slender stalks to be crowned by a multitude of lilies. In ancient Greece this plant was sacred to Hera, Queen of Heaven, and was said to have arisen from the drops of her breast milk as they fell to Earth during the creation of the Milky Way. One of Mother Mary's many titles is "Queen of Heaven and Earth," and she too is represented by the lily—in fact, her energy is so entwined with *Lilium candidum* that one of the plant's common names is the Madonna Lily. The English monk and scholar Venerable Bede (673–735 AD) described the white lily as the emblem of the Blessed Virgin, where the white petals symbolize the purity of her body and the golden anthers the beauty of her soul. In Christian symbolism, the lily of mercy balances the flaming sword of judgment and represents purity, innocence, and chastity.

The calyx, or cup, of the lily is particularly distinct—it resembles a trumpet or chalice and evokes feelings of drinking deeply of the Divine. A stone bust of Greco-Roman origin attributed to the first century BCE depicts an unknown Greek goddess emerging from a calyx of a lilylike flower, reaffirming lily's role as a mythic container and birthplace of the Divine. Carl Jung said the lily represents psychic integrity that is no longer pulled apart by effects. The alchemical lily is "incorruptible" and "eternal," "the noblest thing that human meditation can reach."[19]

> **Blending Tip** – Try blending lily absolute with milk thistle fixed oil (see chapter 3). These two plants combined are the essence of the maternal archetype, symbolizing life, care-taking, and the sacred bond between mother and child.

❀ Magnolia (*Magnolia champaca*)

Presiding influence: the moon

Key energies: fullness, abundance, fertility, the divine feminine, lightness of being, soothing, calming, magic, blurring of edges, deep rest, holding the moon in your hand, the uncanny, the deep of night, sealing up the cracks, psychic abilities, saturated, soma

The milky blooms of the magnolia tree are the essence of the full moon, offering wholeness and an opportunity for the fragmented parts of yourself to be healed. The soothing energies of the magnolia flower are said to offer the gift of soma, the ambrosiac drops of the moon, said in the Vedas to be the drink of immorality. This energy is abundant, fertile, soothing, creative, illuminating, and nourishing, and fosters wholeness.

The full moon is credited for its ability to change human behavior, shifting the mundane to the sublime. Magic and moonlight have always gone together to shift the borders of the mind. How can the impossible be done? Magic. It starts by believing in the impossible.

The full moon offers perspective on time and fertility. What is yours now? And what will wax or wane? With the gift of magnolia we are always working toward fulfilment.

....

Blending Tip – Blend magnolia absolute with cloudberry fixed oil (see chapter 3). With its milky white energy, this soothing blend cultivates your internal light. It's the deep rest of night—the moon in your hand—sealing cracks, awakening psychic gifts, and saturating the soul in sacred soma.

....

❀ Myrrh (*Commiphora myrrha*)

Presiding influence: the sun god Ra, the goddesses Isis, Ishtar/Inanna, and Astarte

Key energies: mysteries of the dead, Adonis, Queen Hatshepsut, repentance, long-distance travel, worship, redemption, death, morning, resurrection, veneration, reverence, being elevated

Myrrh is the dried sap or resin of a tree of the *Commiphora* genus. It has been used for offerings and healing since antiquity. This tree grows naturally in the drier parts of Africa, Arabia, Madagascar, and India, and as the demand for this resin grew too great for wild harvesting, plantations were established in southern Arabia. A contributing factor to the popularity of myrrh was the domestication of camels in the second millennium BCE, allowing large caravans to cross the oceanic Arabian desert, bringing this fragrant resin to Babylon and the port cities of Judea and Phoenicia. From there myrrh was shipped all over the ancient world.

Queen Hatshepsut of Egypt was so enchanted by myrrh that she sent an expedition to the fabled land of Punt* not only to bring back some of the resin, but also to collect thirty-one living trees, making this one of the oldest records of tree transplantation. Daily worship of the sun god Ra included burning golden resin at dawn, myrrh at noon, and at sunset a combination of frankincense, honey, and wine, symbolic of perfect harmony. Myrrh is an ingredient in the famous temple incense blend known as *kyphi*, used in embalming and deification mysteries of the dead in ancient Egypt.

In Greek mythology, Adonis, the lover of Aphrodite, was said to have been born from the heart of the myrrh tree. We still use Adonis as a metaphor to suggest that someone is impossibly handsome. Ovid describes how Adonis's mother, Smyrra, was transformed into this tree as part of her repentance for an incestuous relationship with her father: "Though she has lost her former senses with her body, she still weeps, and warm drops trickle down from the tree. There is merit, also, in the tears: and the myrrh that drips from the bark keeps its mistress's name, and, about it, no age will be silent."[20]

---

*The land of Punt is fascinating in that the location was kept secret such that no maps showing its location have ever been found, although it is well-documented by Hatshepsut and King Sahure, among others.

Myrrh was used to venerate the Great Mother in her various forms: Isis (Egypt), Ishtar/Inanna (Mesopotamia), and Astarte (Phoenicia). References to myrrh are found throughout the Bible. At Mount Sinai, God commanded Moses to have frankincense and myrrh blended with spices into fine oils for anointing and consecration: "Do not make any incense with this formula for yourselves; consider it holy to the Lord" (Exodus 30:37). Nicodemus brings "a mixture of myrrh and aloes" with which to prepare Jesus's body for burial (John 19:39). The Lord commanded Moses to blend liquid myrrh, cinnamon, calamus, and cassias in olive oil to be the sacred anointing oil for the Ark of the Covenant, the altar, and the priests (Exodus 30:22–29). Upon visiting the Baby Jesus, the Magi offered frankincense, symbolic of his divinity; myrrh, to indicate his future death on the cross; and gold, to honor him as king. To this day myrrh is an important part of the Catholic Mass (the distinctive incense blend consists of myrrh, frankincense, and benzoin). It holds the energy of redemption, death, morning, resurrection, reverence, and being elevated.

The Catholic faith is a liturgical faith. It makes use of all five of our senses: sight, sound, smell, taste, and touch. This is certainly by design as each sense aids us in availing ourselves of the salvific grace flowing from the Holy Sacrifice of the Mass. This is precisely why every effort should be used to employ all of our senses whenever possible during the celebration of the sacred liturgy.[21]

Blending Tip – Try blending myrrh absolute with safflower oil (see chapter 3) and applying to your beard to bring out your inner Adonis. Myrrh absolute blended with black currant fixed oil (see chapter 3) carries the energy of redemption, death, mourning, and resurrection. It is also deeply supportive during the grieving process, helping to navigate the loss of a loved one.

❀ Narcissus (*Narcissus poeticus*)

Presiding influence: Narcissus

Key energies: self-love, submitting to the Divine, an inflated sense of self-importance (narcissism), garrulousness, an excessive need for admiration, disregard for others' feelings, subterfuge, an inability to handle criticism, sense of entitlement, growth, the ego misused and misunderstood, transmogrify, water, the emotions, divine inner marriage, melted by love, the hidden fire, discovering oneself

The myth of Narcissus, as told by first-century Roman poet Ovid in his *Metamorphoses*, is rich with details that help us understand the energy of this flower. It is not just a simple story of a boy selfishly consumed with himself, but rather it describes a journey toward genuine self-love, submitting to the Divine, the divine marriage, and the complexity of this kind of journey.

With a narcissistic personality disorder, a person has an inflated sense of self-importance. This includes an excessive need for admiration, disregard for others' feelings, an inability to handle any criticism, and a sense of entitlement. It is a total focus on oneself instead of other people, concepts, the Divine, and nature. This disorder represents the extreme end of the spectrum, although if we are honest with ourselves, who among us has not sometimes been needy, vain, a little narcissistic, hostile, dependent, cold and withdrawn, manipulative, selfish, or afraid? Narcissus is a guide for working with these kinds of energies.

The basis of this myth involves a beautiful youth of divine origin, unable to give love to another, who falls in love with his own reflection in a pool of water, not realizing it is actually himself. His difficulty is often attributed to being ensnared in his own distorted ego, and his eventual transformation is attributed to the dissolution of the small self, or ego, facilitated by the warming fire of love, which allows him to experience the wholeness of the true self.

One of the more fascinating aspects of working with the ego happens when what you cannot or will not face within yourself (because it disrupts your more flattering self-image) is projected outward onto situations and other people. Since the energy you find so disturbing is now "out there," you don't have to face it "in here." This is not a conscious act, which is why projection is so powerful, because it's hard to imagine that what we are reacting to "out there" actually originated "in here." Said another way:

> When I was a child, I spake as a child, I felt as a child, I thought as a child: now that I am become a man, I have put away childish things. For now we see in a mirror, darkly; but then face to face: now I know in part; but then shall I know fully even as also I was fully known. But now abideth faith, hope, love, these three; and the greatest of these is love. (1 Corinthians 13:11–13)

Often an immature ego needs to be in relationship with others and exterior situations so it can clarify and define what is occurring inside; this is frequently a sloppy process.

Narcissus was a child of a river god and a nymph, born of water. Water is the element that houses the emotions and the unconscious in the physical body, and the unconscious is always trying to become conscious and the emotions understood and refined. This is one of the gifts of narcissus absolute: to mindfully use this flower is to become self-aware and understand your impulses and internal forces.

Upon his birth, Narcissus's mother sought out a seer, "being consulted as to whether the child would live a long life, to a ripe old age, the seer with prophetic vision replied 'If he does not discover himself.'"[22] This thought-provoking statement suggests that truly knowing yourself and loving yourself is a form of self-knowledge that will lead to a death of some sort—in this case, the death of Narcissus's distorted ego. An interesting aspect of a healthy ego includes a full and rich understanding of your true self that allows you to engage in right relationship, not only with yourself, but with others as well.

This comes to pass as Narcissus first encounters himself in "an unclouded fountain, with silver-bright water, which neither shepherds nor goats grazing the hills, nor other flocks, touched, that no animal or bird disturbed not even a branch falling from a tree. Grass was around it, fed by the moisture nearby, and a grove of trees that prevented the sun from warming the place."[23] Narcissus, born of water, now encounters a pure water source not touched by any earthly thing or even by the sun. The sun is a common symbol for understanding, clarity, and divine light. The fountain represents a divine mirror that allows Narcissus to start the process of understanding his true nature, and so now his work begins: "He is seized by the vision of his reflected form. He loves a bodiless dream. He thinks that a body, that is only a shadow. He is astonished by himself, and hangs there motionless, with a fixed expression, like a statue carved from Parian marble."[24] He is seized by the vision of his reflected form. In the following verses, Narcissus's journey of self-discovery begins, allowing the pure rays of understanding to melt away the constructs that have deluded and bound him.

Vedanta teaches the same concept:

Deluded by his ignorance, a man mistakes one thing for another. Lack of discernment will cause a man to think that a snake is a piece of rope. When he grasps it in his belief, he runs a great risk. The acceptance of the unreal as real constitutes the state of bondage. Pay heed to this, my friend. The Atman is indivisible, eternal, one without a second. It is eternal made manifest by the power of its own knowledge. Its glories are infinite. The vale of tamas hides the true nature of the Atman, just as an eclipse hides the rays of the sun. When the pure rays of the Atman are thus concealed, the deluded man identifies himself with this body, which is non-Atman. Then rajas, which has the power of projecting illusory forms, afflicts him sorely. It binds him.[25]

Narcissus did not possess the ability to be in right relationship with the world around him or even with himself. He literally did not know how. This is not just a cautionary tale about being selfish and egocentric; rather, it is an exploration into understanding what the ego is, what a healthy ego's role is, and learning that truly loving and seeing yourself is a powerful portal to freedom.

Let's explore from a western and an eastern tradition the complex task of being able to perceive the ego. Neither tradition spells this out in a simple manner; it's as if you are encouraged to look out of the corners of your eyes and use your heart's ability to "see," as if to look too directly at it would cause the concept to move out of view.

Narcissus says,

Fool, why try to catch a fleeting image, in vain? What you search for is nowhere: turning away, what you love is lost! What you perceive is the shadow of reflected form: nothing of you is in it. It comes and stays with you, and leaves with you, if you can leave! . . . I am enchanted and I see, but I cannot reach what I see and what enchants me—so deep in error is this lover—and it increases my pain more, that no wide sea separates us, no road, no mountains, no walls with locked doors. We are kept apart by a little water![26]

Let's take a moment to look at the energy of water:

Water represents the unconscious journey of the soul into deeper awareness and wisdom. No act of will can make the soul take this journey; it can only happen after much searching and questioning. It is also a precondition of this experience that some kind of wounding has taken place. It is through the pain and endurance of the wounding that wisdom comes, at which point the individual can cross the lake to the island of healing and protection. It is a natural state of surrender that allows the inner self to travel across the emotional sea to the otherworld.[27]

Narcissus goes on to say,

> I am he. I sense it and I am not deceived by my own image. I am burning with love for myself. I move and bear the flames. What shall I do? . . . As he sees all this reflected in the dissolving waves, he can bear it no longer, but as yellow wax melts in a light flame, as morning frost thaws in the sun, so he is weakened and melted by love, and worn away little by little by the hidden fire.[28]

One of the greatest obstacles in life is the misused and misunderstood ego. Ego—or rather, one's mistaken view of the "I"—is a common cause of problems and suffering both internal and external. The ego is an illusory belief in a solid, concrete, separate entity, independent and disconnected from any other phenomena. If understood this way it's only natural that the ego becomes an insurmountable barrier between oneself and the rest of the world, with no possibility of true communion, interaction, and relationship, not only with others but also with the true and authentic Self. This is a barrier that needs to be dissolved, and in this tale Narcissus is weakened and melted by love and the hidden fire. This suggests that a divine act is taking place. The aim is not the annihilation of the ego, but the dissolution of the false ego. When this occurs, we open to all possibilities that present themselves, and above all we come to realize that we are infinitely more than what we believed we were when we identified with the small ego. Once you are released from the bonds of egocentrism, you can begin the work of engaging the deep self, the authentic self, with the world around you and with others in a nourishing, wholesome way.

Working with these energies, what is dissolved is the hardened, contracted ego that pursues its own selfish agenda. This allows the healthy ego to emerge. A robust, healthy ego is required to navigate daily life; moreover, it is one of the most dynamic vehicles for coming to "know thyself." According the Vedas, self-knowledge—that is, knowledge of the higher Self—is the highest perfection.

In the Western sense of *solutio*, an alchemical concept that pertains to the water element, meaning the return of matter to its original undifferentiated state, the dissolution of the hard, dry soil of the conscious ego through engagement with and fertilization by the fluid unconscious is a necessary requirement for transmutation to take place. This is another way of saying that surrendering the personal ego to your inner divine Self and the power of love is a process of growing awareness. It describes the experience of moving from duality to nonduality, moving from the small self to the cosmic and the mystical. You may have noted as you read this that the energy of softness is required for this task. If you yearn to be in right relationship with your ego and melt all barriers to love both within and without, harshness will not do.

Softened, Narcissus now arrives nearly at the end of his journey. "He laid down his weary head in the green grass, death closing those eyes that had marveled at their lord's beauty."[29] His sisters, the water nymphs, lamented and let down their hair for their brother, and the tree nymphs also lamented. "And now they were preparing the funeral pyre, the quivering torches and the bier, but there was no body. They came upon a flower instead of his body, with white petals surrounding a yellow heart."[30]

With the gentle energy of the Divine melting all barriers that kept Narcissus from experiencing love, and for the first time seeing and knowing himself, his transmutation takes place. The death of his small ego, his merging with the Divine, and his unification within the divine marriage is symbolized by his transmogrification into the beautiful narcissus flower.

· ·

Blending Tip — Blend narcissus absolute with passion fruit fixed oil (see chapter 3) to awaken the dormant divinity within, helping you become a living mediator between Heaven and Earth. Another blend worth exploring is narcissus and guava. Guava seed fixed oil (chapter 3) improves refined personal expression and clears the heart chakra while narcissus absolute ignites the divine fire of love.

· ·

❀ Oak Wood (*Quercus robur*)

Presiding influence: Zeus, Mars, Silvanus (Roman god of the forest)

Key energies: internal power, exploratory nature, nobility, oracle tree, strength in hardship and the wisdom to find your way, the hero's journey, masculine strength, archetype of the king, decisive action, Father Sky, the balance between nurturing caregiver (the feminine) and heroic warrior (the masculine), finding the balance between stoic strength and self-care

The common oak tree is anything but common; this magnificent, pioneering tree sends its seedlings into open grasslands rather than shady forests. The growth pattern of oak speaks to its internal power, exploratory nature, and nobility.

Ethnobotanist Fred Hageneder notes:

> The ancient Gauls and the Romans associated the oak with Mars Silvanus, the god of agriculture and healing. The oak was an important presence in the farmyard, where it had a nurturing role. It was with reluctance that the oak god resorted to arms, but Mars was nevertheless eventually transformed into a war deity and the cultural history of the oak reflects this transition from the plough to the sword.[31]

Zeus's sacred tree is the oak, often portrayed in mythology as an oracle tree. In the myth of Jason and the Argonauts, their ship, the *Argo*, was built at Dodona, the location of Zeus's oracle grove, and was made from a sacred oracle oak tree. The myth of Jason and the Golden Fleece is a coming-of-age story in which fighting against seemingly impossible odds, a boy triumphs and grows into a man.

The role of oak is no different today. It offers the vibration of strength in hardship and the wisdom to find the way. Of all the trees that could have been used to build Jason's mythical vessel, only oak had the vibration to carry him on his hero's journey, which centered on the Golden Fleece, which symbolizes spiritual knowledge. In the beginning of his quest, Jason has the strength and creativity to outwit his opponents, but as the journey progresses and gets more difficult he finds that he must turn to the divine feminine to reach his goal.

Hageneder notes that oak lore has two sides: "the caring, paternal qualities, and the ability to fight ruthlessly when justice demands it."[32] Jungian analyst Jean Shinoda Bolen states that Zeus "was the first of the Greek sky gods to be protective, generous, and trusting toward many of his sons and daughters,"[33] while still being rooted firmly in his masculine strength, as he is the archetype of the king, or Father Sky in Western culture. The lightning bolts he hurls as weapons remind us of oak trees, which are struck by lightning more often than any other type of tree but seem to sustain less damage as a result.

This tree has a beautifully masculine energy, balancing the nurturing caregiver and the heroic warrior. I would venture to say that the feminine from which Jason required assistance was his own feminine/intuitive aspect. On the first part of his journey, the masculine aspect of his mind provides all the strategy he needs, but as his journey becomes more difficult he requires a deeper form of knowledge. The oak, which was hewn from the oracle forest, symbolically and vibrationally allows him to access his deep intuitive wisdom, which is his feminine side.

Oak balances the poles of nurturing caregiver and heroic warrior and assists in finding the balance between stoic strength and self-care. This allows you to complete your own personal hero's journey by accessing all that you are. Use oak to access your inner wisdom or use in conjunction with oracle tools such as tarot cards, runes, or the I Ching.

Blending Tip – Blend oak wood absolute and sunflower fixed oil (see chapter 3) to cultivate inner strength, a bold exploratory nature, and a sense of nobility. This blend channels the wisdom of the oracle tree, providing resilience in hardship and guiding you along the hero's journey. With the power of masculine strength and the archetype of the king, this blend helps you stay your path. Apply to your solar plexus to awaken this energy.

❀ Orris Root (*Iris pallida, Iris florentina*)

Presiding influence: the Greek goddess Iris

Key energies: rainbows, messages, luminous incubator, first cause, fingers of time; past, present, and future; the form behind the form, focus on a point in time, colored threads of light in your psychic space, living dispositions, spaciousness, energy cluster that dictates behavior, untie the knot, give thanks

Orris root is the rhizome of the iris flower. The brightly hued flowering head of this plant is named after the Greek goddess Iris, a messenger of the gods. Her vehicle is the rainbow, which allows her to travel from Heaven to Earth, bringing messages and thereby allowing gods and humans to communicate. Iris guides the spirts of women and girls to the afterworld; to ensure their safe passage, irises are placed on the grave, a tradition still practiced in modern-day Greece.

Orris root encompasses Heaven, Earth, and the afterworld. It is stable and self-contained. Swirling within this absolute are multihued strands of time and memory; it is full of energy—dynamic, expanding, and divergent. A luminous incubator, it is primordial, an ovum in a sea of sperm. It recounts the daily birth of the sun out of eastern waters, supported by the breath of spirit coaxing light and form to emerge. It is the eye opening in a blink with the ability to truly see. It is the mysterious center, the vessel that holds space and allows the fingers of time to weave storylines into being and then to undo these same threads.

Physiologically the iris is what gives the eye its color and the ability to see the multitude of hues that make up life that are simply not just black or white. The aqueous humor is the clear fluid that fills the space between the lens and cornea; this fluid bathes and nourishes the lens, bringing certain perceptions into sharp focus.

Time is the indefinite, continued progress of existence and events in the past, present, and future, regarded as a whole and existing in both the dreaming and waking states. This is where one starts to ponder the form behind the form, behind the form.

Pierre Teilhard de Chardin (1881–1955), a scientist, paleontologist, Jesuit priest, and all-around inspirational human being, describes this phenomenon:

> First, I noticed the vibrant atmosphere which formed a halo . . . [that] radiated into Infinity . . . in which could be seen a continuous pulsing surge. . . . *The whole Universe was vibrating.* And yet when I tried to look at the details one by one, I found them still as sharply drawn, their individual character still intact. . . . This scintillation of beauties was so total, so all-embracing . . . so swift, that it reached down into the very powerhouse of my being, flooding through it in one surge, so my whole self vibrated to the very core of me, with a full note of explosive bliss that was completely and utterly unique.[34]

I had a similar experience that opened me to understanding in a different way. I have been asking my whole life for nature to allow me a more intimate way to know her. This was her response:

> When it finally happened, it was unexpected, and I was broadsided. I was sitting on my bed reading *Jane Eyre* when all of a sudden, before my waking eyes, luminous yellow twin buttercup fairies about the size of my thumb appeared and laid down these words in my mind: "*We are here to heal you.*" They then entered my body through my chest area, and I saw many interconnecting light lines in different hues against an indescribable background. My awareness was enfolded in this light, in what I am guessing is my energy body, and then *true bliss* filled my body. I had read about the sensation of bliss, but until this moment I had never felt it personally. I can testify, it is beyond words.[35]

The Divine meets you at the same level as your consciousness, and my prayer at that time was not so much to understand the universe as a whole but rather to understand the role of the plant kingdom and

Mother Nature within this matrix, and how this applies to the subtle complexities of being human. It makes sense to me that my teachers would be fairies.

Orris root has an interesting role to play in this paradigm. She gifts you with the ability to focus on a point in time, to see it clearly without confusion—be it past, present, or future—and then to use it as an anchor point for further examination.

It has been my experience that you cannot will an experience such as what's described above; it happens spontaneously at the most unexpected time, when the Divine finds that you are ready. Often it comes as colored threads of light in your "psychoid" space (the middle space between psyche and matter), each strand holding information at a specific moment in time and recorded within are living dispositions. Living dispositions are karmic actions set in motion that run on calcified energy tracks—on autopilot—that one's mind does not regulate. They feed off the energy given to them, but it's not mindful, and they can dictate behavior. Living dispositions do not come into being by their own accord but instead they are created by external events impacting you or they are generated internally. Where this gets fascinating is when they take on a life of their own and continue to operate in your subtle body. This in turn creates behaviors, often unconscious behaviors, that get played out in your life as automatic actions. How they orchestrate you depends on what is recorded on these light strands.

What you are looking for at this point is spaciousness; you need time to be suspended as you delve into a "first cause"—first exposure or feeling of "I want that!"—that creates a way of being. This may take some practice, and to help you along I suggest anointing the center of your forehead (the physical location of the psychoid space) with orris root absolute and borage fixed oil (see chapter 3). Once you've done this, close your eyes, let your mind relax, and wait for the light strands to appear. When they do appear, pluck the most vivid one with your mind's eye and follow it. Here you will find the nexus—a link between multiple elements or points, often acting as a central hub that holds a behavior or living disposition. Feel into this energy cluster. Is it something wonderful that you are so happy is operating within you? If so, give thanks and carefully examine each thread or the aspects that contribute to the whole. If you are curious about how this affects your behavior, follow the threads and see what aspects of your life they influence.

If what you find does not support your well-being, it is time to untie the knot. The more you do this, the easier it will be. In essence what you're doing is exploring and becoming conscious of the successive stages of a behavior, retracing it to its root. Once you are holding this nexus in your psychoid space, do nothing—just feel and listen. If this knot is discordant, most likely it was caused by inner contradictions—the friction of opposites rubbing against each other that some part of you cannot reconcile. I frequently see my hands holding the knot of light, the energy complex, and I allow myself to be informed about what energies or actions are contained within. Words arise in my mind, accompanied by bodily sensations and emotions. At this point it is easy to understand and label. This is an important aspect—you need to be able to label what you find or your mind cannot process it. Once you have a clear understanding what each thread contains, visualize in your mind's eye untying the knot.

Since you are working with energy and energy is never lost, you need to repurpose it. If you just ask the living dispositions that are contained within the threads of light where they would most benefit you, and you hang on to them energetically and follow them, they will show you. As you carefully unpack each experience, you can apply what you have learned to other aspects of your life.

How you know you've been successful in repurposing contrary energy is when you are no longer triggered by situations attached to the energy knot. The friction is gone. You can be smack-dab in the middle of what used to be a triggering situation and feel emotionally neutral, or you may even get a powerful insight into the situation. This causes compassion to arise.

Exploring a positive energy complex often leads to a profound knowledge and a desire to act on your new insight. No matter what becomes conscious, this kind of internal processing is empowering and fascinating, and can even be life-changing.

....

Blending Tip – Apply orris root absolute and borage fixed oil (see chapter 3) to the center of your forehead to facilitate the inner journey described above.

....

❀ Rose Otto, White (*Rosa alba*)

Presiding influence: Venus, the Virgin Mary, Cybele, Isis
Key energies: purity, innocence, light, secretive, alchemical, magic, undoing, sub rosa

Since Earth first became fertile, the wild rose and her myriad cultivated offspring have borne witness to the complexity of human life, soothing our souls, elevating our spirits, and marking rites of passage. Speaking to the proud as well as the humble, white roses are the very essence of purity, innocence, and light. They crown the victor and pay homage to the martyr. They have symbolized royal blood and nations. Above all, rose is love in all its heavenly and earthy tones. The white rose in particular represents the Virgin Mary, who is known as the Mystical Rose of Heaven. It is also sacred to Venus (it is said all roses were white until Venus pricked herself and drew blood, bringing red roses into the world) and celebrated by artists. Botticelli famously depicted Zephyr gently drying Venus with his warm breath scented with roses as the goddess is birthed from the ocean.

Devotees of the Anatolian mother goddess Cybele honored her and her retinue by shadowing them with a snow of roses. Humorously in Lucius Apuleius's novel *The Golden Ass*, the hero, Lucius, excited to experience the sensations of being a bird, turns to witchcraft, but by an unfortunate miscalculation he finds himself transformed into a donkey. He knows he can revert back into his own body by eating rose petals, but these prove singularly elusive. The roses he requires are always just out of reach until the Egyptian goddess Isis makes them available. She then called Lucius to priestly duty and initiates him into her rites. Many scholars believe this novel is a self-portrait of the author and is valuable for its description of the ancient religious mysteries, including the use of roses to undo magic gone awry, and that Apuleius himself had been initiated into the Isis cult. The idea behind the term *sub rosa*, "under the rose" or secretive, is an alchemical concept involving the entire process of psychic transformation that occurs in the silence of self-containment, as silence is required to enter the womb, or "rose," and within these hallowed folded petals the Self is secretly conceived.

Let us not forget we can use the rose to show love and affection to another person. In the Victorian era, suitors sent bouquets of white roses at the beginning of a courtship. Perhaps the white rose allowed the recipient's heart to warm and open and be ready to receive pure love.

Blending Tip – Apply white rose absolute with guava fixed oil (see chapter 3) to prepare to receive pure love. Blend white rose absolute with black currant fixed oil (chapter 3) to undo curses.

❀ Siberian Fir (*Abies sibirica*)

Presiding influence: the dark forest

Key energies: exotic forces that are outside the inhabited constructs of daily life and thoughts; on the edge of one's mind are magical forces, a call to action, a quest; traversing through uncharted territory; being soul sick and in need of healing; a true path; confronting fears, worries, and inner demons; being guided and set free from past influences; the journey; loneliness, silence, entanglement, healing, regression, loftiness, obstruction, spontaneous growth, decay, knowledge, the second half of life

The forest, even when saturated with sunlight, is ever-moving and alive within the continuum of light and dark. Shadows play with the light, creating images that inflame our imagination, offering dark places that are a refuge for small things that want to be hidden from sight. Here plants can only grow in an eternal twilight. The Siberian fir can grow to over a hundred feet and live up to two hundred years, creating homes for fauna and flora alike. Its timber is used to build homes and heat these homes, making it possible for humans to live in harsh environments. At one time whole forests of these trees encased villages, towns, homesteads, and castles within their vast reaches. We are far more "civilized" now and must travel great distances to find an unbroken forest to experience what our ancestors must have experienced.

The forest holds very real physical dangers if one has not prepared adequately. Cold, wet, harsh weather, bears and wildcats, lack of food if you do not know how to hunt or forage, and the danger of getting lost and not finding your way out.

Mythically, the dark forest, with all its exotic forces, exists outside of daily life and mundane thoughts. But situated at the edge of one's mind or in the deep, dark forest are magical forces. In fairy tales, the protagonist who lives at the edge of the forest is called to action with the dreamlike appearance of an unusual presence or an enchanted animal emerging from the forest. Here is where the hero's journey begins. Common themes are loneliness, silence, entanglement, healing, regression, loftiness, obstruction, spontaneous growth, decay, and knowledge. You may meet a kindly fairy, a devouring hag, a sorceress, a libidinous satyr, wild animals, a wise magician or shaman, helpful elves, friendly animals or plants that speak, and perhaps even an angel.

We seek the forest when we are soul sick and in need of healing and a true path. We confront our fears, worries, and demons by hiking and camping in remote places, seeking answers to our questions. We go there as we would to a place of worship, to be filled with light, joy, and beauty, and to be taught by nature. This quest can be literal or can take place purely on a subtle level.

Katherine Arden's brilliant novel *The Bear and The Nightingale* is set in medieval Russia and features the heroine Vasilisa, who finds refuge in the forest, with its many nature spirits, plants, and animals, and where she learns how to escape a life that does not feed her wild soul.

> The Forest was Quiet on the cusp of winter, the snow thicker between trees. Vasilisa Petrovna, half-ashamed and half-pleased with her freedom, ate her last half honeycake stretched out on the cold limb of a tree, listening to the soft noises of the drowsing forest. "I know you sleep when the snow comes," she said aloud. "But couldn't you wake up? See, I have cakes."[36]

Her journey is an adventure she gladly undertakes even though it is filled with difficulties and setbacks. But what hero's journey is not? Her journey is blessed with grace and unexpected support as she jumps in feet-first, driven by faith, desire, and an inner knowing that she must be doing what she is doing, while not exactly knowing what the outcome will be.

Many spiritual and psychological journeys begin, as Dante's did, in the dark forest of psychic wilderness. It is horrible, tangled, and wild, and even the memory of it instills fear. Dante imagines a scary forest as a metaphor for sin. While he seeks a way out of the forest, he meets three beasts—a leopard, a lion, and a wolf—who force Dante back into the dark forest. The three beasts are allegories for the three different sins: the leopard represents lust, the lion pride, and the wolf avarice. In Canto 1 of *Inferno*, he writes:

> *Midway upon the journey of our life*
> *I found myself within a forest dark,*
> *For the straightforward pathway had been lost.*
> *Ah me! How hard a thing it is to say*
> *What was this forest savage, rough, and stern,*
> *Which in the very thought renews the fear.*

Because the forest has no set routes and is ever-changing, anything is possible. All questions asked can be answered, all problems can be resolved, all aspirations reached, as long as you forge forward. As Robert Frost writes in "A Servant to Servants,"

> *He says the best way out is always through.*
> *And I agree to that, or in so far*
> *As that I can see no way out but through*

The only way out is through, and this journey has many forks in the road. Each time the path splits, one road seems to lead back to the place where we started (seeming safety), while the other takes us through the dense forest. We hope that the destination on the other side of the forest is what we're looking for, although we cannot guess how far off it is, what we might meet along the way, or what exactly *is* on the other side. We might start to worry that the treasure we seek, the enticing vision in our mind, is all an illusion. I would say take heart and forge on—it is always best to stay the course, because the supposedly safe way back to where we started is the true illusion. It's the path to a life that is deeper that we seek; it's about tuning out the noise of the outside world and listening to that still inner voice in the quiet of the dark forest.

. . . .

Blending Tip – Blend Siberian fir absolute with safflower fixed oil (see chapter 3) for a guiding light, helping you navigate the dark forest with new sight and strength.

. . . .

❀ Spanish (Genet) Broom (*Spartium junceum*)

Presiding influence: the Wise Woman archetype

Key energies: uncanny energy, sorcery and magic, homemaking, thresholds, the beginning and the end, the journey in-between, heroine's journey, spiritual authority

The word *broom* comes from the plant *Spartium junceum*, a small, deciduous shrub that was once used to make many early sweeping devices. Right from the get-go, brooms were considered women's tools, and this ubiquitous household item became a powerful symbol of female domesticity. "Jumping the broom" at weddings, a custom more common in the African American community, is said to seal the union. In Christian ceremonies the broom handle represents God, while the bristles signify the couple's families. In similar pagan ceremonies it is said that the broom handle represents the male phallus, while the bristles represent female energy.

Brooms represent thresholds—the beginning and the end, and importantly the journey in-between. Many households and businesses mark the start of the day by sweeping the floor; life then occurs in a task-driven way—lessons are learned, challenges are met, then the end of day is brought to a close by sweeping the floor once again. In Disney's 1940 classic *Fantasia*, the sorcerer's apprentice, Mickey Mouse, tries to shirk his duties and enchants a broom to life to do his work for him. Soon all goes terribly wrong as he is out of his depth and is literally drowning in the chaos he has created due to skipping steps in his training in his desire to jump ahead to the end. Before all is lost, the sorcerer appears and sets all back to order, and Mickey has to start all over again from the beginning. In the fairy tale *Baba Yaga and Vasilisa the Brave*, the broom marks the beginning and the end of Vasilisa's tasks (her learning). Unlike Mickey, she stays the course and faces her difficulties head-on, and as a result she reaps a great reward, demonstrating that broom can be a powerful ally on the heroine's journey.

Broom, the plant, is associated with uncanny energy, sorcery, and magic. In folklore, brooms are witches' tools. The earliest known image of witches on brooms dates to 1451, when an illustration appeared in the manuscript of French poet Martin Le Franc's *Le Champion des Dames*, which translates as "The Defender of Ladies." In the drawing, one woman soars through the air on a broom and the other sits astride a stick. The inscription above their heads identifies them as Waldensians, a Christian movement that began in twelfth century France which sought a return to simplicity and was a forerunner of the Reformation. Waldensians were threatened with heresy by Church authorities in 1215 for allowing preaching and consecration of the sacrament by any layperson, including women.

From maintaining a home to owning a direct relationship with spiritual authority, women have the divine birthright to follow their own path. This oil not only facilitates that journey but also provides practical steps to help navigate it—the heroine's journey. For those who are practicing witches, this plant is a powerful familiar.

Blending Tip – Blend broom absolute with black currant fixed oil (see chapter 3) to tap into uncanny energies and fully own your sovereignty. This blend amplifies the right to control your life and make decisions without outside interference—to govern yourself with autonomy, self-mastery, and inner authority.

❀ Spinach (*Spinacia oleracea*)

Presiding influence: Venus, Osiris, Green Tara

Key energies: abundance, love, growth, the color green, spring and summer, lushness, richness, flourishing, thriving and plenty, cultivating crops, symbiotic love relationship, the middle way, heart chakra, green-eyed jealousy, the Great Mother

The word *spinach* is derived from the Persian word *ispanai*, meaning "green hand," while the term *chlorophyll*, the pigment responsible for anything green in the plant world, is derived from the Greek for "green" and "leaf." Green is the essence of life, and spinach is the embodiment of this energy. The color green is found midway in the spectrum and is made up of two colors, yellow and blue. Yellow brings wisdom and clarity, while blue promotes peace. Green's basic qualities are balance and harmony. The thylakoids in spinach cells are what in part give spinach its green color;

medieval artists used to extract green pigment from spinach to use as ink or paint.

The miracle of green spreads softly as spring kisses awake a winter-worn world and sleeping seeds, pulling light, earth, and water together in a miraculous act of birth. We as a species depend on this holiest of acts, the emergence of new, green plant life that produces the oxygen and food we need to survive. This green energy is linked to the creative fertilizing power of new birth; resurrection is symbolized by the seeds of possibility buried deep in the earth, unknown until the rain falls, sprouting new shoots throughout the land. Verdant abundance brings the energy of lushness, richness, flourishing, thriving, and plenty.

Spinach is an excellent oil for ushering these energies into your life. U.S. currency is printed in the color green, earning the slang term *greenbacks* to refer to our paper money. For cultivating abundance and renewal, work with the aspect of spinach that is expressed as "the Egyptian god Osiris—green of skin—the god of resurrection and cultivation of crops, of whom it was declared, 'the world waxes green in triumph through him.'"[37] Osiris is also credited for teaching people how to gather wild fruit, train grape vines, and ferment foods.

> Reigning as a king on earth, Osiris reclaimed the Egyptians from savagery, gave them laws, and taught them to worship the gods. Before his time the Egyptians had been cannibals. But Isis, the sister and wife of Osiris, discovered wheat and barley growing wild, and Osiris introduced the cultivation of these grains amongst his people, who forthwith abandoned cannibalism and took kindly to a corn diet.[38]

Green is the primary color of the plant kingdom. It symbolizes growth and therefore change. Plants teach us about cycles and about transformation from one state to another. A series of resurrections occur throughout our lifetime: spring or a new morning that brings playfulness, hope, the planting of new ideas, innocence, and the feeling of awakening to the world anew and anticipating what the day will bring. In the summer or at high noon, green represents the energy of productivity, of getting the job done and empowering the mind. In its aspect of fall or twilight, green gifts the energy of bringing your energy inward, tying up loose ends, finishing projects, gathering your harvest or the fruits of your labor, and getting ready to rest. In its aspect of winter, or night, green represents the gifts of deep rest, sleep, hibernation, rejuvenation, dreaming, communing with deep mysteries, and shedding what is no longer useful from your previous cycle before you awaken and start anew. We live these cyclic energies seasonally as well as daily as we are reminded when and how to be a child, an adult, and an elder, and accept the responsibilities involved in each of these cycles.

In arid cultures where green plants are akin to life itself and not easily coaxed into being, the phrase "to do green things" means to do positive, life-affirming actions, whereas "doing red things" implies destructive actions. Just as green is complementary on the color wheel to red, the fresh moistness of green is often juxtaposed with the fiery heat of red.

Green in many ways is the energy of the middle way or the joining of forces. The heart chakra, whose color is green, is the middle of the seven chakras, bridging the gap between the upper and the lower chakras and representing our ability to love and connect with others. Green is found midway in the color spectrum. Green strikes the eye in such a way as to require no adjustment whatever, and is, therefore, the middle way.

The goddess Venus is the lover of the fiery Mars; she is often depicted soothing his more destructive impulses. In the Renaissance painting *Mars and Venus United by Love*, which we'll revisit in chapter 8, Cupid binds Mars, the god of war, to Venus, the goddess of love, with one of his love knots. This painting celebrates the civilizing and nurturing effects of love, as milk flows from Venus's breast as Mars' warhorse is restrained. Perhaps surprising to those who associate Venus with the pinks and reds of Valentine's Day, the Goddess of Love has historically been associated with the color green, and she is the patroness of gardens, vegetation, and vineyards.

The heart chakra, *anahata*, is a radiant green, illuminating and teaching love from the inside out, gifting all forms of love: unconditional, universal, romantic, and divine. The female buddha, Green Tara, represents the enlightened air element (air produces the heart chakra and is a smoky green color); invoking her is the purest expression of air, which rules higher love and compassion in action. She is the Mother of All Buddhas and is associated with fertility and the growth and nourishment of plants, flowers, and trees.

According to color theorist Lillian Verner-Bonds:

Green aids the memory, which makes it an important healing colour. Most physical and mental illnesses result from events in the past. Green can release these traumas . . . Green energy has to do with [the] pushing back of boundaries, of growing beyond what is known. Because green is connected to the heart it must develop relationships with things around it, but it also needs a degree of control and power, which may be supportive or destructive.[39]

On the destructive side, Shakespeare famously addresses this aspect of green in *The Merchant of Venice* when Portia exclaims, "How all the other passions fleet to air, as doubtful thoughts, and rash-embraced despair, and shuddering fear, and green-eyed jealousy!" And in *Othello*, the villainous Iago warns, "O, beware, my lord, of jealousy; It is the green-eye'd monster which doth mock the meat it feeds on."

The buddha of all-accomplishing wisdom, Amoghasiddhi, is green, and it is taught that if you meditate on his green color your jealousy will be transformed into wisdom.

On the nurturing side, Shashti, a Hindu mother goddess, is the benefactor and protector of children as well as a deity of healthy and prolific vegetation. Mothers worship her and ask for a long life and well-being for their children. One of the traditional offerings to her is spinach curry. As I wrote in my book *Vibrational Nutrition*, "Spinach supports nurturing yourself in a healthy way by fostering self-love, self-approval, and the ability for self-care. It's excellent for those who feel motherless, need mothering, or miss their mother's loving energy, as it opens you to the energy of the Great Mother."[40]

One of the newer spinach stories to work its way into the collective consciousness comes from the cartoon character Popeye: "I'm strong to the finich, cause I eats me spinach, I'm Popeye the Sailor Man!" Popeye was created by Elzie Crisler Segar, who in 1929 introduced the character into his existing newspaper cartoon strip, *Thimble Theatre*. Popeye's story represents the journey of incorporating and loving one's tender inner child, as seen in the character's relationship with his ward, Swee'Pea. Finding a supportive and caring way—the essence of spinach energy—to strengthen and stabilize himself enough to overcome hardship, as represented by the character Bluto the Terrible, finally allows Popeye to connect with his divine inner feminine, as expressed in his relationship with his sweetheart, Olive Oyl. In the end the Popeye story represents doing what you can for others and always following your heart and doing what you think is best.

> **Blending Tip** – Try blending spinach absolute with strawberry base oil to tame base instincts and bring out the gentle, loving aspects of human nature.

❁ Sweetgrass (*Hierochloe odorata*)

Presiding influence: White Buffalo Calf Woman

Key energies: sweet prayers, calling in positive energy, caretaking, removing sorrow from the body, blessings, summer energy, softness, holiness, heartfelt prayers

Every culture to have come in contact with sweetgrass has recognized its sacredness. Its botanical name, *Hierochloe odorata*, literally means "fragrant holy grass." In Northern Europe, sweetgrass was scattered in front of churches on holy days so the heavenly fragrance would be released when people walked over it to enter. In North American traditional cultures, sweetgrass has an auspicious pedigree and is referred to as one of the four sacred medicines (the others being tobacco, white sage, and cedar). I was taught that it should not be used for the removal of negative energies (purification), but instead should be used after a cleansing rite to call in sweet, beneficial energies and spirits and send heartfelt prayers.

In perfumery sweetgrass is referred to as *foin coupé*, or "cut hay," because it has the same beguiling scent as hay being cut and harvested on a warm summer evening. An interesting aspect of this absolute is that sweetgrass is cut and harvested in June and July and allowed to dry naturally in the sun until August. During this process, the grass becomes fragrant as coumarin, the aromatic lactone responsible for its sweet, haylike aroma, which is only liberated when the plant material is cut and dried. The finished product offers a sweet, faintly herbaceous scent with jamlike notes of fig and prunes. Some even claim it smells like the sweet breath of young bovines.

Blending Tip — I like to blend sweetgrass absolute with fig fixed oil (see chapter 3), as it amplifies and enriches the figgy, jammy notes. Folklore recommends applying it to the stomach and lower back after giving birth to receive blessings for the mother and the newborn. It is equally supportive of those who have suffered a miscarriage, as it removes sorrow from the body.

❀ Violet Leaf (*Viola odorata*)

Presiding influence: Mother Mary, Archangel Gabriel, fairies
Key energies: modesty, being humble in nature, devotion, dare to be happy with me, gentleness, childhood blessings, mothers-to-be

One beautiful creation story goes like this: Violets first blossomed when

Archangel Gabriel told Mother Mary (also known by the title "Viola Odorata," meaning "Our Lady of Modesty") of her son's coming birth. Due to the way the violet came to be, this flower has become an emissary for the energy of modesty, humility, and devotion. The Archangel Gabriel's name means "God is my strength." Gabriel brings messages to humankind from the Divine. He also brings aid in all areas related to children, helping during conception, pregnancy, childbirth, and child-rearing.

Fascinatingly, the Greeks tell a similar story. Violets first came into being to protect one of Artemis's nymphs, who like her mistress had pledged to stay a maiden. Out of compassion for her vows, Artemis turned her into a violet to shelter her from Apollo's relentless pursuit. This tale illustrates the energy of modesty and devotion that is attributed to violets.

During the Middle Ages, violets and their leaves went by the charming name "heart ease." In the Victorian language of flowers, white meant modesty, whereas the color violet expressed the idea that "my thoughts are occupied with love," coupled with the invitation to "dare to be happy with me."

This flower vibrates to the energy of delicate love, affection, modesty, faith, nobility, intuition, dignity, mystical awareness, inspiration, spiritual passion, and sovereignty. It is a patron of children and those gentle of heart. It also helps us access the gentler side of fairies.

Blending Tip – Violet absolute whispers, "dare to be happy with me." Dragon fruit fixed oil (see chapter 3) opens you to a world of delight—bringing amusement, fascination, and wonder. Apply this blend over your heart and that of your beloved to amplify this joyful, enchanting energy.

2

Essential Oils

Steam-Distilled or Expressed Plant Extracts

The mind I love most must have wild places, a tangled orchard where dark damsons drop in the heavy grass, an overgrown little wood, the chance of a snake or two, a pool that nobody fathomed the depth of, and paths threaded with flowers planted by the mind.

KATHERINE MANSFIELD

Essential oils are volatile concentrated plant extracts that retain the natural scent of their source. Each essential oil has a unique composition of chemicals, and this variation affects the oil's smell, absorption, and effects on the body. See chapter 1, "About Botanical Extractions," to review the various methods of extraction—in the case of the essential oils discussed in this chapter, most are created via steam-distilled extraction (except for citrus, which is commonly cold-pressed).

This chapter speaks to aspects of the body, mind, and emotions that are impacted by the essential oils included in this chapter. This information, presented in a snapshot format, will allow you to explore different effects of these plants on both the subtle and the physical bodies. Each of these plants displays a rich and multifaceted personality that may offer so much more than what we've profiled here, so take the time to get to know each plant and see what magic it wants to share with you.*

Basil, Sweet (*Ocimum basilicum*)

Subtle gifts: This oil vibrates to the heart chakra, allowing you to bridge the mundane and the Divine to foster love of all types, as well as forgiveness and compassion. Basil essential oil sharpens the mind and helps you think quickly to be able to figure out how to achieve your goals and ambitions. It is associated with the element of air, so there is a degree of fickleness to this oil. Be mindful when using to not rush head-in once your first ideas pop up, as this can lead to impulsiveness or even recklessness in how you use your newly gained knowledge. Instead, allow your ideas to percolate so you can develop a heart-based strategy that allows you to overcome obstacles and difficulties.

Physical gifts: antidepressant, anti-infectious, antimicrobial, antiseptic, antispasmodic, antiviral, cephalic, emmenagogue, expectorant; treats acne, eczema, infections, itchy insect bites, shingles, coughs, sinus infections/congestion, muscle aches, joint pain, PMS

Bergamot (*Citrus bergamia*)

Subtle gifts: Bergamot essential oil is liquid sunshine. It helps you value simplicity and overcome the tendency to try too hard or think too much, which can make things more complicated than they need to be. Resting in simplicity helps you develop a sunny outlook and a feeling of contentment and serenity.

Physical gifts: antiseptic, anti-depressant, antispasmodic, astringent analgesic, antidepressant, antifungal, anti-infectious, antimicrobial, diuretic,

---

*Remember that gardenia absolute can support creating your own deeper knowing of and relationship with each of these plants and oils. See the gardenia blending tip on page 45.

reduces fever and redness in skin; effective against gingivitis, sore throat, vaginal itching, fungus infections, lost appetite, flatulence, acne, psoriasis, eczema, sadness, cold sores, nerve and muscular pain, oily skin, shingles, colds and flu; heals scar tissue

Caution: Be mindful of sun exposure while using this oil; it can make your skin more sensitive to sunlight, increasing the risk of sunburn or irritation. Wait at least twelve hours after applying before sun exposure.

Black Pepper (*Piper nigrum*)

Subtle gifts: The name of this essential oil in Sanskrit is *marich*, meaning "sun." As its name signifies, this oil holds vast amounts of solar energy, which illuminates the mental body (ayurveda teaches that the mental body is produced by the third chakra). Black pepper essential oil applied on the third chakra allows you to release and transform rigid patterns held by the mind, bringing the knowledge that you do not have to repeat the past and lighting the way to seeing new solutions to old problems. This oil also brings the gift of refining an idea into its best expression and living in integrity. It enhances living by your personal code of conduct and is excellent for cultivating the precision that is needed to be a specialist.

Physical gifts: antiseptic, antispasmodic, expectorant, analgesic, antineuralgic, hemostatic; effective against colds, sore throat, headache, diarrhea, urinary tract infections, stomach cramps, small intestine health, rheumatism, neuralgia, earaches, psoriasis, acne

Blood Orange (*Citrus sinensis*)

Subtle gifts: Blood orange teaches you how to share your gifts and talents and overcome self-consciousness to allow your natural charisma to shine forth. It brings the gifts of being happy, emotionally regenerated, and strongly self-confident, thereby cultivating your inner sparkle, radiance, and exuberance.

Physical gifts: carminative, expectorant, heart tonic, disinfectant; treats weak digestion, gallbladder blockage, bladder and kidney disorders, fever, gingivitis, cellulite, dry skin, aging skin, anxiety, sadness

Caution: Be mindful of sun exposure while using this oil; it can make your skin more sensitive to sunlight, increasing the risk of sunburn or irritation. Wait at least twelve hours after applying before sun exposure.

Blue Chamomile (*Matricaria chamomilla*)

Subtle gifts: This sagacious oil helps you cultivate a profound knowledge of any subject you are focused on. It helps you understand ideas from past eras, supports you in opening to guidance from your higher Self and from spiritual guides, and stabilizes this connection, allowing you to communicate your discoveries. It is a very good oil for writers and artists, as it instills wisdom and advances good communication and an expansive worldview.

Physical gifts: anti-inflammatory, immune-stimulant, analgesic, antispasmodic, sedative, emmenagogue; effective against inflamed skin, leukocyte formation, arthritis, headache, insomnia, irritability, menopause, digestive problems, liver and spleen congestion, anger, tantrums, burns

Cardamom (*Elettaria cardamomum*)

Subtle gifts: This motivational essential oil stimulates creativity, opening you to the unexplored part of your psyche that bring new perspectives and understandings. It is an incredible oil for dissolving the patterns of being inflexible, judgmental, and contrary; in turn, this shift opens you up to the ability to work in collectives in a joyful manner, encouraging enthusiasm and confidence.

Physical gifts: stimulant, expectorant, carminative, stomachic, diaphoretic, aphrodisiac; effective treatment for colds, cough, loss of taste, indigestion, impotence

Cedar, Eastern White (*Thuja occidentalis*)

Subtle gifts: This tree offers a sense of our interconnectedness, strengthening our perception of the web of light shared by all beings and all particles and the union of past, present, and future. Cedar brings wholeness to seeming duality and combines all energies, uniting all that was, is, or could be. When we lose our awareness of this connection in our lives, we feel isolated, lonely, and bereft. Yet the energy is there—we just need to open to it. Cedar oil lightens and frees you from low vibrations, energetic burdens, and parasitic energies on the subtle level. It encourages supportive friendships and community-building.

Physical gifts: thins mucus, making it less thick and sticky and easier to cough up, removing it from the ears, nose, and throat to relieve respiratory conditions such as a chesty cough, catarrh, and bronchitis; anti-infectious, antiviral (especially against cold sores and plantar warts), insecticide, analgesic; heals scars

Caution: *For external use only*! Cedar is potentially toxic and neurotoxic and should not be ingested or taken orally. Toxicity symptoms include epileptic convulsions, gastroenteritis, flatulence, and hypotension. Ingesting cedar's thujones can also result in fatty liver disease. *Poisoning has only been reported after oral administration*. Keep out of reach of children. If you have any concerns, speak to a health care provider before using.

Cinnamon Leaf (*Cinnamomum zeylanicum*)

Subtle gifts: This essential oil is very dynamic for pulling you out of the mire of self-defeat, self-pity, self-destructiveness, and not taking care of yourself. It helps you clearly see your negative self-fulfilling prophecies and helps you shift your energy before they come to be. It holds space for you when seemingly no one else wants to, when you feel like the whole world is against you. We all get down sometimes, and this oil helps you properly explore your gloomy feelings so that you can be done with them. This is the type of energy that no one can pull out of you except you and you alone. Cinnamon essential oil is steadfast, practical, realistic, and direct.

Physical gifts: analgesic, antiparasitic, antibacterial, antifungal, anti-inflammatory, antimicrobial, antiseptic, antispasmodic, aphrodisiac, astringent, bactericidal, carminative (relives flatulence), digestive, germicide, orexigenic (stimulating effect on the appetite); effective against amenorrhea, anorexia, insect bites, candida, colds, cough, diarrhea, nervous exhaustion, gum disease, influenza, lice, rheumatism, scabies, stomach distention, stress, ringworm, athlete's foot, jock itch, toothache, warts; stimulates contractions in childbirth and improves circulation

Caution: Do not use during pregnancy or if suffering from stomach or intestinal ulcers; may cause skin irritation (use a skin patch test before use); in excess can cause tachycardia, inhibited blood clotting, and may react with certain medications such as diabetes medications or anticoagulant medications; may cause dyspnea (difficult or labored breathing); not for use in the bath.

Citron, Buddha's Hand (*Citrus medica*)

Subtle gifts: This essential oil helps you question your reality, ask the hard questions, pull back the curtains of your life, and start your own unique journey to uncover the truths that are tailor-made for you; calms the mind and helps right irrational states of being

Physical gifts: supports lung well-being; antiarthritic, relieves headache and sluggish digestion

Caution: Be mindful of sun exposure while using this oil; it can make your skin more sensitive to sunlight, increasing the risk of sunburn or irritation. Wait at least twelve hours after applying before sun exposure.

Clary Sage (*Salvia sclarea*)

Subtle gifts: This oil helps you integrate suppressed emotions and liberate deep-seated feelings of anger or sorrow, and if applicable, feelings linked to sexuality that lead to discord and acting out or shutting down. Clary sage warms and thaws out the emotional body and leads the way for the resolution and healing of what needs to come to the surface. It brings beauty and light into your sexual relationships, which fosters bonding and growth on an emotional level. It is a plant of resolution, free-flowing emotions, and positive sexuality.

Physical gifts: antibacterial, antidepressant, anti-inflammatory, antipyretic (lowers fever), antiseptic, antispasmodic, aphrodisiac, astringent, carminative (relieves flatulence), cytotoxic, deodorant, digestive, emmenagogue (stimulates menstrual discharge), hypotensive, nervine, sedative; effective against acne, boils, constipation, cramps, dandruff, oily hair, depression, exhaustion, nervousness, high blood pressure, hyperactive behavior, low libido, lymphatic congestion, migraine, muscular aches, nervousness, premenstrual tension, stress; supportive of adrenal glands and kidney health and useful in menopause

Elemi (*Canarium luzonicum*)

Subtle gifts: This fascinating resin takes its name from an Arabic term meaning "above and below," and not surprisingly, elemi essential oil is dynamic for connecting the mind and spirit and for supporting an understanding of the micro-/macrocosm relationship. This in turn allows your own higher guidance to open you up to different perspectives on life, supporting you in taking actions that allow true growth. It is also helpful for exploring your experience of self.

Physical gifts: immune system tonic, promotes wound healing, effective against chronic bronchitis, colitis, diarrhea, exhaustion, muscular pain, parasites, rheumatic pain, sinus infections, stress, varicose ulcers

Caution: Avoid during pregnancy.

Frankincense (*Boswellia carterii*)

Subtle gifts: This remarkable essential oil opens you to the ability to read energy in your environment so that you understand how best to react in the moment from an evolved state of mind. This oil also brings the gifts of refinement in speech, helping you to find the right words for yourself and to use words to affect your environment. It allows you to tap into your inner muse for inspiration, mysticism, and authentic self-expression.

Physical gifts: alterative (favorably altering the course of an ailment), analgesic, rejuvenative, anti-inflammatory, disinfectant, antiseptic, astringent; effective against bronchitis, colds, sinus infections, wrinkles

---

Boswellia

Boswellia carterii is a type of frankincense from Somalia that is often confused with *Boswellia sacra* (see chapter 1), but they are distinct species and as such they have distinct energy signatures. *B. carterii* is typically extracted through steam distillation to create an essential oil, while *B. sacra* lends itself beautifully to being an absolute.

Grapefruit (*Citrus paradisi*)

Subtle gifts: Grapefruit essential oil is helpful for when you are trapped in the authoritarian powers of others and cannot figure out how to break free. It will help you dissolve those bonds, counter any self-doubt, and find the energy to move forward into a more supportive environment.

Physical gifts: stimulant, carminative, diuretic, lymphatic, digestive, nervine; effective against digestive problems, obesity, water retention, liver and gallbladder issues, cellulite, depression

Caution: Be mindful of sun exposure while using this oil; it can make your skin more sensitive to sunlight, increasing the risk of sunburn or irritation. Wait at least twelve hours after applying before sun exposure.

....

Blending Tip — Blending grapefruit essential oil with okra fixed oil (see chapter 3) can help release you from limiting situations and guide you toward greater autonomy.

....

Jasmine (*Jasminum grandiflorum*)

Subtle gifts: In Vedic thought this oil promotes psychic abilities and helps make the mind open and insightful, especially when experiencing non-ordinary states of consciousness. Traditionally, jasmine essential oil has been used for making the mind sensitive to the frequency of mantras, so it can be of benefit for chanting, affirmations, or prayer work. It has a refined and sensual quality that increases sensitivity.

Physical gifts: cooling, moisturizing, nervine, antibacterial, aphrodisiac, antidepressant; effective against hypersensitivity, headache, fever, excessive sun exposure; supports lymph health, sooths dry skin, and promotes healthy sexuality

....

Blending Tip – Jasmine blended with red raspberry fixed oil (see chapter 3) helps to regulate hypersensitive emotions and promotes psychic abilities, making the mind open and insightful, allowing easier navigation through life.

....

Kumquat (*Fortunella japonica*)

Subtle gifts: Kumquat oil moves you toward honest, meaningful connections with people, allowing you to notice the frustration that arises when you're ensnared in shallow, empty, or obligatory relationships, teaching you how to shift this stuck energy by seeking greater depth in yourself and in other people. Ultimately it allows you to get past protective facades.

Physical gifts: astringent, antiseptic, purifying; relieves sluggish digestion, dark skin spots, fine lines

Caution: Be mindful of sun exposure while using this oil; it can make your skin more sensitive to sunlight, increasing the risk of sunburn or irritation. Wait at least twelve hours after applying before sun exposure.

Lavender (*Lavandula officinalis*)

Subtle gifts: Lavender harmonizes more aspects of the human condition than any other essential oil. This plant's remarkable oil encourages you to deeply engage with the world, sharing your unique gifts and your light. It heals feelings of being overly delicate, withdrawn, or fearful and brings spiritual growth by helping you integrate your experiences, which brings an expanded awareness and perspective. It is healing, soothing, and cushioning.

Physical gifts: antifungal, antibacterial (including *Sarcina* genus, involved in dental decay), antimicrobial; an effective treatment for acne, amenorrhea, anorexia, burns, cellulite, colic, cough, cystitis, dandruff, dermatitis, slow digestion, earache, eczema, flatulence, halitosis, headache, hypertension, nervous indigestion, insect bites, insomnia, migraine, nausea, psoriasis, scars, sinus congestion, sores, sprains, stress, sunburn, nervous tension, spider veins, ulcers

Lemon (*Citrus limon*)

Subtle gifts: Lemon is of two minds, both very valuable. On the one hand it dispels darkness through merriment. Gaiety is the means to purify that which shackles your joy. Lemon dissolves this in ripples of laughter. On the other hand, this fruit teaches fulfillment in finding nourishment from a spiritual source, which brings inner security and joy. Goals and desires are reached, and this brings a sense of completion and satisfaction. Lemon accomplishes this by helping you gather all of your energy and intellectual focus and then directing it toward your intended goal or desire. It is a plant of deep purification, versatility, and clarity of mind.

Physical gifts: antiarthritic, antifungal, anti-inflammatory, antimicrobial, antiseptic, antispasmodic, antitoxic, antiviral, astringent, bactericidal, cicatrizing, detoxifying, reduces fever; helps balance the skin's sebum and is effective against warts, dark spots, varicose veins, colds, flu, cellulitis, muscle tension, ring worm; offers general immune support

Caution: Be mindful of sun exposure while using this oil; it can make your skin more sensitive to sunlight, increasing the risk of sunburn or irritation. Wait at least twelve hours after applying before sun exposure.

Lime (*Citrus aurantiifolia*)

Subtle gifts: This essential oil is beneficial for energetic cord-cutting and detaching from the collective. Use it to enhance your perception of the truth of any situation, which allows you to release any illusions that keep you ensnared in a projected reality. It is an oil of release, detachment, and freedom.

Physical gifts: cooling, drying, carminative, expectorant, stimulant, diuretic, antiseptic, antispasmodic, antidepressant, tonic, antiviral; effective treatment for poor digestion, lymph congestion, gallbladder congestion, liver congestion, lung congestion, weight gain

Caution: Be mindful of sun exposure while using this oil; it can make your skin more sensitive to sunlight, increasing the risk of sunburn or irritation. Wait at least twelve hours after applying before sun exposure.

Mandarin Orange (*Citrus reticulata*)

Subtle gifts: This citrus aids in inner-child work, allowing you to address deep-seated fears so that latent abilities are brought to the surface. It permits you to see how you are perceived by others, thus allowing you to see yourself more clearly so that difficulties and struggles can be viewed in a clear light. It is supportive in counseling situations when you are working with deep emotions, childhood memories, and associated bodily sensations.

Physical gifts: cooling, drying, calming, antispasmodic, nervine, digestive; addresses insomnia

Caution: Be mindful of sun exposure while using this oil; it can make your skin more sensitive to sunlight, increasing the risk of sunburn or irritation. Wait at least twelve hours after applying before sun exposure.

Marjoram (*Origanum majorana, Marjorana hortenis*)

Subtle gifts: Marjoram brings the energy of what Scandanavians call *hygge*, a coziness and comfortable conviviality accompanied by feelings of wellness and contentment. It is a warm embrace, the perfect cup of tea, sitting by the fire with a book, a soft pillow, a warm bowl of soup on a winter's day. Use in times when you are in need of comfort and being held and uplifted on an emotional level. Marjoram is an herb of comfort, peace, and contentment.

Physical gifts: antibacterial (especially against type 2 herpes simplex), antifungal, carminative (relieves flatulence), diuretic, digestive, laxative, nervine (supports the nervous system); encourages only healthy cells to grow, not scar tissue; cephalic (i.e., "related to the head" and used to treat various mind/brain disorders like weak memory); effective against arthritis, rheumatoid arthritis, bronchitis, bruises, chilblains (the painful inflammation of small blood vessels in the skin that occurs in response to repeated exposure to cold), colic, diarrhea, hyperactivity, hypertension, leukorrhea (vaginal discharge), PMS, respiratory infections, sinusitis, muscle spasms, migraines, sprains, mouth ulcers, vertigo; lowers high blood pressure, promotes vasodilation, supports the autonomic nervous system

---

The "Herb of Happiness"

Known colloquially by several monikers, including "joy of the mountains," marjoram is predominantly warming and sedating. Seventeenth-century English botanist Nicholas Culpeper recommended it for "cold griefs," deep bone or muscle aches, while sixteenth-century English herbalist John Gerard recommended it "for those who are given to over-much sighing." It was traditionally believed to help curb excessive sexual impulses. It is said this plant gets its scent from the goddess of love, Aphrodite, to whom it is dedicated and who touched it with tenderness and brought its scent into the world.

Neroli (*Citrus aurantium*)

Subtle gifts: This refined essential oil is a delight! Neroli brings the energy of pure love and lightness of being by melting away sorrows and bringing a peaceful, stable calm. This oil is indispensable for healing trauma from childhood abuse or anytime you are in an emotional crisis or suffering from sadness, shock, or upset; in such cases neroli fosters a sense of hope and leads you out of fear. Neroli opens you to the love within yourself and the freedom of allowing that love to flow freely. It is a plant of spirituality and serenity.

Physical gifts: antidepressant, antiseptic, antispasmodic, aphrodisiac, antibacterial; promotes good muscle tone, treats spider veins, sensitive skin, and stretch marks, and improves the tone and elasticity of skin

Oakmoss (*Evernia prunastri*)

Subtle gifts: A species of lichen, this plant's vibration releases you from clinging to old fears, letting you move forward without carrying old baggage, giving you the ability to stay in the present and act in the present. With the release of old fears, the energy drain that has been occurring to keep these fears alive is returned in a form that nourishes one's growth and well-being. Oakmoss is a plant of inner peace. It releases you from feeling tired, sapped, and unable to stay present. This oil has the energy of the Old Man of the Forest.

Physical gifts: warming, sedative, calming; awakens naturalistic impulses; relieves stress and frigidity

> **Blending Tip** – Try blending oakmoss essential oil, Siberian fir absolute (see chapter 1), and cloudberry fixed oil (see chapter 3) to explore your internal labyrinth.

Orange, Common (*Citrus sinensis*)

Subtle gifts: The common orange brings out your hidden desires and dissolves frustration, self-consciousness, and low self-esteem, allowing you to bask in the warm glow of happiness.

Physical gifts: carminative, expectorant, heart tonic, disinfectant; addresses weak digestion, gallbladder blockage, bladder and kidney disorders, fever, gingivitis, cellulite, dry skin, aging skin, anxiety, sadness

Caution: Be mindful of sun exposure while using this oil; it can make your skin more sensitive to sunlight, increasing the risk of sunburn or irritation. Wait at least twelve hours after applying before sun exposure.

Patchouli (*Pogostemon cablin*)

Subtle gifts: This essential oil offers the gift of self-containment, allowing you to enjoy being alone with yourself in a content and relaxed state; this in turn gives rise to having a large store of energy so you can get things done. Patchouli can be very supportive in helping you reach your goals, from clarifying what you desire to having the tenacity to do what is needed to reach them. It helps you overcome fatigue and feeling downhearted. A very sensual oil, it offers poise, lucidity, and serenity.

Physical gifts: warming, regenerative, fungicidal, decongestant, antidepressant, aphrodisiac, antiseptic, tonic; effective treatment for acne, eczema, cracked and chapped skin, impetigo, seborrhea, dandruff, yeast infections of the mouth and vagina

Peppermint (*Mentha piperita*)

Subtle gifts: This essential oil encourages you to avoid extremes and in doing so it opens the door to achieving the impossible. Peppermint oil makes this possible by teaching at an energetic level the art of staying in the flow when an outcome is impossible to predict, allowing you to keep a cool head and observe events unfold with detachment until you see the most auspicious path, and then jumping in with both feet! Peppermint reminds you that life is always in flux, and energy can be rechanneled at any given time toward a desired outcome as long as you remain poised, present, and cool-minded. It is clarifying, awakening, stimulating, and penetrating.

Physical gifts: analgesic, anesthetic (topical), antiacid, antibacterial, anti-inflammatory, antifungal, antimicrobial, antiviral, digestive, expectorant, hepatic, insecticide, rubefacient, sedative, stimulant, vasoconstrictor, vasodilator; effective treatment for congested breasts, bruises, nasal inflammation, colds, cramps, dermatitis, diarrhea, exhaustion, fever, flatulence, gallbladder congestion, swollen gums, halitosis, headache, heartburn, indigestion, influenza, insect bites, itching, kidney congestion, liver congestion, lumbago, mental fatigue, migraine, nausea, rheumatism, ringworm, scabies, sciatica, shingles, sinus infections, toothache, vertigo; helps dry up lactation and raises the libido. Peppermint oil is an apoptotic essential oil, meaning it can either sedate or stimulate depending on the action needed. Applied externally, peppermint initially constricts the capillaries, causing cooling of the skin. After some minutes it then has a rubefacient effect of dilating the capillaries, bringing blood and warmth to the surface of the skin.

Caution: Not for use in first trimester of pregnancy or while breastfeeding, as it may reduce milk production; not for use in children under two years old; avoid with epilepsy and when using homeopathics, as peppermint can neutralize their effects. A 2 percent dilution rate and skin patch test is recommended. Not for use in the bath.

Petitgrain (*Citrus aurantium*)

Subtle gifts: This oil grants discernment, the ability to judge well in all things.

Physical gifts: antiarthritic, anti-infectious, anti-inflammatory, antiseptic, antispasmodic; helps balance excessive perspiration and greasy hair and skin; effective against asthma, colds and flu, hay fever, respiratory infections, shallow breathing, joint inflammation, candida, ringworm, athlete's foot, chronic fatigue syndrome, mental exhaustion, PMS, menopause

Caution: Be mindful of sun exposure while using this oil; it can make your skin more sensitive to sunlight, increasing the risk of sunburn or irritation. Wait at least twelve hours after applying before sun exposure.

Pine (*Pinus sylvestris*)

Subtle gifts: Pine is a key essential oil for restoring the heart when your emotions have hardened. This loving oil releases you from old wounds, letting you move forward without carrying the baggage of the past, bringing the ability to experience your emotions in real time versus playing out echoes from the past. This shift allows your emotional body to be nourished and replenished, bringing growth, inner peace, a strong sense of well-being, and the ability to engage in loving relationships. The quest of Pinocchio, the boy who was carved from pine, was to understand what was required for him to become a "real" boy. Pine offers the gift of self-love, self-forgiveness, and trust.

Physical gifts: warming, drying, expectorant, diaphoretic, antiseptic, supports blood and plasma health; effective against colds, bronchitis, lung problems, sinus issues, hair loss, depression

Caution: May irritate sensitive skin.

Pink Pepper Seed (*Schinus molle*)

Subtle gifts: This spicy essential oil encourages your erotic, rapturous nature and plants love in your body. This gives rise to ecstatic sexuality and supports the healing of shame, body image issues, frigidity, and feelings of vulnerability. It is a plant of inner trust, inner warmth, and expressiveness.

Physical gifts: warming, antiseptic, antiviral, stimulant, supports circulation; treats arthritis, muscular aches, and stiffness

Pomelo (*Citrus grandis, Citrus maxima*)

Subtle gifts: This essential oil, extracted from the peel of the fruit, assists those with latent teaching abilities, allowing this gift to blossom. This may express itself though writing, teaching in a classroom setting, or working with students one-on-one. If you are an established teacher, this essential oil allows you to hone your craft further and innovate.

Physical gifts: treats muscle pain and aches, lung issues, fatigue, loss of vitality, bruising, acne

Caution: Be mindful of sun exposure while using this oil; it can make your skin more sensitive to sunlight, increasing the risk of sunburn or irritation. Wait at least twelve hours after applying before sun exposure.

Grapefruit's Fun Uncle

Pomelo is the largest citrus fruit (6 to 10 inches in diameter) and an ancestor of the grapefruit. It is also known as shaddock, and its botanical name, *Citrus maxima*, means "the biggest citrus."

Red Spikenard (*Nardostachys jatamansi*)

Subtle gifts: Red spikenard addresses subconscious traumas. It is grounding, but not in a dulling way; it allows you to gain control of your life and stabilizes you when you are feeling unsafe in your physical body. Use this oil to shunt the energy from your upper chakras to your first chakra to ground those energies for practical use. Red spikenard is beneficial for those on a spiritual path, to balance the mundane with the elevated, as in the Zen saying "Before enlightenment, chop wood, carry water. After enlightenment, chop wood, carry water." This oil is excellent for grounding spirituality and accessing body wisdom as well as ancient information.

Physical gifts: anti-infectious, anti-inflammatory, bactericidal, fungicidal; addresses sluggish circulation, anxiety, insomnia, headache, hyperactivity, migraine

---

One of the Rarest Essential Oils

A member of the honeysuckle family, spikenard grows mainly in Himalayan countries (China, India, Nepal). Its use goes back to ancient times, to the early Egyptian, Hebrew, and Hindu civilizations, which used it as a perfume ingredient and in spiritual rituals, while the Bible describes Mary anointing the feet of Jesus with spikenard before the Last Supper.

Rosemary (*Rosmarinus officinalis*)

Subtle gifts: This oil is a heavy hitter that teaches how to wield personal power. Rosemary sharpens the intellect, logic, and will. It teaches leadership and integrity, courage and self-worth, consciousness and refinement—and let us not forget *remembrance*. Rosemary balances the third chakra. The name rosemary comes from the Latin *ros*, meaning "dew," and *marinus*, meaning "sea," translating to "dew of the sea," reflecting its Mediterranean origins and fresh, invigorating scent.

Physical gifts: anti-inflammatory, relieves pain and muscle soreness, promotes hair growth, strengthens hair follicles, reduces dandruff and scalp irritation, enhances memory and concentration, reduces mental fatigue as well as indigestion and bloating, strengthens digestion, improves circulation, reduces inflammation in blood vessels, may help lower blood pressure

Caution: Avoid during pregnancy, especially in the first trimester, and with epilepsy or a history of seizures. Rosemary may interact with blood thinners (like warfarin) and diabetic medications, affecting blood pressure and blood sugar levels. It could also increase lithium toxicity. Use high dilution rates when applying it to the skin, as it may cause irritation. Avoid using it for children under two years old.

Sandalwood (*Santalum album*)

Subtle gifts: This wise tree brings an inner awareness and a sense of ease when engaging your higher consciousness. This is helpful for gaining insights into blockages on your spiritual path, whether internal or external, so you can gently process them at the deepest level. Ultimately, sandalwood breaks down illusions, helping you align with your true self. This is an excellent oil for meditation, spiritual practice, and healers. Sandalwood is associated with enlightenment, meditation, and connection with the Divine.

Physical gifts: anti-inflammatory, anti-infectious, antimicrobial, antispasmodic, astringent, bactericidal, cicatrizing, diuretic, expectorant, insecticidal; effective against infections of the mouth and genitals, cramps and muscle spasms, bronchitis, sore throat, compromised immune system

Tangerine (*Citrus tangerina*)

Subtle gifts: Tangerine helps you grow into adulthood when there's been a habitual pattern (either self-directed or having been forced on you) of staying in a child's energy, such as with the Peter Pan syndrome. Tangerine offsets sadness, fear, and irritability.

Physical gifts: cooling, diuretic, nervine; treats insomnia, rheumatism; supports liver, stomach, and gallbladder health

Caution: Be mindful of sun exposure while using this oil; it can make your skin more sensitive to sunlight, increasing the risk of sunburn or irritation. Wait at least twelve hours after applying before sun exposure.

Vanilla (*Vanilla planifolia*)

Subtle gifts: This sweet-smelling essential oil is highly viscous, and its physical form reveals many of its energetic traits. It helps create strong emotional bonds and encourages you to follow your heart. It gives rise to passion, positive sexuality, wildness, and touch as a form of communication. It helps heal emotional conflicts, oversensitivity, bitterness, hostility, insincerity, and resentment. It gives rise to being unselfish and truly understanding what is required to be in a balanced partnership.

Physical gifts: warming, moisturizing, tonic, calming, relaxing; softens anger and all rough edges; a mild stimulant during menstruation

Vetiver (*Vetiveria zizanioides*)

Subtle gifts: This rich essential oil brings the gifts of being grounded and centered in yourself. This in turn cultivates strength, honor, and a strong mind-body connection. If you are struggling with loss of purpose and trying to find the right direction, this is an excellent plant to aid you in finding the right path forward. It is a plant of integrity, protection, and serenity.

Physical gifts: antiarthritic, antifungal, anti-inflammatory, antimicrobial, antiseptic, antispasmodic, antiviral, bactericidal, expectorant, nervine; treats inflammation, dry skin, irregular breathing, muscle aches, arthritis, ringworm, athlete's foot, chronic fatigue syndrome, PMS, menopause

....

Blending Tip – Blend vetiver essential oil with Siberian fir absolute (see chapter 1) and diffuse to help you navigate your life and find the right path forward.

....

White Birch (*Betula lenta*)

Subtle gifts: White birch is an expression of the divine feminine. It brings light into darkness and provides deep purification, emotional succor, protection, and a profound sense of calm. It expands your appreciation of beauty and your own inner radiance as a reflection of that archetype. In Russian folklore as well as in Norse and Germanic cultures, birch is called the "Lady of the Forest." Many cultures attribute qualities of nurturing, mothering, renewal, and protection to the white birch tree. The nourishing, caring birch is an age-old symbol of the White Goddess, and the Germanic rune *berkana*, "birch," stands in part for protection.

Physical gifts: vasodilator; nourishes blood flow by cooling action followed by warming action, thereby treating aches and pains of the muscles and joints such as arthritis, backache, sprains; rubefacient; effective against cramps, colds, congestion, fever, gout, inflammation; purifies the blood; removes toxins from the body; potent germicide

Caution: Do not take orally or use during pregnancy. This essential oil mainly consists of methyl salicylate, so it should not be used by anyone allergic to aspirin or who is taking blood thinners or who has a low blood-clotting ability. Avoid with epilepsy and Parkinson's disease. Not for use with children or with the frail. Do not use in the bath.

Birch Bark Writing

In antiquity, birch bark was often used in place of paper to write on. The oldest surviving Buddhist texts, dating as far back as the first century BCE, are preserved on long rolls of birch bark and are known as the Gandharan Scrolls, so named for having been written in Gandhari, an early regional Indic language that is long extinct. The Rig Veda, a foundational Hindu text that is part of the Vedas, was originally an oral text, not written, so no complete manuscript exists or has probably ever existed. The oldest surviving manuscript, which dates back to 1040 CE, is a transcription written on birch bark that was discovered in Nepal.

During the Viking Age, about 800 to 1500 CE, information was inscribed on birch bark. This practice also occurred in North America, where birch bark scrolls were used as writing sheets. A notable example is the Ojibwe people of the Great Lakes region, who made birch bark scrolls called *wiigwassabak* on which ceremonial practices and teachings were recorded; these scrolls date back four hundred years and were found preserved in caves. There is some secrecy involved in their preservation today due to their sacred nature. This points to why birch bark is so enduring due to its potent essential oils, which render it resistant to decay and insect attack thanks to the presence of suberin and betulin. This bark is pliable and can be readily bent and rolled but not folded.

Even today, the bark of the birch tree is used in India and Tibet to record sacred mantras. This is called *written japa* and is a powerful variation of silent japa, the meditative repetition of a mantra or a divine name. It entails repeatedly writing a mantra on paper, birch bark, or tree leaves.

White Lotus (*Nelumbo nucifera*)

Subtle gifts: White lotus holds the vibration of the entire path of enlightenment and is a powerful teacher and guide. This radiant oil first stimulates you at the unconscious level, bringing the desire to become actualized, and then supports this path as your budding consciousness learns the lessons offered from each chakra. Of course, the ultimate goal of this oil is to usher you into a state of enlightenment. This is an excellent oil to reach for when you cannot quite name what has you stuck, but you need relief, as lotus supports your whole life journey and circumstances. It is a plant of growth of soul and spirit.

Physical gifts: treats morning sickness and nausea, headache, tightness in the chest area, and assists when feeling despondent.

3

Fixed Oils

The Carriers for Blending

Our hearts irrigate this earth.
We are fields before
each other.

St. Thomas Aquinas,
from "We Are Fields Before Each Other,"
translated by Daniel Ladinsky

Fixed oils, also known as base or carrier oils, are pressed from the fatty portions of a plant or botanical such as the seeds, nuts, or kernels (see chapter 1, "About Botanical Extraction"). Since they are "fixed," they do not evaporate, unlike absolutes and essential oils, which are volatile oils and will evaporate upon contact with air.

You can blend fixed oils with essential oils and absolutes or use them alone for their rich gifts. Some of these oils are intense in energy and viscosity. If you find this to be the case, dilute with a fractionated coconut oil 50/50 or even more. I personally like my tomato seed oil diluted with 25–75 percent fractionated coconut oil. Fractionated coconut oil is a *neutral energy*, so it will not interfere with the vibrations of other carrier oils.

What Is Fractionated Coconut Oil?

Fractionated coconut oil is so-named because it is a fraction of the whole oil in which the long-chain fatty acids are removed so that only the medium-chain saturated fatty acids remain. This gives it a long shelf life, as it won't go rancid like unrefined oils. It is also capable of handling high heat, which makes it easier to work with than solid coconut oil. Fractionated coconut oil is sometimes sold as MCT (medium-chain triglyceride) oil because it consists mainly of medium chain caprylic and capric acids. You will see fractionated coconut oil included in many of the blend recipes in this book. It is a scentless, energetically neutral addition, used to enhance slip and glidability.

Almond, Sweet (*Prunus amygdalus var. dulcis*)

Subtle gifts: Sweet almond oil addresses the fear of aging to make the passage of time sacred and not solely experienced through the physical body. It opens you to the complex beauty of your true self and a strong inner vitality.

Physical gifts: Almond oil is a rather stable and light, readily absorbed emollient oil high in monounsaturated oleic acid and linoleic acids and rich in vitamin E. This oil rates high in its ability to retain moisture and prevent water loss through the skin by creating a light, occlusive, protective film for the stratum corneum, the outermost layer of the skin.

Apple Seed (*Pyrus malus*)

Subtle gifts: Apple gives rise to a greater understanding of yourself and the environment by accessing the unfolding but unused aspects of the self. It connects the conscious mind with the unconscious for growth and deepens the creative impulse that leads to beauty here on Earth.

When cut lengthwise, an apple reveals a near-perfect five-pointed star, with each point containing a seed; this design expresses the tenet "As above, so below," the microcosmic-macrocosmic principle.

Physical gifts: Apple seeds possess a high concentration of protein and amino acids such as magnesium, potassium, phosphorus, iron, and calcium, and a lower content of amygdalin, alpha-linoleic acid, oleic acid, and linoleic acid. Apple seed oil activates collagen, the protein that stimulates the cells of the lips and skin, providing a youthful plumpness. Collagen production lowers as one ages, which weakens the cells and can result in fine lines and the appearance of a lack of vibrancy; this oil provides softness and elasticity. Additionally, it has a high content of antioxidants that eliminate free radicals, delay signs of aging, and protect against UV damage.

Apricot Seed (*Prunus persica, Prunus armeniaca*)

Subtle gifts: Apricot seed oil balances mood swings and extreme emotional states. It promotes an exchange between the mental and the emotional bodies and facilitates the reconciliation of internal conflicts and strong negative emotions that have been stored in the body. It empowers you to take responsibility for your life and make the changes necessary for your health and well-being. It also fosters delight in life itself.

Physical gifts: This oil is excellent for mature skin due to its emollient, nurturing, and revitalizing properties. Its high vitamin E content provides free-radical protection from oxidation of cell membranes. It is an anti-inflammatory, soothing, and supports the protective barrier function of the skin due to its beta-sitosterol content. This plant is unique in that it has one of the highest concentrations of vitamin B_{17} (also known as laetrile) in the plant world, which is why it has been promoted as an anticancer compound. You may want to consider this oil as an addition to blends to address skin cancer and those with a high risk for skin cancer.

Avocado (*Persea gratissima*)

Subtle gifts: Avocado oil facilitates intimacy by granting the gift of positive touch. It harmonizes the body and mind by dissolving emotional tensions and the negative influences of past pain that cause you to turn inward and harden against love that is offered. It offers shelter when feeling overwhelmed with emotions and allows you to become more vulnerable to others without fear.

Physical gifts: This oil is pressed from the fruiting body or the flesh that surrounds the seed or pit, similar to olive oil production. The oil is composed of 20 percent essential unsaturated linoleic acid and a generous 12 percent of rare palmitoleic acid. Avocado oil has a number of healthful unsaponifiable compounds: vitamins A, B, and E; proteins and amino acids; and a small amount of phospholipid lecithin. This oil supports a healthy stratum corneum, the outer layer of the skin, and increases water-soluble collagen content in the dermis, the middle layer of the skin. When your skin lacks soluble collagen, it appears aged and thin. The phytosterol content of avocado oil supports collagen and skin structures, helping to prevent age spots and cell-wall weakening, while calming inflammation, regenerating tissues, and protecting the barrier functions of the skin. Avocado oil is also high in the carotenoids that protect against UV rays.

Blackberry Seed (*Rubus fruiticosus*)

Subtle gifts: This oil is excellent for healing the compulsion to sacrifice yourself while trying to live up to the expectations of others. It offers strong support and protection against gossip and what I call "helpful meddling," where someone says or does something that's to your detriment, and indeed causes hurt, but claims it's to benefit you.

Physical gifts: This oil is light and easily and deeply absorbed. It is high in phytonutrients and essential fatty acids, including linoleic acid (60 percent) and alpha-linolenic acid (15 percent). Its vitamin E tocopherol and tocotrienol compounds, beta-sitosterols and carotenoids, and lutein content makes this oil anti-inflammatory and free radical–scavenging, as well as soothing, nourishing, and protective to all layers of the skin. Its high vitamin C content helps to slow skin aging and supports production of collagen while smoothing blotchy areas and wrinkles, and reducing enlarged pores.

Blending Tip – Blend sunflower seed and blackberry oils for protection against gossip and its hurtful actions.

Black Currant Seed (*Ribes nigrum*)

Subtle gifts: This oil helps you become still and focused so you can look for answers within instead of rushing around asking questions and seeking counsel from others. It supports you in finding answers in the cave of your own heart. It remove dense, dark energy from the subtle body and brings in light.

Physical gifts: Black currant oil protects against environmental aggressors and reinforces your skin's barrier. It is high in vitamin C and gamma-linolenic acid (GLA), an omega-6 fatty acid that is vital for healthy cells and is a building block of the immune system. It is capable of penetrating the tissues easily, supplying fatty acids and nutrients not only to the skin, but to the joints and muscles as well, helping to repair the effects of stress on the body.

Blueberry Seed (*Vaccinium corymbosum*)

Subtle gifts: Blueberries are perfectly round with a five-pointed star shape that is formed at the blossom end of the berry. The blue skin the berry is wrapped in is the rarest color on earth. Blue evokes otherworldly feelings and a sense of the wild blue yonder and sky-driven horizons pulling us ever forward into the future. Blue evokes the deep blue sea, a fascinating watery realm that expresses a reality that rivals the most vivid imagination; this color is almost as unknown as outer space. The color associated with the fifth chakra, *vishuddha*, is a radiant blue; this grants the throat center the gifts of clarity of speech, wit, improvisation, and the ability to express your truth and engage with your inner muse. Blue is linked with eternity, the star-filled skies, the beyond, and supernatural beauty; it promotes detachment from earthly concerns. Mother Mary is draped in a celestial cloak that displays the blue vault of heaven.

The Rarest Color in Nature

The color blue has various associations. The Hindu god Shiva, the Destroyer, is blue. He reminds us that all beginnings must have an end, that all that is born must die, and that all that is must cease to be. Blue is cooling, calming, and promotes restful sleep. We say we are feeling "blue" to describe melancholy, which explains the blues as a musical art form that is neither completely sad nor completely happy. Pablo Picasso's paintings from his Blue Period show the disenfranchised in states of lethargy and despair, all painted blue to show lack in some form. In contrast, the artist Henri Matisse, in his painting *The Dance*, used what he called "the eye-smacking color scheme of a sapphire-blue sky" to create a sky that is the bluest of blues to express joyful exuberance, as dancers dance hand in hand, expressing an effortless ease.

Physical gifts: This oil has extremely high levels of antioxidants, high in linoleic acid (40 percent) and alpha-linolenic acid (25 percent), allowing it to deeply nourish the skin's layers. It is also rich in phytosterols, carotenoids, and vitamin E, effectively delivering nutritional benefits to protect the outer layer of the skin and repairing damage, including scar tissue and free-radical damage. Blueberry seed oil regenerates tissues, smooths fine lines, and increases the elasticity of the skin and slows down the aging process. Additionally, blueberry seed oil alleviates pain from burns and is believed to help epithelial tissue regenerate more quickly. Its significant level of antioxidants, including phenolic compounds and tocopherols, are anti-inflammatory and provide additional skin protection. Blueberry seed oil is especially good for dry, irritated skin conditions like eczema and psoriasis.

Borage (*Borago officinalis*)

Subtle gifts: Borage, also known as starflower, is a transcendent seed oil that enhances your ability to have visions, so it therefore supports vision quests and journeying. It brings clarity and brightness to the thought process, helps you to see your path more clearly, and assists you in connecting your inner truth with your newly emerging outer path.

Physical gifts: This oil has one of the highest contents of gamma-linolenic acid, or GLA (25 percent) of any oil. This helps regenerate, firm, and rejuvenate the skin's barrier function, decreasing water loss and maintaining the skin's elasticity. Its linoleic acid content (35 percent) prevents wrinkles and premature aging and fights loss of skin elasticity and dryness. Its wide range of nutrients stimulate cellular activity in the skin while offering anti-inflammatory actions against pain in the joints and soft tissues. Ferulic acid, a powerful antioxidant, protects and soothes damage caused by the sun and weather. An astringent oil, it contains tannins that create a dry feeling on the skin, calming redness and minimizing pore size. Ellagic acid supports the production of collagen, preventing its breakdown and regenerating skin cells.

Broccoli Seed (*Brassica oleracea* var. *italica*)

Subtle gifts: This oil offers the gift of achieving balance, helping you to be responsible and respond to the challenges you face. Broccoli also helps you to "get it right" and clear up loose ends that nag at you internally, like taking care of unkept promises and unfulfilled duties, including those that matter to others. This oil helps you choose your tasks with freedom and joy so your to-do list comes from a place of service. This is accomplished by allowing you to tap into the fullness of your mind and your robust energy.

A Hearty Vegetable of the Cabbage Family

Brassica oleracea var. *italica* refers to a nonheading type of broccoli that will produce multiple small heads throughout the harvest season to bridge the gap between summer and winter vegetables. Sprouting broccoli was cultivated in Italy in ancient Roman times and was introduced to England and America in the 1700s.

Physical gifts: The idea of savory vegetable oils in body preparations may seem odd to some, but many of these oils are powerhouses, both energetically and physically. This oil is roughly 50 percent omega-9 erucic acid, a very long-chain unsaturated fatty acid that moisturizes with a stable, nongreasy, yet effective action, and as such it protects against damage from excess sun exposure. Its sulforaphane content provides additional UV protection by stimulating the production of the enzyme glutathione, a coenzyme antioxidant that all cells make, which acts by continuously protecting cells, neutralizing and eliminating toxins and free radicals. This oil stimulates anti-inflammatory actions in the capillaries, reducing the effects of rosacea by slowing or even stopping new growth in the fine blood vessels of the face. Broccoli seed oil is thick, viscous, and protective, penetrating the cells without leaving an oil residue. It is frequently used in hair treatments (especially good for curly or frizzy hair) and for nonoily skin care.

Buriti (*Mauritia flexuosa*)

Subtle gifts: Buriti oil is from the moriche palm from Brazil and the Amazon basin. The word *buriti* in Brazilian means "Tree of Life," and indeed this oil is its archetype in terms of its ability to awaken knowledge in both the body and the mind.

Physical gifts: Buriti oil is a vivid and rich red-orange, indicating it is one of the best sources of carotenoids and beta-carotene, even more than what's in carrots. This oil has been used traditionally to heal wounds and prevent excessive scarring. Its oleic acid content helps to refresh, moisturize, and rebuild the skin to maintain its elasticity. Buriti oil, when used in small amounts in topical preparations, adds a radiant yellow luster to blends that epitomizes its nourishing nature.

Caution: It is important to note that this oil will stain cloth and porous surfaces but not the skin, where it is absorbed readily.

Cabbage Seed, Red (*Brassica oleracea* var. *rubra*)

Subtle gifts: This oil helps to heal feelings of loss of success or abundance, and the sense that because you didn't succeed in the past you cannot succeed in the future. It supports the need for individuality and a life path that is informed by the soul.

Physical gifts: High in fatty acids, particularly linoleic and alpha-linolenic acids and vitamin E, red cabbage contains anthocyanins, compounds that gives plants their vibrant colors and prevent or inhibit the oxidative damage caused by free radicals, thus reducing oxidative stress. Scientific studies say that including anthocyanin-rich sources in the diet such as red cabbage lowers the risk of a wide range of neurodegenerative diseases.[1] This oil is light in texture and provides intense hydration without leaving the skin feeling slippery. Deeply moisturizing, it can slow down visible signs of aging.

> **Blending Tip** – Try blending red cabbage seed oil with prickly pear oil as you plan the next steps in your life.

Cantaloupe Seed (*Cucumis melo*)

Subtle gifts: This oil teaches the concept of accepting the shadow side of those you love or have close bonds with, which is a natural part of being human, and how important it is to allow others their own time to process and work with whatever energy they are struggling with in order to bring about true change.

Physical gifts: This oil is rich in vitamins A, B_6, C, and E, as well as potassium, caffeic acid, ellagic acid, and superoxide dismutase, or SOD, the body's smart antioxidant enzyme that protects the cells from highly reactive, cell-damaging free radicals, making it useful as an antiaging ingredient that helps prevent wrinkles, fine lines, and age spots. Promising studies are emerging that look at cantaloupe seed oil for its role in addressing ultraviolet radiation, oxidative stress, sunburn, and rashes. It can even induce a significant visual reduction of cellulite on the thighs and has a potent antipruritic (reduces itching) activity.

Cashew Nut (*Anacardium occidentale*)

Subtle gifts: This oil offers the gift of finely honing your ability to discern the subtle levels of truth, ultimately broadening your viewpoint.

Physical gifts: Cashew nut oil contains proanthocyanidins, copper, and vitamin C, which eliminate free radicals and maintain elastin and collagen in the skin.

> **Blending Tip** – Try blending cashew nut fixed oil with petitgrain essential oil (see chapter 2), which also holds the gift of discrimination, to amplify your ability to see what is actively being hidden from you in any situation.

Cherry Kernel (*Prunus avium*)

Subtle gifts: This oil has a cheery "cherry" radiance from the inside out, allowing you to feel authentically happy to be who you are and celebrating all that it entails.

Physical gifts: Cherry kernel oil contains alpha-eleostearic acid (12 percent), a conjugated fatty acid that plays a role in prostaglandin production in the body, prostaglandins being compounds with hormonelike effects. Cherry kernel oil has been shown to slow tumor growth in animal tests. High in vitamins A and E and alpha, delta, and gamma tocopherols and tocotrienols, it softens, moisturizes, and protects the skin cells from UV rays.

Caution: Prostaglandins can promote uterine contractions, so this oil should not be used if you are pregnant.

Chia Seed (*Salvia hispanica*)

Subtle gifts: This oil teaches the art of self-sufficiency. It supports you in creating a thriving life built on a foundation of your own hard work. Chia also teaches the art of tenacity and keeping with your goal, even after setbacks, until you hit the mark. *Chia* means "strength" in the Mayan language, and the chia plant certainly lives up to its name. This desert plant is not only drought-tolerant, it is known as a "fire-following" plant, meaning that it is one of the first to reappear after a devastating wildfire. Remarkably adaptable, chia plants can self-pollinate if the bees or butterflies don't do their job. They will self-sow in the autumn and have no known vulnerabilities to pests or diseases. Digest this phrase with mythic eyes: *fire-following plant*. What life circumstances have left you feeling so scorched that a fire-following plant would be required?

Physical gifts: Chia seeds are exceptionally high in the omega-3 essential fatty acids (up to 60 percent). These are balanced with omega-6 fatty acids (21 percent), amino acids, and vitamins and minerals, including zinc. A powerful anti-inflammatory and antioxidant, chia seed oil is a natural choice for treating skin tissues such as acne and preventing scarring from the lesions.

Cloudberry Seed (*Rubus chamaemorus*)

Subtle gifts: A wild plant found in northern regions, cloudberry helps you see and act from the indestructible light of purity that resides deep within. This oil is cold-pressed from the seeds of this luminous berry found deep in the Nordic marshes and wet meadows, where it grows in peat-rich moors in damp and freezing conditions. It helps you learn to grow by surrendering to your inner vision. It encourages you to exchange low self-esteem with an awareness of your inner value, helping you to open to the true source of your being and reflect it out into the world for others to see and benefit from.

Physical gifts: Cloudberry seed oil is rich in vitamin C, which stimulates the production of collagen, the skin protein that promotes the renewal and growth of skin cells and forms protective tissues in the body. It is also high in vitamin E, carotenoids, phytosterols, and ellagic acid, which protect against free-radical damage brought on by damaging sun rays and other environmental factors like pollution. With its distinctive, well-balanced profile of omega-3, -6, and -9 essential fatty acids, it deeply moisturizes and helps regenerate the skin cells, delaying and preventing fine lines, wrinkles, and other signs of aging.

Coconut (*Cocos nucifera*)

Subtle gifts: Coconut oil promotes endurance and perseverance for completing tasks, which in turn helps you manifest your full potential. It provides strong, steady energy and the ability to welcome challenges and be solution-oriented.

Physical gifts: Lauric acid, a medium-chain saturated fatty acid, makes up close to 50 percent of coconut oil. Lauric acid converts to monolaurin, a compound able to destroy viruses and kill harmful bacteria and protozoa. Before sun exposure became something to be afraid of, coconut oil was the go-to remedy because often oils produced from plants that grow in tropical areas contain compounds that protect the skin from the sun's rays, allowing natural vitamin D formation to take place in the skin layers. Coconut oil reduces the potential for stretch marks, as this oil helps the skin grow and expand without tearing. In its unrefined virgin form it is a saturated oil that has film-forming properties that protect the skin. Fractionated coconut oil (or MCT oil that stays liquid—see box at the beginning of this chapter) makes an effective lightweight moisturizer for your face and lips. It is quickly absorbed into the skin, leaving it feeling not greasy but hydrated and enriched. It is also good for hydrating dry, heat-damaged hair.

Blending Tip – Try blending coconut oil with cabbage seed oil and wheat germ oil when in a difficult work (or other) phase and you need support to complete the cycle and get to the finish line.

Corn (*Zea mays*)

Subtle gifts: Corn expresses fertility and being "earthed," rooted and grounded in life. Corn oil supports alignment with earth energy, opening one to the cornucopia that life offers. It helps usher in abundance on all levels, especially the joy and pleasure associated with the feminine. Corn supports increased creativity and birthing creative projects. It is useful for fostering friendships based on mutual support and growth by creating synergy, which means that joining with others you can achieve goals larger than what you can achieve alone.

Physical gifts: This golden oil helps keep the epidermis hydrated and can be used for dry, mature, or sun-damaged skin. It repairs the skin's lipid barrier, soothes irritation, and fights against harmful bacteria.

Cranberry Seed (*Vaccinium macrocarpon*)

Subtle gifts: This oil's gifts are simple but profound: it promotes inner discipline and stimulates the right balance of flexibility and restraint.

Physical gifts: Cranberry seed oil is a rich yellow color, alerting us to its provitamin A carotenoid (the most common of which is beta-carotene) content, which is turned into vitamin A by the body's metabolic processes. This oil is high in polyphenols, carotenes, quercetin, anthocyanidins, and proanthocyanins, giving it the ability to protect against oxidation and free-radical damage. Tannins give this oil a light feeling and provide antibacterial properties, while beta-sitosterol eases redness and itching from inflammation and repairs and regenerates tissues. This oil is well-rounded and supports elastin and collagen formation, diminishes blemishes and acne, while providing relief from dryness, scaling, and itchy and irritated skin conditions.

Cranberry Seed, Arctic (*Oxycoccus palustris*)

Subtle gifts: This oil helps you take stock of your life: what do you need to do to create an emotional and physical state of satisfaction? What goals or desires does this entail? This includes the physical rewards and comforts that come from fulfilling your wildest dreams. This oil opens your view so you can see the connections you need to make and the relationships you need to foster. This is not the energy of instant gratification, but rather it is the life you have worked so hard to build, with long-sought security and well-being coming together. It endows you with the ability to rest in comfort and share your bounty with those you love and care for.

Physical gifts: Arctic cranberry differs from the more common variety of cranberry eaten in the fall and winter; they are smaller and grow in the wild, in peat bogs and the moist forest areas of the Arctic tundra. High in tocotrienols and gamma-tocotrienol, Arctic cranberry oil has a near-perfect ratio of omega-3, -6, and -9 essential fatty acids. Deeply moisturizing and rejuvenating, it offers antiaging properties that are ideal for dry skin.

> **Blending Tip** – Using a blend of Arctic cranberry seed oil and sheep's milk (see chapter 4) helps you grasp the necessary actions and stay committed, creating a safe, abundant life. This blend embodies the energy of long-term goals.

Cucumber Seed (*Cucumis sativus*)

Subtle gifts: The cucumber plant is a creeping vine from the melon and pumpkin family whose original home was India, where it has been cultivated for over four thousand years. It is associated with the moon and brings the energies of fertility and merriment, and provides a cooling physical as well as subtle energy. This plant can be understood as nature's form of Rescue Remedy. I have found that cucumber offers broad-spectrum relief from difficult emotional states. It renews and refreshes the physical body from exhaustion, illness, and shock that drains one's prana, and deeply supports reengaging in life.

Cool as a Cucumber

Cucumber is associated with the god Vishnu, the preserver of the universe, especially in his form as Krishna, the god of protection, compassion, and love. On Krishna's birthday, celebrated in August, households in India are decorated with ripe cucumbers in his honor as a celebration of divine love, or *bhakti*, when the love of human souls is given over completely to the Divine. The Mahāmrtyuñjaya Mantra (the Great Death-Conquering Mantra) translates something like this: "We worship the three-eyed one who is fragrant and who sustains all living beings. May he liberate us from [samsara] death. May he [Lord Shiva] lead us to immortality, just as the cucumber is released from its bondage [attachment to the plant], [so shall we]."

In Japanese folklore, a *kappa* is a mischievous, magical creature that inhabits fresh water, about the size of a ten-year-old child, yellow-green in color, with fish scales instead of skin and a tortoise shell on its back. On the top of its head is a hollow indentation called a *sara* that is filled with water. If the water spills, the kappa loses its magical powers. When encountering a kappa you want to trick them into bowing low, thus spilling their water. If you refill their sara, you may request a boon and it will be granted out of gratitude. Due to repaying this debt the kappa teaches the knowledge of bone-setting and healing salves. A kappa's pranks can be harmless, like making noises similar to flatulence or trying to peek up a lady's dress, although some are more malevolent and can drown livestock and people, kidnap children, and steal one's life force. There is one sure remedy to placating them—offer them cucumbers!

The cucumber has been featured in the works of numerous artists. Robert MacBryde (1913–1966), a Scottish modernist painter, featured this plant in a work called *Still Life with Cucumber*, an image used for a ration book cover during the post–World War 2 era. MacBryde favored fruits and vegetables, especially those with phallic associations or those that are full of seeds. Cucumber is both, beckoning fertility and abundance back to the land and to life.

American poet Robert Haas (U.S. poet laureate from 1995 to 1997) celebrated the cucumber in his "Poem with a Cucumber in It":

> If you think I am going to make
> A sexual joke in this poem,
> you are mistaken.

He instead describes the setting of the sun:

> Sometimes from this hillside just after sunset
> The rim of the sky takes on a tinge
> Of the palest green, like the flesh of a cucumber
> When you peel it carefully.

Physical gifts: Cucumber is unusually high in phytosterols, compounds that strengthen the skin's barrier function and help maintain its moisture and elasticity. High in omega-6 linoleic acid (65 percent), it is helpful for treating problematic skin conditions like eczema and dermatitis. It is a good source of vitamin C and antioxidants, aiding in blood flow, reducing puffy areas with regular use, including the eye area. High in silica content, it strengthens the skin and hair, providing structure and support.

Daikon Radish Seed (*Raphanus sativus*)

Subtle gifts: Daikon, whose name means "large root" in Japanese, ranges in size from six inches to three feet. It is beneficial for those who feel guilty or helpless because others are suffering and they are not, especially when it's not apparent what to do or how to help, when there is nothing within your power to offer aid.

Physical gifts: This oil has the dramatic effect of improving the barrier function of the skin significantly over a period of only a few hours, resulting in a soft feeling within minutes of application as the skin is moisturized and the oil is well-absorbed. This oil has a recommended shelf life of only six months to a year. It is frequently used as a replacement for silicone in hair care and cosmetic products due to its high erucic acid (34 percent) and gadoleic acid (10 percent) content, both being long-chain unsaturated fatty acids.

Date (*Balanites aegyptiaca*)

Subtle gifts: This oil opens your eyes to seeing and feeling life as a lover, the way ecstatic poets like Rumi and Hafiz experienced life itself as the beloved. This allows you to embrace life in all of its aspects, extending yourself joyfully and participating fully in what life offers you and drinking it in.

Physical gifts: Date oil has been used traditionally in the treatment of rheumatism as well as conditions that affect the reproductive system that involve sex hormones and fertility. Date kernel oil possesses antioxidant, anticancer, antimicrobial, and insecticidal properties. This oil has been used for centuries for skin hydration, for stimulating the production of collagen, and for promoting suppleness and firmness of the skin. It is a regenerating and restorative oil, repairing damage caused by oxidative stress and stimulating the body's own restorative response.

> **Blending Tip** – It was said that Cleopatra bathed in saffron-infused mare's milk before taking a lover to bed. You most likely cannot get your hands

on mare's milk, but you could try substituting goat's milk (see chapter 4) to open you to your wild and sensuous nature—add one tablespoon macerated saffron oil and one tablespoon date oil to a half cup goat's milk, swirl into your bathwater, submerge, and be opened!

. . . .

Dragon Fruit Seed (*Hylocereus undatus*)

Subtle gifts: This dazzling, usual, crimson-colored fruit is the product of a night-blooming cactus also known as *pitaya*, or moonflower. It offers an invitation to enter the archetypal Garden of Earthly Delights, a place where you can play with magic and experience delight while here on Earth, opening you to discoveries that fascinate, astonish, and bring wonderment.

Physical gifts: This oil has a good antiaging effect, supporting smooth, firm skin. It is rich in antioxidants and unsaturated fatty acids, including omega-3 and omega-6, two fatty acids that help control inflammation.

Fig Seed (*Ficus carica*)

Subtle gifts: The sticky-sweet, delicious, urn-shaped fruit of the fig is what is known as a *syconium*, which is an enlarged stem tissue or inflorescence consisting of an inverted cluster of tiny fleshy flowers that bloom entirely in the dark. Just considering this you can delight in how awesome nature is. Fig seed oil opens the higher channels of the mind to decode the memories of your deepest origins to reveal the inner fruit and nectar that's stored in your soul. In essence you become the alchemical holy vessel, gaining access to your deepest knowledge and essence.

Physical gifts: One of the oldest recorded plants harvested for multiple use, fig provides a moisturizing oil rich in alpha-linoleic acid, an essential fatty acid, as well as phenols and flavonoids, antioxidants that protect the skin from oxidative damage. This oil brightens dark spots and stimulates the skin's natural collagen production. Exceptionally rich in vitamin E and teeming with antioxidants, it can help diminish the appearances of wrinkles and fine lines.

Mutualism in Nature

All fig trees are pollinated by very small wasps of the Agaonidae family. When a female wasp dies inside a fig, an enzyme known as *ficin* in the fig breaks down her carcass into protein.

When it comes to fig pollination, it's what's inside that counts. An immature fig emits a tempting odor to signal that it's ready to be pollinated. Attracted by that scent, the female fig wasp burrows deep into the fig, tunneling a passageway for herself so narrow that she loses her wings and pieces of antennae in the process. She won't need them. She will die in the dark interior of the fig after her life's work there is done. Once inside, she moves from flower to flower, laying her eggs and spreading the pollen she has brought with her from the fig where she was born. The flowers she pollinates will soon produce seeds; the eggs she lays will hatch, her larvae feasting on the tissue of their small, silent nursery.

This is a beautiful, rhythmic example of how two different organisms create a synergy that meets each other's needs at just the right time to produce a beneficial overall effect. Figs offer a snug nursery where fig wasps can lay eggs and raise their young. In turn, the wasps distribute fig pollen, enabling the plant to make seeds and reproduce. Theirs is a unique relationship, one of the best examples of mutualism in nature, where both organisms and the wider ecosystem benefit.

Blending Tip – Try blending fig seed oil with gardenia absolute (see chapter 1) to work further with the energy of mutualism. Fig seed oil will open the higher channels of your mind to reveal what's stored in your soul, while gardenia supports you in this process by mirroring back to you the reflection of your higher Self in nature.

Goji Berry Seed (*Lycium barbarum*)

Subtle gifts: This oil prepares the mind to make it pliable and absorbent when studying ancient wisdom traditions like Buddhism, Vedanta, ayurveda, and so on.

Physical gifts: Rich with skin-enriching vitamin C, vitamin A, omega-6, palmitic acid, and stearic acid, goji berry is an antiaging oil with restorative properties for all skin types, especially for dry or mature skin. It smooths wrinkles, enhances skin elasticity, and evens out skin tone, leaving the skin feeling silky soft. Exceptionally high in essential fatty acids, especially omega-6 linoleic acid, this exquisite oil protects and repairs the skin by stimulating intracellular oxygenation, helping to restore the vital balance of water and fats in the hydrolipidic film of the skin. As it is light in texture, it is ideal for use around the delicate eye area. Vitamin E neutralizes fat-soluble free radicals and helps protect cell membranes from lipid oxidation, thereby maintaining skin elasticity and firmness. Goji berry penetrates deep into the skin, stimulating blood circulation and raising skin metabolism, thereby accelerating cell turnover, helping to even out skin tone and lessen melanin deposits such as age spots and freckles.

....

Blending Tip – I teach the philosophical aspects of yoga, and often my students are eager to learn but the concepts are foreign enough to them that even though they are listening and paying attention, they do not grasp the information right off the bat. I support them by using goji berry oil on the first day of class; I blend it with sandalwood, blue chamomile, and lemon essential oils and apply it to the third eye, the back of neck, and the wrists of my students. I've observed a noticeable effect in the absorption and application of information.

....

Grapeseed (*Vitis vinifera*)

Subtle gifts: This luscious fruit brings soulfulness and an expression of incredible depth that creates a sense of softness toward the human experience. It is not a quest for perfection, but instead a practice of exploring what it means to be fully human. It is growing to love the seemingly disorderly and paradoxical aspects of human incarnation and staying within that process without shutting down, until the rich gift of experience has bloomed. This oil expresses aspects of the soul.

Physical gifts: Grapeseed oil is pressed from the seeds of grapes after the juice is harvested. Oils from harvesting varietal wine grapes such as merlot, cabernet sauvignon, Riesling, and chardonnay are available. High in vitamin E, grapeseed oil provides chlorophyll and antioxidants, as well as an abundance of vitamins, minerals, and the flavanol proanthocyanin, all of which strengthen collagen and maintain elastin, the connective tissues in skin and joints. Especially high in the omega-6 linoleic fatty acid (76 percent), grapeseed oil makes for a light oil that penetrates the skin layers. This oil has toning and astringent properties that tighten pores and tone skin tissues. It is very effective for washing your face.

Guava Seed (*Psidium guajava*)

Subtle gifts: This oil balances the emotions and cleans the heart chakra, easing tension and anger stuck in the energetic heart. It improves personal expression, confidence, creativity, and the love of beauty and the arts.

Physical gifts: Guava seed oil is noncomedogenic and high in essential fatty acids such as linoleic acid, phenolics like chlorogenic acid, and phytosterols (stimasterol, beta-sitosterol, and campesterol) and vitamins E and A, making it an ideal oil for addressing acne and blemishes. Due to its high antioxidant activity it helps offset signs of aging such as dark spots. Early studies have shown that it can promote wound healing, as it increases the migration of keratinocytes, which are skin cells.

. . . .

Blending Tip — Try combining, guava seed oil with fleur de sel finishing salt (see chapter 4); the resulting salt scrub enhances your appreciation of the arts. Use before going to the ballet, theater, opera, or symphony. I recently used this blend before attending a concert with the violinist Joshua Bell playing Dvořák, which enhanced my experience, making it all the more ecstatic.

Jojoba, Golden (*Simmondsia chinensis*)

Subtle gifts: This oil supports the highly sensitive, spiritual person to be able to cope with the mundane. It brings a sense of ease and security. It is grounding and helps you participate in daily life and relationships without feeling overwhelmed.

Physical gifts: This plant is native to the Sonoran Desert of Arizona, Northern Mexico, and arid California. Although referred to as an oil, jojoba is actually a liquid plant wax with remarkably similar properties to our skin's sebum, the oily secretions the skin produces to protect itself. Jojoba has an outstanding shelf life and molecular stability for up to twenty years. It grows in semidesert areas, in ecosystems where heat and dryness would kill most plants. This resilient plant produces oil in the form of a liquid wax, which protects the plant by sealing the stomata (the plant's pores) against evaporation during intense daytime heat and equally intense nighttime conditions of cold. Jojoba oil serves a similar function for the human skin, with its exceptional ability to prevent water loss, one of the primary reasons behind skin aging.

> **Blending Tip** – If strongly empathic, blend golden jojoba and raspberry fixed oils before going to crowded places.

Kiwi Seed (*Actinidia chinensis*)

Subtle gifts: This oil supports you to ask your muse for divine inspiration—perhaps when working with the creative spark that exists in your higher imagination or in an aspect of nature or in some ethereal source.

Physical gifts: Kiwi seed oil is nonoily and readily penetrates skin tissues. It is high in omega-3, alpha-linolenic (60 percent), linoleic (20 percent), vitamins C and E, and potassium and magnesium, making this oil anti-inflammatory and hence dynamic for repairing skin damage while nourishing and regenerating the skin layers.

> **Blending Tip** – I have often heard Deepak Chopra say that creativity is one of the most important evolutionary impulses. Try blending kiwi seed oil with blood orange essential oil (see chapter 2) to let yourself shine from the inside out with a luminous display of unique talents.

Mango Kernel (*Mangifera indica*)

Subtle gifts: This oil promotes sexual bonding and the ability to put into action what you're feeling in your heart. It stirs the energy of desire and passion and couples it with an eagerness to bond and create with another, ultimately allowing a couple to share beautiful, mutually helpful energies.

Physical gifts: Mango kernel oil is high in caffeic acid, making it a powerful antioxidant and fungicide. Mangiferin, a polyphenol specific to mango, is antioxidant, antifungal, and strongly anti-inflammatory. The tannins in the oil create a dry feeling that provides an astringent effect. It is also high in vitamin C, thereby moisturizing, repairing, and revitalizing the skin layers to give the skin a soft, silky feel.

Milk Thistle (*Silybum marianum*)

Subtle gifts: Milk thistle is inherently discerning. It will embrace, protect, or enforce boundaries as required. The ancient Greek botanist Dioscorides claimed that the root of milk thistle dispels melancholy and causes one to be merry, and according to Yorkshire Flower Essences (see Resources), milk thistle brings more light and love into one's life.

This can be understood in the context of Chinese medicine, which says the liver houses the emotion of anger, and because milk thistle heals the liver on the physical level, it can clear the dark energies of anger and melancholy. The spiny edges on this plant's abundant, swordlike leaves that surround the tender bloom protect the vulnerable flower. This suggests the person who keeps others at a distance but who in reality has a soft heart. This thistle is associated with self-protection, boundaries, impenetrability, severity, resilience, and difficulties.

Physical gifts: Milk thistle oil is an important liver herb. It is the byproduct of the extraction of silymarin, a hepatoprotective active substance used to treat liver failure and liver poisoning. Silymarin's flavonoid properties protect and regenerate damaged cells and can detoxify and restore the liver to normal functioning. Silymarin is a flavonoid complex, an antioxidant, and a membrane-stabilizing compound. The oil retains some measure of this compound, and how much depends on the extraction and refining process used. Milk thistle also contains polyunsaturated fatty acids, mainly linoleic acid (up to 65 percent). The plant's healing properties are abundant, including phytosterols such as beta-sitosterol, stigmasterol, and campesterol, as well as phospholipids and squalene. It is also high in vitamin E and antioxidants that nourish and repair damage to the skin and body. It treats skin suffering from chronic inflammation, including psoriasis, constitutional dermatitis, and acne. In addition, holy milk thistle oil is rich in minerals and the trace elements magnesium, zinc, selenium, and manganese.

Milk of the Madonna

The sweet fragrance of milk thistle's purple blooms welcomes pollinators, who feed and rest on this plant and gather golden pollen, which ensures propagation of the species. Milk thistle provides a nursery for painted lady butterflies, who lay their eggs on their thorny fortress, which keeps them safe until they hatch. The wee caterpillars who eat the leaves become big caterpillars that go through a metamorphosis to eventually become butterflies. During the Renaissance it was believed that butterflies on thistles are a sign of resurrection—once free of their chrysalises, they represent redeemed souls. According to author, teacher, mineral expert, and Reiki master Nicholas Pearson, "One of thistle flower['s] . . . gifts is the ability to trust your own inner authority." He adds, "It empowers you to take the reins for your own well-being."[2] One important aspect of this energy is understanding boundaries—what to let in and what to keep out.

According to the Bible, thistle came into being to punish humankind. After the expulsion from Paradise, God told Adam, "Cursed is the ground for your sake; in toil you shall eat of it all the days of your life. Both thorns and thistles it shall bring forth for you, and you shall eat the herb of the field" (Genesis 3:17–18). However, as Mother Nature is wont to do, she set about righting this wrong and rewriting the narrative. Eventually this plant became known as blessed milk thistle, Marian thistle, Mary thistle, and Saint Mary's thistle. These names derive from milk thistle's white-veined leaves, which according to legend contain the milk of the Madonna. According to the ancient doctrine of signatures that teaches that nature provides visual clues as to what functions a plant offers, milk thistle is particularly good at stimulating breast milk production. Truly, like a mother, this plant has the ability to nurture, sustain, and be fiercely protective when needed.

Oat (*Avena sativa*)

Subtle gifts: This oil brings a sense of stability, empowerment, and peace in situations where you feel vulnerable, off-balance, or just in need of an energy reset. It feeds and bolsters that part of your soul that is nostalgic and homesick for a time and place that no longer exists and that you cannot return to.

Physical gifts: A luxurious oil from a common grain that is highly emollient and rich, oat oil soothes and conditions the skin. This plant is classed as a nervine known for its ability to calm jagged nerves and soothe related nervous conditions. It is helpful for irritated and itchy skin conditions and can calm and repair damaged, sensitive, tender skin. High in oleic and linoleic acid, this a great oil to support the stratum corneum, and its saturated palmitic acid content soothes and protects as well.

....

Blending Tip – *Hiraeth* is a Welsh concept that describes a longing for home or missing a time, an era, or a person, including homesickness for what may not exist any longer. This type of soul ache comes up often in my practice, and my favorite blend to feed this nonspecific longing is oat oil blended with marjoram essential oil (see chapter 2), which brings the energy of coziness, comfortable conviviality, and contentment.

....

Okra Seed (*Abelmoschus esculentus*)

Subtle gifts: This oil strengthens you so you're not pressured against your will or overly influenced by the desires of others. It is an excellent plant for healing dominating and submissive relationships.

Physical gifts: Okra seed oil is abundant in essential unsaturated fatty acids, phenolic compounds, catechins and flavonoids, as well as tocopherols. It is traditionally used to reduce dark spots and enhance elasticity and firmness by boosting collagen production. One of my favorite applications of this oil is to wash my face with it. It gently but thoroughly cleanses the skin's surface of impurities and unblocks pores. My method is simple: I use a quarter size or more of the oil, rub it gently over my entire face, including my closed eyes (it will remove eye makeup and even waterproof mascara), for about a minute, and remove with a warm, wet cloth. While my skin is still moist I then apply a generous layer of whatever oil I need in the moment.

Olive (*Olea europaea*)

Subtle gifts: Olive oil opens you to the frequency of bringing profound knowledge into conscious awareness for practical use. This stone fruit teaches creative visualization and how to harness natural laws so you can manifest your ideas in the world for practical ends. You can use this energy for finding the right actions to bring about intended results. Olive vibrates to the archetype of Athena.

Athena's Gift

The olive has a significant role in our cultural consciousness, as there are living olive trees still producing fruit and oil today that are over a thousand years old! We use the phrase "offering an olive branch" to show peace given and accepted. A dove brought back an olive branch to Noah to signify the end of the flood. Stories abound in the Bible and most ancient texts about using olive oil to anoint animals, sanctuaries, sacred stones, and the heads of men and women, royalty and priests. The story goes that Poseidon and Athena challenged each other on who could offer the most beautiful gift to the people of Athens. Poseidon offered a fast, strong horse to help the people in their battles. Athena, on the other hand, struck a rock with her spear and caused the first olive tree to spring forth. Thanks to the olive tree's fruit, the people could illuminate the night, medicate wounds, and feed themselves with her gift. Zeus, judging the more peaceful gift, the olive tree, to be more beneficial, gave the victory to Athena, who became the patroness of Athens.

Physical gifts: Olive oil is very stable and can tolerate some exposure to heat and light. Its oleic acid content supports the natural breathing process and sebum production of the skin, aiding in repairing sun-damaged tissues. Its phytosterols provide humectant properties, attracting moisture to the skin and soothing very dry skin. A major source of plant-based squalene, a common lipid produced by skin cells (shark's liver is the most dynamic nonplant source), it lubricates the skin, prevents the evaporation of moisture, is a natural emollient and protective agent, and supports the delivery of oxygen to skin cells while removing waste.

Onion (*Allium cepa*)

Subtle gifts: Onion's many layers allow you to access the many layers of your being, letting you explore your vast energies. Do you want to work with a specific aspect of yourself? Clear a painful memory? Revisit a feeling? This vegetable is a gateway to any part of yourself, positive or negative, that you need to get at—all you need to do is set your intentions as to where you want to go and why.

Physical gifts: Onion oil has strong antioxidant, anti-inflammatory, and antimicrobial properties. Its quercetin content reduces redness, itching, and inflammation in damaged skin; it also restores skin barrier function, increases hydration, and reduces water loss. In addition to quercetin, onion produces allicin, which is a sulfur-containing volatile compound that kills the bacteria that causes acne, reduces swelling and inflammation, and improves blood circulation. These beneficial effects allow the skin to receive more nutrients. Ayurveda recommends using this oil as a scalp treatment to stop hair loss and stimulate hair growth. I have seen a rise in shingles in my clients recently, and onion oil has an affinity for helping this most plaguing condition on both the physical and subtle levels.

Papaya Seed (*Carica papaya*)

Subtle gifts: This oil aids in spiritualizing the emotions, especially the loving energies that connect you with another person. It aligns the energies of the second chakra with those of the heart and crown chakras.

Physical gifts: This oil is high in oleic acid (70 percent), palmitic acid (16 percent), and vitamins A and C. It contains the enzyme papain, which clears the skin of debris and dead cells, making it an ideal oil for exfoliating and fading dark spots. In general it nourishes and strengthens tissues, facilitating fresh, glowing skin, making this oil an ideal match for mature skin. It is also a dynamic full-body massage oil, as its anti-inflammatory properties soothe muscle soreness and cramps.

Passion Fruit Seed (*Passiflora edulis*)

Subtle gifts: This oil helps you remember that your truest mission is to reflect the dormant divinity within your being, allowing you to be a living mediator between Heaven and Earth so that the budding passion of the soul can be understood and realized.

Physical gifts: High in vitamin C, passion fruit contains calcium and phosphorous, minerals that support a healthy nervous system. Its linoleic acid content (77 percent) makes it light and easily absorbed. This plant has been used traditionally for calming the nervous system, relieving stress, and for sleep disorders. Its anti-inflammatory, antispasmodic, and sedative properties make it an excellent choice for massage as well. It benefits aging and dry skin prone to cracking.

Peach Kernel (*Prunus persica*)

Subtle gifts: A ripe peach shimmers on a peach tree, displaying the vibrant hues of the second chakra, making it evocative of feminine gifts. Peach kernel oil vibrates to the energy of the muses, the goddesses of the arts, and incites the gift of artistic expression. The precious gift of the peach is to open you to the memory of the muse in your own heart and the joyous expression that flows from this wellspring.

Physical gifts: High in boron, a nutrient necessary for maintaining bone and joint health, peach kernel oil is rich in vitamins E, A, and some B. Primarily composed of oleic acid (60 percent) and linoleic acid (30 percent), the feel of this oil is very light, penetrating, silky, and smooth. It is wonderful for antiaging treatments and for those with unusually sensitive skin.

> **Blending Tip** – Try blending peach kernel oil with kiwi and passion fruit oils before any inspired endeavor and feel the creativity start to flow.

Pineapple Seed (*Ananas comosus*)

Subtle gifts: Pineapple brings joy, playfulness, communion, and bonding among friends and opens the heart to kindness, gratitude, and playfulness. It brings out childlike qualities, alleviates stress, and encourages wonderment, honesty, availability, openness, and finding commonality. If you feel like you're locked in a humdrum routine and don't see the magic and beauty of life all around you, this fruit contradicts the heaviness, adding sparkle to everyday experiences.

Physical gifts: Pineapple is a dynamic source of bromelain, an alkalizing ingredient with anti-inflammatory and antiaging properties that can reduce swelling and redness in the skin, as well as improve the skin's overall texture and appearance. It also acts selectively on aged skin cells to break them down, showing a nice peeling effect.

> **Blending Tip** – Try blending pineapple seed oil with dragon fruit and cherry oils to feel deliriously happy and experience life with wonder.

Pistachio Nut (*Pistacia vera*)

Subtle gifts: This oil opens the heart to a wider spectrum of experiences and heightens your intuition for more immediate and sensitive relationships with others.

Physical gifts: Pistachio nut oil is nongreasy and easily absorbed by the skin, providing moisturizing and softening effects and limiting water loss. It is noncomedogenic, which means it doesn't build up on the skin. This oil has a natural resistance to oxidation and rancidity, thanks to antioxidant compounds in the nuts that help extend the shelf life of homemade products containing essential oils, absolutes, and butters.

Blending Tip – Try blending pistachio nut oil with avocado oil to enhance your ability to use touch as a means to express how you feel without words.

Plum Kernel (*Prunus domestica*)

Subtle gifts: The push-pull of self-love and the complexity of this dynamic is the weft and warp of this oil. It supports you to authentically love yourself, to see yourself without distortions, and develop trust. This oil helps when you are struggling with self-doubt, unable to appreciate your true worth and underestimating yourself. It brings an open-minded, fresh approach to life and teaches boldness to those who hide their light under a bushel.

Physical gifts: A favorite aspect of this oil is that it smells of marzipan, a real treat for the nose. It boasts a generous amount of vitamin E and is high in oleic acid, with linoleic and palmitic acids in lesser quantities. This oil is nourishing for all skin types.

Blending Tip – Try blending plum kernel oil with narcissus absolute (see chapter 1) to dispel any distortions of self that hinder you from being in relationship not only with others, but with your true self.

Pomegranate Seed (*Punica granatum*)

Subtle gifts: I owe much to this fruit, being one of my major plant allies for navigating my interior life in conjunction with my exterior life. Pomegranate is the fruit of Persephone, daughter of Zeus and Demeter and Queen of the Underworld; she is the personification of vegetation and the seasons of spring and winter. This fruit has a rough exterior containing off-white membranes (representing, Kore, the maiden aspect of Persephone); this pith cradles vibrant purple or red seeds that are difficult to access (her Queen of the Underworld aspect). This fruit is a clear example of the doctrine of signatures, meaning the way a plant looks helps explain its function. Using this oil allows you—not unlike Persephone—to divide your energy in a balanced way between the two realms, your personal interior life that only belongs to you, and your expression of yourself out in the world. The underworld is a very soulful place, where fertility begins and where the goddess lived as queen for part of the year, nurturing that seed. The other part of the year she lived above ground in her role as Kore, the maiden, where she personifies spring, when her latent interior expressions blossom. In this expression of yourself, as with the vibration of pomegranate, you can grow anything: relationships, family, inner work, artistic expression, and so on.

Physical gifts: What does this oil *not* do? High in punicic acid (75 percent), it is a highly nourishing fatty acid for the skin, able to balance pH and condition the skin's surface. The fatty acid is anti-inflammatory, antimicrobial, and cell-regenerating, helping to increase the elasticity of the skin and repair sun and weather damage. Punicic acid is an omega-5 fatty acid and its long-chain, supersaturated fatty acids with three conjugated double bonds are an unusual form that causes this oil to feel thick, rich, and luxurious on the skin while effectively delivering the oil's beneficial properties to the tissues. Pomegranate seed oil offers a rich array of phytohormones, phytosterols, flavonoids, and polyphenols, the antioxidative properties that deeply penetrate and protect against free-radical damage in the skin tissues. Gallic acid heals wounds and soothes burns, while ellagic acid protects and rebuilds collagen and provides thickness to the skin. Early research has shown promise on cancer tissues, breast tissue in particular having favorable results.

Poppy Seed (*Papaver somniferum*)

Subtle gifts: This oil helps you interact with the spirit world and achieve altered states of consciousness.

Physical gifts: Poppy seed oil is obtained by pressing the seeds of the opium poppy flower. The alkaloids found in the pods, flowers, and stems are absent in the seeds, which contain trace amounts if any, although this oil still holds the holographic imprint of this plant's famous properties. A rich source of linoleic acid (70 percent) and oleic acid (16 percent), it offers general moisturizing properties. *Note*: This oil requires refrigeration to keep from oxidizing.

Prickly Pear Seed (*Opuntia ficus-indica*)

Subtle gifts: The brilliant red-to-purple colored tuna, or fruit, of the paddle cactus allows you to stay centered and act out of a sense of inner calmness, taking a breath and assessing a situation rather than getting angry or afraid about things that have happened and circumstances you cannot change in the present. This helps you to not freeze in fear and shut down or come from a reactionary place that might feel satisfying in the moment but can cause you more personal damage in the long run. Pause. Breathe. Assess. Act.

Physical gifts: High in linoleic acid, omega-6 and -9, amino acids, zinc, polyphenols, betalain, and vitamin K, the oil of the prickly pear fruit eases inflammation and calms irritations. Its powerful antiviral and antibacterial properties treat acne, and it reduces pores and the dark circles under the eyes as well as fine lines and wrinkles. It is also effective for sunburn relief.

. . . .

> **Blending Tip** – Blend prickly pear seed oil with water buffalo's milk (see chapter 4) to avoid freezing in fear (as in the "fight-or-flight" response) or reacting impulsively. This blend encourages you to be thoughtful and reflect on what you're exploring.

. . . .

Pumpkin Seed (*Cucurbita pepo*)

Subtle gifts: This oil is a gateway to the ocean of archetypal memory, a direct line to your ancestors, and can connect you to the spiritual echo of past lives—not only yours and that of your family line, but to the universal wellspring of all who went before you, allowing you to see how we are linked to the past and how we are still driven by many of the same primal fears, desires, and needs faced by the first humans. The wisdom and teachings of our ancestors are freely available to us if only we ask.

Physical gifts: This oil is thick, dark in color, and has a strong nutty scent that I personally like. The oil is high in in vitamins and essential fatty acids, especially linoleic acid (55 percent), zinc, copper, manganese, caffeic acid, and tocopherols, which act as free-radical scavengers, protecting against oxidation and cell damage. Its vitamin A content helps to reduce redness and itching and acts as an anti-inflammatory.

Blending Tip – To make this thick oil easier to work with, make a 50/50 blend with fractionated coconut oil (MCT), as its neutral energy lets you focus on the energy of whichever oils you may be working with—in this case, pumpkin energy. MCT also improves the viscosity of the blend.

Quinoa (*Chenopodium quinoa*)

Subtle gifts: This oil promotes holistic thinking and the ability to perceive the physical world and physical life with spiritually clear thoughts so as not to get weighed down by an overly mundane worldview.

Physical gifts: Rich in essential fatty acids, minerals, and amino acids known to be highly emollient and replenishing to the skin, quinoa oil is also a source of antioxidant tocopherols, a potent anti-inflammatory complex that replenishes the barrier function of the epidermis and combats premature tissue damage. It supports the growth of collagen, the protein that maintains the strength and firmness of the skin. This oil is high in linoleic acid (60.1 percent), oleic acid (20.5 percent), palmitic acid (9.8 percent), and alpha-linolenic acid (6.5 percent).

Raspberry Seed (*Rubus idaeus*)

Subtle gifts: This oil offers a refuge if you're an empath who identifies with the emotions and other energetic states of those around you to an uncomfortable extent. It encloses your aura and creates energetic boundaries to protect you from others' extremes so you can enjoy only the exchanges you wish to engage in.

Physical gifts: High in omega-3 (25 percent) and omega-6 (52 percent) as well as antioxidants and phospholipids, this oil has a relatively stable shelf life. It is also rich in vitamin E and provitamin A (a provitamin being any substance that once ingested is converted by the body into a vitamin). Preliminary studies have also been done for this oil's use as a broad-spectrum UV-A and UV-B sunscreen, as initial claims say it has an SPF between 28 and 50 when it is used undiluted on the skin. This oil is outstandingly light and absorbs quickly, creating a dry yet softly moisturized feeling.

Safflower (*Carthamus tinctorius*)

Subtle gifts: This oil encourages you to stand on your own two feet, to recognize your own wisdom, to depend on your own personal strength, and to acknowledge and work with your own good qualities. In this case, wisdom can mean knowing when you need help. Safflower oil helps you see and make connections with the support you need. This applies not only to the mundane world but also to the solar creative life force that supports serendipitous events. You may want to incorporate this fatty oil into your absolute and essential oil blends to usher in miracles and move into the light, to pass on blessings and to provide service from a place of strength.

Physical gifts: The safflower plant shines bright like the sun, resembling a thistle with tufted flowers in brilliant yellows, oranges, and reds. Ayurveda deems this oil beneficial for all dosha types, particularly kaphas. From a Vedic perspective, safflower is warming and lubricating; it fortifies the whole system, builds tissues, soothes bodily membranes, and activates the digestive fires.

....

Blending Tip – To shine brilliantly from the inside out, blend safflower and sunflower base oils with labdanum absolute (see chapter 1).

....

Strawberry Seed (*Fragaria ananassa*)

Subtle gifts: The vivid red berry with no thorns, skin, or pips—one of the first sweet fruits of the year—is evocative of love, sensuality, fertility, and abundance, while the plant's pristine white flowers speak of purity of mind and emotions. Strawberry grants softness, innocence, and a new beginning in which all is possible.

Physical gifts: Rich in palmitic acid, stearic acid, oleic acid, linoleic acid, and alpha-linolenic acid, this oil is lightweight, absorbs quickly, and is noncomedogenic; it improves skin tone, skin elasticity and luminosity, and promotes the production of collagen.

Nature's Fauvism

Strawberry is nature's original expression of the early twentieth-century art form known as *fauvism*, a painting style that favored the pairing of complementary colors on the color wheel, such as the red of a plant's berry and the green of its leaves. *Fauvism* means

> "the wild beast" and originally was meant as a jab, referring to the color choices that were savage and wild. Novelist Charles-Louis Phillippe declared in a letter written in 1897 concerning this movement: "What we need now are barbarians . . . One

must have a vision of natural life. . . . Today begins the era of passion. Fauvism, similarly, grew out of this new spirit of joyous, pagan affirmation and represented a return to natural reality."[3]

Strawberry, true to this energy, encourages a return to an untrammeled state, a naturalness, a juicy aliveness. This plant gets its name from an Anglo-Saxon word meaning "spreading berry" due to its abundant, sprawling shoots that grow from the mother plant. As I write in my book *Vibrational Nutrition*, "Strawberry encourages being adventurous and daring and willing to take a risk and stretch for things out of your reach and getting them. It facilitates going headfirst and trusting the Divine to deliver and offers wonderful encouragement to venture out of your known environment and experience the wonders of the world and its treasures."[4] Let your curiosity lead you, let your adventures ripen you, dare for wonder to be your guide!

Sunflower Seed (*Helianthus annuus*)

Subtle gifts: Sunflower can help you develop your personal power and manifest love in action. It heals relationships with men in general and addresses intense self-effacement and low self-esteem on the one hand, or overly hard-hitting masculinity and arrogance on the other. It spiritualizes the ego, allowing your personality to radiate out. It addresses the kind of superiority that is reflected in the attitude of "my way or the highway." Use this oil to help heal the energy around misogyny, narcissism, cruelty, and punitiveness. It helps you value viewpoints that differ from your own and opens you to a radiant emotional life. Sunflower expands your ability to create order and experience moderation; it is good for self-discipline, helps develops the left brain, and expands appreciation of the classical arts. This plant's vibrational signature indicates that it heals the shadow issues associated with the negative traits of this plant's ruling deity, the sun god Apollo: problems communicating, difficulty with intimacy, narcissism, hostility, cruelty, punishment, and secret-keeping.

Physical gifts: The sunflower is one of the few flowers that offer "meat" in the form of its delicious seeds, which are highly nourishing. Sunflower seeds are a good source of magnesium, and numerous studies have demonstrated that magnesium helps reduce the severity of asthma, lowers high blood pressure, prevents migraine headaches, reduces the risk of heart attack and stroke, and offers many other benefits. Sunflower is also high in linoleic acid and vitamins E, A, and D. When used topically it treats bruises and sprains. It leaves the skin feeling smooth and nongreasy.

The Sun Embodied

This oil is the embodiment of form, law and order, and the sun; as such it resonates with the sun, personified as the Greek god Helios. The word *sunflower* in fact comes from the Greek *Helianthus*—*helios*, meaning "sun," and *anthos*, meaning "flower." It is Roman mythology that provides us with the story of the origin of the sunflower, as recounted in Ovid's *Metamorphoses*, in the account of the transformation of Leucothoë.

The sun, as Helios, visits the Babylonian princess Leucothoë, coming into her room disguised as her mother, sending her servants away before revealing his true form. I am he "who measures the long year, I am he. I see all things, earth sees all things by me, I, the world's eye. Trust me, you please me." Although she is afraid, his sudden brightness and beauty melts all her worries and she "submits" to his amorous advances. Leucothoë's sister Clytie finds out, and in a jealous rage she tells their father, who in "his pride and savagery buried [Leucothoë] deep in the earth, she praying, stretching her hands outward towards Sol's light . . . [her father having] piled a heavy mound of sand over her." Buried, she cannot lift her face or move her limbs, which are "crushed by the weight of the earth." Clytie, meanwhile, is transformed into a sunflower, or heliotrope. "They say her limbs clung to the soil, and her ghastly pallor changed part of her to that of a bloodless plant: but part was reddened, and a flower like a violet hid her face. She turns, always, towards the sun, although her roots hold her fast, and altered, loves unaltered."[5]

To further understand the sunflower it's important to explore the sun god Apollo (as a form of Helios, who is the personification of the sun itself). Jean Shinoda Bolen writes in *Gods in Everyman*,

> Apollo could see clearly from afar and observe the details of life with an overview perspective; he could aim for a target and hit it with his bow and arrows or create harmony with his music. As an archetype, Apollo personifies the aspect of the personality that wants clear definitions, is drawn to master a skill, values order and harmony, and prefers to look at the surface rather than at what underlies appearances. The Apollo archetype favors thinking over feeling, distance over closeness, objective assessments over subjective intuition. The man [individual] who most closely conforms to the Apollo archetype has attributes that will hold him in good stead in the world. He can succeed in a career and can master a classical art form easier than most people can.[6]

The sunflower was depicted in the Victorian language of flowers as indicating one who blindly follows the sun; thus the sunflower was used as a symbol of infatuation or foolish passion. This interpretation is reflected in the myth of Clytie and Helios/Apollo and speaks of unhealthy infatuation or power-over behavior. Not all cultures used the sunflower to depict foolish love, however. The Aztecs worshiped the sunflower, placing its image, often made of gold, in their temples, and crowning princesses in their bright yellow flowers. The sunflower is associated with the third chakra, the energy center that radiates the positive qualities of personal power, consciousness, action, self-worth, and will. Notably, the third chakra is traditionally understood as the intellectual center of the body, from which linear intelligence springs, producing what in ayurveda is the *pitta* body type, which is known for fiery intelligence and will.

Blending Tip – Try blending sunflower base oil with narcissus absolute (see chapter 1) to heal the energy around unrequited affection, foolish passion, communication struggles, difficulty with intimacy, narcissism, hostility, cruelty, punishment, and secret-keeping. This blend promotes emotional balance and healthier connections.

Tomato Seed (*Solanum lycopersicum*)

Subtle gifts: This oil, first and foremost, teaches togetherness in many forms, be it a loving family, a robust community, the dance of a love relationship, a passion, or even courtship. This fruity vegetable is all about the heart. A part of this dynamic is this plant's ability to help you to be open to differences and new circumstances and joyfully embrace them.

Physical gifts: With its rich content of nutrients and essential fatty acids, particularly omega-6 linoleic acid, tomato seed oil is powerfully calming, with anti-inflammatory effects that can reduce the redness associated with acne. The carotenoids present in tomato have an active role in scavenging free radicals and increasing collagen production, which helps heal skin issues and repairs damage that's already occurred, making the skin look younger and fresher. It lessens pock marks, acne scars, and sun stress.

Watermelon Seed (*Citrullus vulgaris*)

Subtle gifts: This oil fosters a positive sense of self and allows you to see the beauty of your life and not just focus on what you would like to change; this allows you to rest in the sweetness of the present moment.

Physical gifts: Also known as *ootanga*, *tsamma*, and *kalahari* melon, the first record we have of this plant is found in five-thousand-year-old Egyptian hieroglyphs. Watermelon originated in the Kalahari Desert. The juicy plant oil derived from this fruit's seeds has been traditionally used for cooking as well as for skin and hair care. A very light oil that absorbs well and is used for distressed skin, it dissolves excess sebum in pores, repairs damage to the cells, and reduces pore size. High in linoleic acid (up to 65 percent), B vitamins (especially niacin), and magnesium and zinc, it is a highly stable oil with a long shelf life and can therefore be added to recipes to help preserve products. This oil is suitable for the very young.

Wheat Germ (*Triticum aestivum*)

Subtle gifts: Wheat germ oil brings coherence within the physical form and restores a sense of vitality, facilitating the ability to move into life with ease. It offers nurturing, growth, parenting, and patience. Wheat germ provides the energy to keep growing in even the most inhospitable conditions, and along the way to learn many lessons that will allow you to mature as your project, idea, or self grows and stretches into the finished product, as age alone does not create maturity or enable creative problem-solving. In so doing, it helps you develop patience and pleasure in the process and overcome any tendency to procrastinate.

Physical gifts: Wheat germ oil is the farmer's friend, protecting the skin against sun and wind damage. Its squalene (1 percent), linoleic acid (55 percent), and vitamin E content improves the circulation close to the skin's surface and strengthens connective tissues, helping to maintain the skin's elasticity.

Saturn Can Be Your Friend!

Poor Saturn, it seems many people have a strained relationship with his principle, which teaches us the value of real time and the importance of constructively working with delays and overcoming hardships and limitations in life. Wheat germ oil vibrates to the planet Saturn, the Lord of Time, as well as to Demeter, the goddess of the harvest. In their book *Mythic Astrology Applied*, Ariel Guttman and Kenneth Johnson describe Demeter:

> There are several goddesses that may be regarded as "earth goddesses," particularly Gaia. . . . But Demeter is an offspring of Gaia—a granddaughter actually. Gaia is the quintessential "Earth Mother"; she is the earth itself. Ceres/Demeter, two generations removed, represents the fruits of Mother Earth—the flowers, the fields, and the food. Ceres/Demeter is primarily concerned with the growing of things and how things are nourished to provide that growth."[7]

Just as Demeter teaches us the principle of growth as a labor of love, nurturing, and parenting, an equally important factor in understanding wheat is time. Wheat has traditionally been a symbol of patience and the fruition that comes as a result of long, hard work; no major civilization has thrived without a grain to fortify it.

Wheat represents the prolonged attention needed to accomplish very large goals in a step-by-step manner. I appreciate Saturn (I have a double Saturn ring on my right hand), as he teaches us about maturity, boundaries, limitations, practicality, and, as a byproduct, creative problem-solving. We are told that "Saturn likes productivity and abhors stagnation or procrastination."[8]

Saturn, the Lord of Time, was the Roman deity who presided over agriculture and the harvesting of crops. Cronus was his Greek equivalent, and he too ruled the harvest. Agriculture is intrinsically linked with the seasons and time, such that the two cannot be separated. One of the most important Roman festivals, Saturnalia, celebrated Saturn during the winter solstice, around the time when winter grain was sown.

4

Other Tantalizing Tidbits

Macerated Oils, Milk Baths, Plant Butters, and Unrefined Salts

Butter and milk are milked from the living cloud; the navel of Order, the ambrosia is born.

RIG VEDA 9.74.4

Tantalizing by definition means to excite one's senses or desires. This chapter explores some truly sumptuous offerings from nature that are sure to dazzle and delight your senses! Macerated oils, milks, plant butters, and unrefined salts are carriers, or bases, that you can use to create blends with the absolutes, essential oils, and fixed oils in this book. Approach these carriers the same way you would the other oils featured in this book—blend for the properties that best support your goals. Allow your imagination and intuition to help you create fantastic blends—luxurious milk baths; scrubs and soaks with salts; unguents, body oils, and creams made with macerated oils and plant butters.

Macerated Oils

Macerated oils are vegetable oils to which other plant material has been added. These botanical oils are prepared via slow, low-temperature maceration (also known as *infusion*) to avoid potential heat damage during processing.

Making Macerated Oils

Macerated oils, also known as infused oils, are carrier oils that are used like a solvent to extract the therapeutic properties of a certain plant. The traditional way of doing this involves putting dried plant matter and a base oil in an airtight container such as a glass jar and placing it in a warm or sunny location for up to three weeks. This will gently heat the oil to extract many of the plant's properties. During the time you are macerating you can from time to time replace the macerated plant material with new plant material so you can continue to extract more therapeutic properties into your base oil. Macerated oils can impart beautiful fragrances into skin-care products depending on the plant being macerated.

If creating your own macerated oil the following plants make excellent choices to add to a base oil, using any of the fixed oils listed in chapter 3, which you can then macerate over a period of weeks. These macerated plant oils listed here are also available for retail purchase.

Banana (*Musa paradisiaca*)

Part used: peel

Subtle gifts: This phallic fruit helps you understand the role of sexuality and how male and female energies are intertwined on the subtle level, making it helpful for those exploring the alchemical concept of the divine marriage on the symbolic level or even literally, as in the sexual practices like tantra.

Physical gifts: Banana is good for acne-prone skin; it soothes inflammation and irritation, reduces the appearance of scarring, and balances the skin's natural moisture and oil production. It diminishes stretch marks and promotes the growth of new skin while boosting its suppleness. Its astringent, anti-inflammatory, and antioxidant properties help tighten lax skin. As well, it is good for treating dry, frizzy, damaged, and brittle hair without leaving a heavy, greasy film. It reduces dandruff, strengthens the hair, and may reduce hair loss while enhancing growth.

Daisy (*Bellis perennis*)

Part used: flowering top

Subtle gifts: Daisy supports seeing the big picture, how all the small parts create the whole. This makes for a wholesome, joyful oil bringing serenity and sunshine to your soul.

Physical gifts: Daisy oil is used in folk medicine for healing bruises, relieving muscle spasms, and treating arthritis and nerve pain such as sciatica.

Ginkgo (*Ginkgo biloba*)

Part used: leaf

Subtle gifts: Gingko fortifies the mind and offers support when you feel mentally foggy or overwhelmed and brings focus when you are exhausted and need support. It allows you to tap into ancient memories and supports the mental body in all ways.

Physical gifts: *Ginkgo biloba*, also known as maidenhair tree, occupies a unique biological niche between ferns and trees. It is one of the oldest plants in existence, dating back as far as two hundred million years, around since the time of the dinosaurs. Currently the oldest maidenhair tree in the world is 3,500 years old and is found in China. The leaves of the ginkgo have been used in medicinal formulations for more than five thousand years. It is high in alpha hydroxy acids and other antioxidant compounds such as vitamins C and E, making it ideal for reducing the appearance of scars and hyperpigmentation. It is also an ideal face cleanser, as it removes makeup effectively and supports a glowing complexion.

Orchid (*Anacamptis morio*)

Part used: flower

Subtle gifts: Orchid offers the vibration of romance, sensuality, sexuality, and fertility. This can be for attracting in a new love relationship or for revitalizing the relationship you are already in if it's become lackluster. This is a dynamic oil to use to energetically prime your body to conceive; both partners should use it.

Physical gifts: This oil is remarkably nourishing and soothing and can improve the skin's elasticity and promote cell regeneration, making it an excellent choice for mature, aging skin. It is helpful for relieving skin conditions such as psoriasis and eczema. Orchid macerated oil also promotes new tissue formation, accelerating healing and healthy skin growth. It possesses anti-inflammatory, antibacterial, and antifungal properties and is a useful germicide that can prevent or eliminate infections. Orchid oil is also wonderful as a hair treatment.

Potent Sexual Energy

Orchid has a potent sexual energy and historically has been associated with fertility. Specifically, in ancient Greece orchids were associated with virility. Greek women believed that if the father of their unborn child ate fresh, large orchid tubers, the baby would be a boy. If the mother ate small orchid tubers, she would give birth to a girl. Pliny the Elder was a first-century AD Roman naturalist and philosopher who claimed that even holding the roots of an orchid would stimulate one to ecstasy.

The Latin word for orchid is *orchis*, which comes from the Greek *orkhis*, meaning "testicle," because the orchid's twin bulbs resemble testicles. The Romans believed that orchids came into being when satyrs, male nature spirits with ears and a tail resembling those of a horse as well as a permanent, exaggerated erection, spilled their seed on the earth.

Saffron (*Crocus sativus*)

Part used: stigma of the flower, called saffron "threads"

Subtle gifts: Almost more than any other plant, saffron is noted for its distinctive brilliant yellow color. Saffron smells the way it looks—just gazing at saffron you feel the sun rising and setting. It's a liminal experience! It reaches into the realm of gold, the incorruptible and everlasting, and into the realm of blood, vigorous, active, and mutable. The effusiveness of saffron brings arousal to the physical and the subtle bodies; it rouses the second chakra and evokes the tantric unity of opposites. Saffron is a sacred fragrance representing the sacred Flower of Life made incarnate.

Physical gifts: Saffron is used today in a multitude of ways to support the physical body. It balances all dosha types, and according to ayurveda it balances the nervous system, promotes digestion, and quiets the mind. It is considered an alterative, a substance that will gradually restore the proper function of the body and increase health and vitality. It addresses menstrual pain and irregular menses, menopause, impotence, neuralgia, lower back pain, rheumatism, cough, asthma, and chronic diarrhea. Recent studies have confirmed that saffron has "potent antioxidative effects that may benefit autistic behaviors."[1]

Caution: Do not use during pregnancy.

Sensuality and Spirituality

Roman brides wore the *flammeum*, the saffron-colored veil of Aurora, the goddess of dawn. Homer describes the goddess Eos as *krokopeplos*, "clad in saffron," the yellow-red color of the garment of dawn, the part of the day she rules. In Mesopotamia, saffron was regarded as the color of divinity, while Buddhist monks wrap themselves in saffron-colored robes as a reminder of the light of truth that leads to enlightenment.

In Minoan culture an entire religion flourished based around the crocus flower and its stigmas. In one fresco, a goddess, perched on a rock, has injured her foot and her blood runs into the crocus flower and makes the stigma red. In Greek myth there are two stories of the immortal boy Crocus, one of love and one of heartbreak. In the first tale, Crocus was the beloved of Hermes, and one day while playing together a terrible tragedy struck. Crocus was hit on the head and mortally wounded. The heartbroken Hermes transformed his love into a flower, while three drops of blood that had fallen from the head of Crocus became the stigma of the flower. In the second tale, Crocus was in love with the nymph Smilax, but she did not love him in return. The gods took pity on Crocus and transformed him into the saffron flower to relieve his grief, while Smilax was transformed into a noxious bramble.

Aristophanes described saffron as a "sensuous smell," while it is believed that Cleopatra bathed in saffron-infused mare's milk before taking a lover to her bed (see the date oil blending tip in chapter 3). Dioscorides recommended mixing saffron with myrrh for a multitude of disorders. In Assyria it was used for treating stomachache and urinary disorders, while Egyptians favored it for infections, inflammation, diarrhea, and even as a contraceptive, and Pliny the Elder said that saffron increased the efficacy of all medicines.

Milk Baths

Milk does not fully dissolve essential oils and absolutes in bathwater; although it disperses somewhat, you are still left with a floating, milky oil residue that adheres to the skin. Reactions to citrus fruit oils in the bath seem to be quite common. To overcome this, blend a half cup to one cup of milk of your choice with a tablespoon (or more) of one of the fixed oils listed in chapter 3 to support the overall vibration or energy you are blending. Remember, less is more when adding essential oils and absolutes. I frequently take milk baths with milk alone, with only salt added, or salt and fixed oils added to the milk base.

Milk is high in lactic acid, and as such it is a natural exfoliator that leaves the skin silky smooth. You do not need to rinse off after a milk bath—let your skin drink the goodness in!

Milk embodies the soothing energies of the moon and has been said to offer the gift of soma, the ambrosic drops of the moon—meaning you should read its energetic gifts mythically: it is abundant, fertile, soothing, creative, illuminating, nourishing, fostering, and provides wholeness.

Ayurvedic physician David Frawley, director of the American Institute of Vedic Studies, says that milk has a sattvic nature, meaning it promotes the qualities of intelligence, virtue, and goodness, and creates harmony, balance, and stability. He says, "It is light, (not heavy) and luminous in nature. It processes an inward and upward motion and brings about the awakening of the soul. Sattva provides happiness and contentment of a lasting nature. It is the principle of clarity, wideness, and peace, the force of love that unites all things together."[2]

Milk baths have a rich history; Cleopatra was not the only one to indulge in this luxurious practice. Roman Empress Poppaea and French Queen Marie Antoinette also enjoyed the benefits. Floral absolutes infused in milk, blended into warm water—what could be more refined and uplifting?

Using these elements together, it is simple to create a ritual bath. It's a gentle ritual of beauty and spiritual cleansing, nurturing both body and soul. It's a time for relaxation, stress relief, renewal, and insights. Water, considered a gateway to the emotional and collective unconscious, acts as an amplifier, while the addition of milks, plants, and minerals deepens the experience. This sacred time invites focused intention and profound work, free from distractions like phones and laptops. Set a sacred space by turning off overhead lights, lighting candles, and playing music that nourishes the soul.

Most health food stores and farmers markets offer fresh milks: cow, goat, and sheep—and, if you're lucky, camel, water buffalo, and/or yak (see also Resources).

I offer some example bath blends to prime your creativity, although you may blend milk with any oil or salt to create the story you want in your bath!

Camel's Milk

Primary energy: motherly/fatherly love

Energetically, camel's milk brings the energy of caretaking by the archetypal Mother and Father. This succor opens you to being whole such that you experience feelings of unconditional love, trust, hope, healing, fortitude, and resourcefulness. This kind of nurturing encourages a joyful, loving patience with your process, in which you allow universal intelligence to direct you to where you need to be while opening you to the full spectrum of experiences in their many colors and shades.

Camel's milk has been consumed by humans for more than six thousand years. Nutritionally, it is richer than cow's milk in vitamins C and B, iron, calcium, magnesium, and potassium.

᪥ Gentle Support Bath Blend

½ cup camel's milk
1 cup Great Salt Lake salt
1 drop white rose otto absolute

Add ingredients to a hot or warm bath and blend in a figure eight motion, before submerging and absorbing the following gifts: Camel's milk opens you to a sense of wholeness, bringing feelings of unconditional love, trust, hope, healing, and strength. Great Salt Lake salt carries a similar energy, offering grace, lifting you up, and guiding you on your journey. This can be as subtle as a shift in mood or as powerful as a miracle, protecting you from negativity and helping you navigate inner turmoil. It helps reveal new options and connects you to the loving, supportive energy of the universe, all enhanced by the gentle presence of white rose otto absolute.

Cow's Milk

Primary energy: Mother Earth

Cow's milk represents Mother Earth herself. In her aspect of spring or a new morning, she brings playfulness, hope, the planting of new ideas, innocence, and the feeling of awakening to the world anew and anticipating what the new day will bring. In her aspect of summer or high noon she brings the energy of productivity, getting the job done, and empowering the mind. In her aspect of fall, or twilight, she gifts the energy of bringing your energy inward, tying up loose ends, finishing projects, gathering your harvest or the fruits of your labor, and getting ready to rest. In her aspect of winter, or night, she brings the gifts of deep rest, sleep, hibernation, rejuvenation, dreaming, communing with deep mysteries, and shedding what is no longer useful from your previous cycle before you awaken again. We live these cyclic energies seasonally as well as daily as we are reminded when and how to be a child, an adult, and an elder, and accept the responsibilities involved in each one of these cycles.

⊗ Butterfly Bath Blend

1 cup cow's milk
¼ cup Icelandic sea salt
1 drop cyclamen absolute

Add ingredients to a hot or warm bath and blend in a figure eight motion, before submerging and absorbing the following gifts: Cow's milk teaches us to honor the cyclical nature of life, embracing the responsibilities of each phase. Icelandic sea salt helps us surrender to natural forces beyond our control, aligning with their transformative power to allow natural ending and new beginnings. Combined with cyclamen absolute, which holds the energy of the butterfly, this synergy supports deep transformation and growth.

Goat's Milk

Primary energy: Pan, primordial god of the wilds, sexuality

> *Step into a heaven where I keep it on the soul side*
> *Girl, please me, be my soul bride*
> *Every woman has a piece of Aphrodite*
> *Copulate to create a state of sexual light . . .*
> *I mingle with the gods, I mingle with divinity*
> 　　　　　　　　　　　　RED HOT CHILI PEPPERS,
> 　　　　　　　　　　　　"BLOOD SUGAR SEX MAGIK"

Goat's milk helps you understand the forces of nature in their raw, unbridled, uncultivated forms. This vibration is especially beneficial if you're afraid to camp, walk nature trails away from the city, swim in a lake, and so on. It's also beneficial for anyone who is working to release engrained puritanical energies that have led to shame, or anyone who suffers from panic attacks. According to archetypal psychologist James Hillman, panic attacks are often due to not being able to integrate your inherent wildness into the fabric of ordinary "decent" life. Opening to your inherent wildness allows you to draw succor from nature and be revitalized so as to develop the more vigorous aspects of yourself. This milk also deepens your natural sexual impulses, allowing you to revel in these energies and thereby touch your divinity.

Pan, God of the Wild

The goat is a strong theme in Greek mythology. Pan, primordial god of Earth, the wilds, and sexuality, is half man and half goat. His name simply means "all." In some myths he is known as Earth Father. Notably, it is common not to have a temple dedicated to a god or goddess; instead, natural settings such as grottoes, clear lakes, meadows, woods, and caves are his places of worship. He offers the boon of helping you tap into your body's wisdom so that you can get out of your head and into your instinctual self.

Pan's Consort Bath

½ cup goat's milk
2 tablespoons macerated orchid oil
1 tablespoon macerated banana oil

Add ingredients to a hot or warm bath and blend in a figure eight motion, before submerging and absorbing the following gifts: Goat's milk awakens and deepens your natural sexual energies, inviting you to connect with your untrammeled essence. Orchid oil is a potent force and the embodiment of sensuality. Banana oil reveals the subtle dance of male and female energies, guiding you to understand their harmonious intertwining.

Sheep's Milk

Primary energy: security and stability

Sheep's milk brings the energy to create the resources that make your physical life comfortable—food, warmth, and shelter as the basis of all life, along with the safety and physical security that are needed to thrive. Sheep's milk encourages you to take stock of the general security and stability of your life. If any aspects such as finances, health, or home need to be shored up, sheep's milk will provide the creative ingenuity and strength to do just that. From this place of security you will have the fertile ground needed to plant anything in your life that you would like to grow.

Inviting Abundance to Enter Your Life

Sumerian mythology is rich with deities associated with sheep. Duttur is the Sumerian pastoral goddess of ewes, milk, and the art of crafting dairy products. She is the mother of Dumuzi, an ancient Mesopotamian king with godlike powers who is associated with shepherds and a thriving flock, and who was the primary consort of the fertility goddess Inanna, the Queen of Heaven and Earth. We find in the myth of Inanna the timeless story of Mother Earth watching over us and taking care of us. Her promise is to make the world fertile to produce what sustains us and keeps us safe.

I have a certain softness for the hymns that read as love songs and blessings from Inanna to Dumuzi. The following is one of my favorite invocations to invite abundance into your life:

> My husband, I will guard my sheepfold for you.
> I will watch over your house of life, the storehouse,
> The shining quivering place which delights Sumer—
> The house which decides the fates of the land,
> The house which gives the breath of life to the people.
> I, the queen of the palace, will watch over your house.[3]

❦ The Satisfaction of Longing

½ cup sheep's milk
1 tablespoon Arctic cranberry fixed oil
4 drops spinach absolute

Add ingredients to a hot or warm bath and blend in a figure eight motion, before submerging and absorbing the following gifts: Sheep's milk embodies the energy of security and stability while Arctic cranberry oil teaches you how to create an abundant life. Spinach absolute, with its essence of green fertility, opens your eyes to the steps and opportunities that can help you build your dream life. Together, they guide you toward fulfillment of desires.

Water Buffalo's Milk

Primary energy: inward journeying

The energy of water buffalo's milk is that of finding the true path. This is very simple: Stop. Listen. Learn. Act. This opens you to being contemplative and journeying inward, meditating on the subject you are exploring and receiving answers not only in your mind, but in every cell of your body. It then helps you act accordingly to achieve your desired outcome.

Strength, Service, Dedication

The water buffalo has traditionally been associated with strength, service, dedication, and connection to Mother Earth. Two important figures from the East, the ancient Chinese philosopher Lao Tzu, and Yama, the Hindu god of death and justice, both have the water buffalo as their "vehicle," or mount; this shows the character of the figure the buffalo carries and the nature of this milk. Lao Tzu was a wise man who served in the Zhou court until it grew progressively more corrupt, and this caused him to leave, as he could not serve such a master. He mounted his water buffalo and rode to the western border of the Chinese empire. Although he disguised himself as a farmer, the border official immediately recognized him and implored him to share his wisdom. What Lao Tzu wrote became the sacred text that we know as the Tao Te Ching, or Book of Changes, the central text of Taoism. The Hindu deity Yama was the first mortal to have reached the afterworld and created a path for all to follow. An offering of water buffalo's milk is traditionally used to ask Yama to help you live a long life.

❧ Of the Earth Bath

½ cup water buffalo's milk
1 tablespoon pumpkin seed fixed oil
3 drops brown boronia absolute

Add ingredients to a hot or warm bath and blend in a figure eight motion, before submerging and absorbing the following gifts: Water buffalo's milk deepens and strengthens your bond with Mother Earth, grounding you in her ancient wisdom. Together, pumpkin seed oil and brown boronia absolute awaken the ancestral memories woven into your being, allowing you to recall the timeless history of the world that resides within your body.

Yak's Milk

Primary energy: time traveling, shamanic journeying

The milk of the yak offers a doorway, a portal in essence, that allows you to travel to other dimensions of time and space, places that might not even exist in our third-dimensional reality. This energy emboldens you to take the first brave steps in this exploration; it connects you deeply to universal energy and provides the ability to ground yourself solidly and safely while you explore.

❧ Between the Stars Bath

⅓ cup yak's milk
3 drops orris root absolute
1 tablespoon blueberry fixed oil

Add ingredients to a hot or warm bath and blend in a figure eight motion, before submerging and absorbing the following gifts: The milk of the yak opens a portal, a gateway to other dimensions of time and space, to realms beyond our third-dimensional reality. Orris root absolute connects you to the threads of time, while blueberry fixed oil awakens your third eye, guiding you on your journey.

Plant Butters

Botanical butters are luscious plant fats that make extraordinary moisturizers on their own and also serve as ingredients in a wide array of skin and lip recipes, giving your creations a rich, creamy smooth, substantial viscosity. These butters are solid at room temperature, making them ideal for thickening up body-care formulations. Plant butters are the perfect base for body creams and lip butters (see "Poetic Lip Butters" in chapter 9). You can blend any absolutes, essential oils, and fixed oils with plant butters to create your own unique formulas. The key is to choose ingredients with energy signatures that, when combined, weave the story you wish to bring into your life. For each plant butter that follows, I have included recommendations of oils that will amplify the energy signature of the butter—you are certainly not limited to this list. You may want to make a product based on its physical properties, scent, or flat-out whimsy.

Babassu Butter (*Orbignya oleifera*)

Primary energy: feminine sexuality

Resonant oils: *absolutes*: aglaia, brown bornonia, damask rose (pink), lilac, spinach; *essential oils*: clary sage, jasmine, patchouli, pink pepper seed, vanilla; *fixed oils*: avocado, date, mango, papaya, peach; *macerated oils*: orchid

Babassu butter supports the more feminine, passionate, exciting dimensions of your personality to unfurl, allowing you to explore and play with these juicy aspects of yourself. This butter is made from the expeller-pressed oil of the kernels of the babassu palm tree, native to the Amazon rainforest. A soft, emollient butter with a low melting point, it supports softer, smoother skin. Our skin naturally contains lauric acid, which also occurs in over 50 percent of the fatty acids found in babassu oil, helping to give the skin plumpness and plenty of moisture. As an added benefit the lauric acid content helps reduce skin irritations.

Cocoa Butter (*Theobroma cacao*)

Primary energy: joy, fun

Resonant oils: *essential oils*: lemon, marjoram, neroli, orange (common); *fixed oils*: cherry, dragon fruit, passion fruit, pineapple, strawberry, watermelon

Cocoa teaches you how to live in joy, making it useful for those who tend to be overly serious or have a somber sense of spirituality. Cocoa butter is extracted from cocoa beans, which are the fatty seeds of the cacao tree. They hydrate the skin, support elasticity, reduce the appearance of wrinkles, and protect against environmental factors like wind and cold. A fun aspect of cocoa butter is its warm, chocolatey scent.

Hemp Seed Butter (*Cannabis sativa*)

Primary energy: shamanic journeying, light-heartedness

Resonant oils: *absolutes*: frankincense, juhi, orris root; *essential oils*: frankincense, grapefruit, white lotus; *fixed oils*: borage, fig seed, goji berry, okra, poppy seed

Hemp seed teaches the art of versatility and the ability to wear many hats. It clarifies issues of willpower and how to innovate in the face of authority or restrictive situations. and brings playfulness and lightheartedness to being on the planet. "Lighten up!" it says. Hemp seed oil is useful for shamanic journeys and vision dreams by cultivating awareness around altered states, bringing clarity and order to journeys between the dimensions. Hemp seed butter consists of the pressed seeds of the hemp plant. It is rich in omega fatty acids, nutrients, and minerals, making it an excellent nourishing oil for cosmetic applications. Hemp seed butter is perfect for most skin types as it can moisturize without clogging your pores.

Kokum Butter

Primary energy: innovative thinking, seeing the big picture

Resonant oils: *absolutes*: black currant, cyclamen, elderflower, hyacinth, labdanum, narcissus, orris root; *essential oils*: basil (sweet), bergamot, black pepper, blood orange, cedar (eastern white), citron (Buddha's hand), lemon, lime, white birch; *fixed oils*: quinoa, safflower, sunflower

This highly emollient butter from the fruit-bearing kokum tree, cultivated in tropical areas of India, promotes new ways of thinking and allows misconceptions to fall away. Strands of light emanate from your spiritual core, extending in all directions. These are your internal rays of light, like a great sun that illuminates the potentials to be found in the cycles of life. As each new experience ebbs and flows, it clears the way to see from a bigger perspective. Follow your path with a free and open mind. The kokum tree is also known as wild mangosteen or red mangosteen. Kokum butter refers to the kokum fruit's seed oil, which is solid at room temperature and pale gray or yellow in color. A hard butter with a high melting point, kokum butter has powerful moisturizing properties yet won't clog the pores. It can be used to treat a variety of skin issues, including acne, minor inflammatory conditions, and dry skin, hair, and scalp.

Macadamia Butter

Primary energy: cheerfulness, serenity, peacefulness
Resonant oils: *absolutes*: lily, magnolia, spinach, violet; *essential oils*: bergamot, kumquat, lavender, pine; *fixed oils*: pistachio

Macadamia butter promotes a sunny, serene disposition and counterbalances the energy of being upset easily. Macadamia nuts grow on large, spreading, broadleaf evergreen trees that typically grow from thirty to fifty feet in height. This nut butter is a good source of antioxidants, which can protect against oxidative stress and cellular damage. It is also high in essential nutrients such as magnesium, iron, and zinc. Ultra-rich yet spreadable, this butter improves hydration and smooths the texture of the skin.

Mango Seed Butter

See mango kernel fixed oil in chapter 3.

Olive Butter

See olive fixed oil in chapter 3.

Shea Butter (*Vitellaria paradoxa*)

Primary energy: courage, purity, honesty

Resonant oils: *absolutes*: rose otto (white); *essential oils*: bergamot, blue chamomile, cardamom, cinnamon leaf, frankincense (*Boswellia carterii*), oakmoss, peppermint, petitgrain, red spikenard, sandalwood, vetiver

Shea butter teaches that rather than pursuing an ideal you should instead focus on achieving results. This butter lends courage to the spiritual seeker, helping to align motivations with purity and honesty, empowering the heart with conviction and common sense in order to reach your goal. Shea nuts grow on the shea tree. Shea butter is an emollient that softens and smooths dry skin and helps reduce skin inflammation. It is traditionally used for acne, burns, dandruff, eczema, and chalky skin.

Unrefined Salts

In the beginning—our beginning—Earth was a watery planet, completely enveloped in a salty primordial ocean. Our bodies still benefit from and indeed crave salts that have not been superheated, processed, and treated—drastic steps that remove the precise electrolytes, trace minerals, and elements our bodies need and that still hold our collective memory.

The Crystal Shapes of Salt

A salt crystal is made up of an orderly array of sodium and chloride ions. This repeating, orderly array is caused by the electrostatic attraction between the negatively and positively charged atoms called *ions*, which forms the salt crystal's distinct cube shape.

In nature, crystals rarely grow evenly and equally in all directions. Instead, many minerals, including salts, appear as clusters of interconnected crystalline regions known as *hopper crystals*. These are the result of anisotropic growth,* creating a structure that resembles a stepped pyramid, or hopper. In the case of hopper-shaped salt crystals, the increased surface area is reported to enhance taste.

Like all crystals, salt exhibits sacred geometry, which provides a template to shape the energy body.

- **Trapezoid:** A trapezoid has four sides. Of these four sides, one pair is parallel, with unequal lengths. The two parallel sides are called the *bases*, while the other sides are called the *legs*. This shape's energy speaks to the beauty that surrounds you and suggests that you focus on that and find more ways to bring that into your life. This shape also asks you to slow down and appreciate what you already have and celebrate the small things.
- **Cube:** A cube has six equal square faces. It brings the energy of solidity, strength, and confined order.
- **Pyramid/hopper:** The pyramid energy signifies movement toward strength and completion. It puts you in contact with the energies of growth, joy, and freedom, reminding you to take stock of where you are in your life path, acknowledge the progress you have made, and reaffirm your commitment to make choices that strengthen and support you in fulfilling your life purpose.

---

*Growth anisotropy (an-ahy-so-truh-pee) describes the condition when growth rates are not equal in all directions. In contrast, when growth rates are the same rate in all directions, growth is isotropic. Anisotropy is a hallmark of plant growth. Almost without exception, cells grow faster in one direction than in another.

Salt baths ease body aches and pains, reduce inflammation, and promote blood circulation, which in turn provides muscles with increased oxygen and nutrients. Salts are a general detoxifier on a subtle and physical level.

Some salts can be quite expensive. To infuse the desired energy signature of a specific salt, blend 2 cups of Epsom salts with 1 to 2 tablespoons of your chosen unrefined salt. Set your intention on the energy you wish to infuse, allowing that specific energy to enter your bath. Epsom salt has a neutral energy and dissolved in water may help the skin absorb magnesium ions, which regulate essential bodily functions such as muscle and nerve function, blood pressure, and inflammation. Of course, you may use only the unrefined salt instead.

Never add essential oils or absolutes directly to a salt soak without a fatty medium like milk or fixed oil. Never add to the bath "hot" oils such as sweet basil and cinnamon; citrus oil; or deeply cooling oils, such as peppermint or white birch. Less is more. I would recommend not more than 4 drops for a full bath, up to 10 drops for a foot soak. If you have a reaction, immediately apply a fixed oil and/or saturate in full-fat milk.

You can use any amount of salt you prefer for a salt scrub, but the key is to thoroughly saturate the salt base with fixed oil. Add a total of 4 drops of essential oils and/or absolutes to ½ cup fixed oil. Moisten skin—in bath or shower—remove yourself from the water and vigorously scrub mixture on body. Then either step back into the shower stream or submerge back into the bath.

Falling under the category of *tantalizing tidbits,* salt baths and scrubs shine when paired with fixed oil allies. Together, they support a healthy body and provide rich, interesting energy signatures to work with.

The salts listed here provide fascinating stories from nature that hold the imprint of the diverse geological landscapes that we often cannot access. The stories are amplified in that traditional salt-making often admixes other local gifts of the earth such as clay, charcoal, and woodsmoke, each helping to weave a complex and beautiful story.

Cyprus Flake Salt

Primary energy: spiritual guidance during times of change
Fixed oil allies: apple seed, cloudberry seed, quinoa, safflower

The process for creating Cyprus flake salt from the Mediterranean Sea around the island of Cyprus is beautiful. Seawater is evaporated using the natural processes of sun and wind, producing a salt brine that is fed into an open evaporation pan. The brine is then slowly heated by the sun until delicate crystals of salt are formed. The unique pyramid shape of this salt as it is harvested is created through the process of solar evaporation of seawater in which the water is channeled into a series of shallow ponds or lagoons and then into large pans, where the water is gradually heated, forming the pyramid shapes of the salt crystals. The process continues until the salt reaches 3 percent humidity, which can take up to two years to complete.

This salt offers spiritual guidance and learning, bringing the energy of transition, freedom, and independence. It helps you foresee and manifest your ideal life with singularly motivated actions. However, this energy can often be instigated by itchy emotions, seeing glitches, and feelings of restlessness that make you want to change. So be ready for movement!

Fleur de Sel

Primary energy: refinement, beauty, the arts
Fixed oil allies: cherry kernel, dragon fruit seed, guava seed, kiwi seed, mango kernel, papaya seed, peach kernel, strawberry seed, watermelon seed

This salt, whose name means "flower of salt" in French, is harvested in the traditional labor-intensive way—in the Guerande, Camargue, and Ré Island regions of France—by passing seawater through a network of dikes and ponds and then harvesting the purest, whitest layer off the top. The fine hollow pyramid crystals are rich in minerals and offer a silken texture with a delicate form.

This salt brings refinement to life, helping you appreciate beauty such as that found in the ballet, symphony, opera, and other classical arts. It stimulates a hunger to try new things, which might manifest as being a tourist in your own town—trying new restaurants, visiting museums you never seem to find time for, or joining a salon purely for the joy of the discussion of ideas.

Great Salt Lake Salt

Primary energy: grace, upliftment, protection
Fixed oil allies: apricot seed, cloudberry seed, milk thistle, passion fruit seed, raspberry seed, sunflower seed

The Great Salt Lake in Utah is salty because it does not have an outlet—tributary rivers are constantly bringing in small amounts of salt dissolved in the river's freshwater flow; once in the Great Salt Lake, much of the water evaporates, leaving the salt behind. This lake is the remnant of Lake Bonneville, a great Ice Age lake that rose dramatically from a small, salty lake some thirty thousand years ago. Due to its high saline content it is impossible to sink in this lake, and instead you bob up and down like a cork.

The energy of this salt is similar in that it offers the gift of grace, buoying your up, helping you on your way. It can be as subtle as a shift in mood or as large as a miracle, or anything in-between. It will protect you from the ill will of others and ignorant behavior, even that which results from your own mistakes and inner turmoil. This salt helps you see options where none seemed to exist before and connects you to the loving and supportive energy of the universe—especially if you feel you do not deserve a break or assistance. It helps you understand that just *being* is enough of a reason for getting support from the universe. This energy does not shield you from learning through mistakes and the learning process that goes with it, but it does offer the grace to make this learning easier. This energy opens your eyes to see what existing support systems are already in place in your life and teaches the right use of those, encouraging you to ask for a helping hand from those you love and trust.

Caution: *For external use only!* The concentrated sea mineral crystals from Utah's living sea are not to be taken internally and should only be used in external applications.

Himalayan Pink Salt

Primary energy: intuition, the power of knowing, logic
Fixed oil allies: cashew nut, goji berry, sunflower

This Jurassic Era pyramid-shaped pink sea salt, some 250 million years old, is known for its healing properties. It is a pure, hand-mined salt found in the pristine foothills of the Himalayan mountains.

The energy of this salt is the power of three: the undivided primal waters of a long-ago sea, the wisdom energy of intuition, and the power of logic operating through you. *The undivided primal waters* refer to pure potentiality, what exists before form. *Intuition* is knowing something in a deeply felt way. This energy is sometimes described as the fire of knowing or a testimony to a truth that cannot be proven or even articulated but is so powerful that it shapes lives and destinies. *Logic* can be understood as the expression of your intuition, dropped into form at a vibration dense enough that the human mind can begin to organize, process, and use the divine information being expressed and act on it.

Icelandic Birch-Smoked Sea Salt

Primary energy: beauty, radiance, succor, calm
Fixed oil allies: grapeseed, oat, okra seed, pomegranate seed

This is a flaky sea salt that is dried over birch smoke according to Icelandic tradition and is produced using only geothermal power. This is done in a small bay in the peninsula of Reykjanes; salt crystals are evaporated by using the heat from natural geysers and electricity produced from geothermal energy. The massive Eurasian and North American plates are slowly pulling apart in the middle of the Atlantic Ocean, and lava and fire pour forth to fill the abandoned space, forming the long mid-Atlantic ridge.

Iceland sits as a peak on this ridge and this salt is the essence of this geothermal energy.

Birch-smoked sea salt expands your appreciation of beauty and your own inner radiance; it brings light into darkness and offers deep purification, emotional succor, protection, and a profound sense of calm. It helps one remain malleable and feel supported as you move through deep inner changes and transformation. It calms and soothes doubts, anxieties, and fears that inevitability arise during times of change. It helps you learn how to surrender to the natural forces that are beyond comprehension and personal control, and in so doing, align with their magical and transformative power, allowing something truly new to emerge.

Japanese Shinkai Deep Sea Salt

Primary energy: kindness, empathy, gentleness, forgiveness
Fixed oil allies: avocado, blackberry seed, cantaloupe seed, cucumber seed, jojoba, pineapple seed, pistachio nut, plum kernel, tomato seed

This salt is the product of the seawater of the Noto Peninsula in Japan, where cold and warm ocean currents intersect, stirring up nutrients from the deep, creating nutrient-rich, life-affirming waters. The energy of this salt is imbued with the soft energy of the Noto Peninsula; it has been described as offering the mouth a feeling of well-rounded tenderness, and it is similarly silky to the touch. The people of Oku Noto are celebrated for their empathy and kindheartedness, justifying the epithet of this little ribbon of paradise: "Noto is a kind land." You can feel the love in every pyramid-shaped grain of salt that is cultivated by the sincere and present people who life here who have carefully nurtured every step of this salt's production.

The gift of this salt is tenderness and life-affirming gentleness, and the healing that can only come from this space. It opens the way to healing the deep wounds of the soul that have resulted from faith betrayed, love dishonored, trust forsaken, and other mortifying actions that fracture the structure of trust and innocence. This salt teaches that the healing balm that is required is forgiveness and letting go of the hurt—a difficult act—allowing one to be renewed and restored. Acknowledging the simple act of letting go of what hurts us makes space for returning to love and compassion. Healing can seem so complex as one navigates the myriad offshoots of the original wounding, navigating through old blocks and resistances, but it is the radical act of letting go that starts the process. The steps to gaining a sense of well-being may be easy or may offer great challenges, but this salt reminds you that the first step starts with you, as healing flows through us and does not originate in us. You are irrevocably changed as this energy courses through you, and this allows you to fully receive the tenderness, joys, and gifts that life has to offer. Once you are filled with this bounty, send your reflection of it back into the world.

Jugyeom Bamboo Salt

Primary energy: strength, resolve, tenacity, flexibility
Fixed oil allies: buriti, chia seed, coconut, corn, cranberry seed, prickly pear seed, wheat germ

This distinctive Korean salt is created by filling a bamboo stem with bay salt produced on Korea's west coast, then sealing it with red or yellow clay and baking it repeatedly in a kiln with pine tree firewood. The salt lumps harden after baking and are taken out and broken apart by hand, resulting in a distinctive irregular shape with a somewhat chunky appearance. During baking, the salt absorbs the bamboo constituents, which bring a distinctive sweetness called the *Gamrojung* flavor. The baking cycle darkens the salt, which results in its distinctive blue, yellow, red, white, and black. Bamboo salt baked at a temperature above 2,730 degrees Fahrenheit produces a unique purple color, which indicates the finest quality.

The energy of bamboo makes the impossible possible by teaching unwavering strength, resolve, and tenacity, balanced with the gracefulness of flexibility; this allows you to adapt to the moment with wisdom. This salt brings focus, clarity, and an overarching understanding of how each small action weaves the larger whole of your reality. It offers special insight if you tend to get enmeshed with others in a nonhelpful way that creates limitations in creativity, competitive behavior, or confines what you are willing to try due to judging yourself against another's accomplishments. This salt imparts strength, valor, and honor that comes from within and does not need to be validated by outside forces. Pine contributes the overlay of self-love and the ability to experience your emotions in real time versus playing out echoes from the past. The overall vibration of this salt is to use all that you are, learn all that you can, and put this into play no matter how many times you stumble as you work toward being the absolute best you can be in any situation.

Kilauea Onyx Sea Salt

Primary energy: dreaming

Fixed oil allies: black currant seed, borage, fig seed, poppy seed, pumpkin seed

This Hawaiian sea salt, with irregularly shaped granules that vary in size and form, has a deep obsidian color and a moist, silky texture. It is solar evaporated with purified black lava rocks to add minerals, then combined with active charcoal to add detoxifying effects. Kilauea onyx sea salt farms are located in the town of Kaunakakai, on the tiny island of Molokai, one of the least developed and most pristine of the Hawaiian Islands.

The energy of this salt invites you into the womb of the Self and the portal to the dreamtime. Entering into inner silence, you will find deep rest and introspection in this hallowed space. Here you can dream into being the next turn of the wheel to be co-created with the Divine. It is also effective for when you become lost in the labyrinth of self, which might present as a malaise of becoming entangled in your own thoughts and unable to find solutions or lost in a self-created isolation that is to your detriment. In such times this salt can act like a midwife and support your return to the light.

Molokai Red Sea Salt

Primary energy: cleansing, purification

Fixed oil allies: apricot kernel, black currant, cantaloupe seed, daikon radish seed

This Hawaiian sea salt produced on the island of Molokai, which is notable for its red dirt, is solar evaporated and combined with red volcanic clay, or *alaea*, to achieve a mineral-rich sea salt with the pristine energy of the deep Pacific. Hawaiians believe that the baked alaea clay, which is composed of more than eighty minerals, provides a variety of benefits, with detoxifying and healing powers. The salt crystal has an irregular shape due to the presence of so many minerals.

This salt is traditionally used for ceremonial purposes such as blessings and purifying seagoing canoes, as well as being an important ingredient in traditional Hawaiian herbal medicine. It cleanses and purifies, helping dispel heavy or dark energy that can overshadow life, so that sunshine and deep radiance can fill your being once again.

Redmond Real Salt

Primary energy: yang, fiery energy, discernment, careful consideration

Fixed oil allies: broccoli seed, cranberry seed (Arctic), olive oil, red cabbage seed

This salt is mined in Redmond, in central Utah, from the remnants of an ancient inland sea. The salt settled to the bottom of the Sundance Sea during the Jurassic Period of the Mesozoic Era, roughly 200 to 145 million years ago. Trapped under five thousand feet of volcanic ash and bentonite clay, it stayed pristine for eons. As time passed, the salt vein was pushed up vertically by tectonic shifts in the Continental Divide, raising it to near-surface level.

This salt brings the active male principle known by many descriptives: yang, fiery, solar, and so on. It fosters the spiritual will to do what is right but difficult, requiring sustained effort both in action and compassion. It encourages the ability to discern truth and protect those in need. It has a crystalizing action with thought when you need to look at a problem from many different angles and not decide in haste, even with immense outside and internal pressures occurring.

Redmond salt is available with or without hickory smoke. The hickory smoke overlay is good for those who wish to change but cannot; it helps the transformation of ingrained, lifelong beliefs that no longer serve us and eases the hardening of fear that clings to untenable ideas and positions.

> **Blending Tip** — Labdanum, saffron, and orris root are all dynamic matches with Redmond Real Salt, with each plant taking the synergy in a different direction. Take a moment to review all the descriptions and then write down where this salt's energy interacts and amplifies the energy of each plant in a unique way.

Sel Gris Salt

Primary energy: relaxing in liminal spaces
Fixed oil allies: black currant, blueberry seed, borage, onion

Sel gris is a French term that translates to "gray salt," and as the name implies, these irregularly shaped crystals have a slight grayish hue. This is due to the harvesting process, in which clay basins are set underwater in the Atlantic Ocean, and once the water evaporates it leaves behind natural salt deposits in which all of the minerals add this grayish hue to the crystals and provide their unique taste: oceanic, with striking minerality due to higher content of iron, calcium, zinc, magnesium, and more.

This salt opens the in-between places and seeks no answers, allowing one to live in a gray quietness.

> **Blending Tip** — Blend sel gris salt with black currant oil and black currant absolute to explore liminal spaces and send your mind growing inward like a root.

PART 2

The Body Ecstatic

Exploring the Body's Energetic Patterns

5

Our Body as Expressed in the Elements

Earth, Water, Fire, Air, Ether

Our hands imbibe like roots, so I place them on what is beautiful in this world. And I fold them in prayer, and they draw from the heavens light.

ST. FRANCIS OF ASSISI

The embodied self encompasses two poles, between which all the different aspects of consciousness function. The element of earth governs the outer self and how we explore this self in the world though our physical body; at the other end of the spectrum the element of ether governs our inner self, the pure I AM presence beyond physicality. These two elements represent two sides of the same coin, two polarities, while the remaining three elements—water, fire, and air—express degrees of energy that exist between these two polarities.

The consciousness of a living being is determined by the frequency of the matter that makes up the body, which is always in flux and manifests different qualities. Being physically incarnate allows us to engage in the play of nature, as no incarnation can be completely worldly or completely spiritual. No matter what level of light or spirituality you attain, you cannot transcend the human experience if you are embodied. Likewise, no matter how terrestrial you think you are, you are always filled with divinity. So, the goal is to experience the balance of spiritual energy and matter working together to create a healthy whole, which furthers curiosity, play, and exploration here on Earth.

An incredibly easy way to access these complementary energies is to work with the five elements, which set the frequencies that give rise to every aspect of the human experience. The five elements are also expressed in nature, specifically in plants, so given our interdependence with nature, we can use her gifts to balance and direct the five elements that comprise our human form.

The Vedic tradition teaches that we are divine beings having a human experience. With this in mind, meditate on the elemental energies and their expressions in plants, as they are energetic gateways that correspond to the spine, our Tree of Life, allowing us to process universal life force frequencies and understand the wondrous energies available to us in incarnate human form.

Each plant distillation in this book represents a snippet of nature and holds a unique frequency that creates and supports a certain state of being. Said another way, plant distillations are a dynamic and fragrant way to entrain your physical matter and bring certain traits to the forefront of your personality to help repattern limiting aspects. You have the ability to arrange and rearrange your deepest self at will with the tools featured in this book.

The five senses—taste, touch, sight, sound, and smell—each provide a unique way to experience and interpret the world. In ayurveda, these senses are referred to as *jnanendriyas*, or gates (this term is also translated as "belonging to knowledge"). The physical senses are portals through which we perceive and understand our surroundings. These gates are also considered the meeting points between the internal and external realms.

My intention here is to introduce this idea in a juicy manner, and not in a clinical manner, and thereby to encourage you to experience your senses as the marvels they are.

In the context of this chapter, sacred shape refers to a yantra, a visual geometric representation of a sound, often known as a mantra.* In the framework of chakras, the simple root yantras featured in this chapter are directly associated with the *bija*, or seed mantra, of each chakra. Yantras are potent tools for organizing energy into specific states of being. To anoint your body with a sacred shape, through this act of resonance you are awakening and bringing all of the primordial energy of the corresponding energy centers to bear. For example, to anoint your body with a square activates the earth element and the root chakra, as each element corresponds to a specific chakra and a specific shape.

Earth: The Foundation of the Food Body

Earth is one of the building blocks of the Annamaya kosha, the physical food body that is the outermost layer of the self. It is in this food body that on a cellular level we hold not only our personal memories but the memories of the entire cosmos. The element of earth corresponds to the lower back and soles of the feet, which provide our support and connect us to the earth.

An aspect of earth can be understood as tribalism in the sense of a hive mentality—thinking and reacting as a group, with patterned beliefs that are inherited from family, community, culture, religion, and the country you were born and raised in. This includes any inherited diseases that have been passed down through your family lineage, such as heart disease or alcoholism, or even behavioral predilections like depression. These patterns are reinforced by lifestyle choices advanced by family or commu-

---

*This book is not focused on only Eastern thought; much like Mother Nature it cross-pollinates ideas from many sources. If you want a stricter Eastern lens, my book *Essential Oils in Spiritual Practice: Working with Chakras, Divine Archetypes, and the Five Great Elements*, is a more faithful exploration.

nity regarding diet, exercise habits, and mental attitudes. From this energy complex you can learn lessons concerning good lifestyle habits and what it takes to create robust health.

A major impulse of earth energy is to seek understanding and meaning through your physical body by using your five senses—touch, sight, sound, smell, and taste. The physical senses allow you to experience the wonders of earthly incarnation, the experience of being alive and embodied. Earth energy creates a desire to heal and grow using the gifts of plants. It supports memory retention, patience, and endurance. Earth energy is a maternal protector; she creates a nurturing place where all can thrive, learn, and grow. Earth is literally a school where we learn refinement of the self. This is the only energy where you can take all the abstract knowledge you have accumulated and put it into action, for it is only here in this physical body that you can practice to find meaning in times of hardship and maintain inner calm and steadiness regardless of external circumstances. Earth is the ultimate testing ground!

Earth exists in the mind as the ego, which is responsible for understanding who we are as an individual self. We identify with our body, its senses and desires, which cause us to act in the world.

Physical Gate: Smell

The sense of smell is the physical gate of the earth element. We take life in through scent. To smell someone is to know someone. Humans prefer genetically dissimilar partners based on scent, as confirmed by a 2019 study that found that humans are able to detect via smell which partners are genetically preferable.[1]

Molecules are invisibly small particles of matter, the diverse building blocks of life that make up things in the material world and give them their substance, qualities, and most cherished secrets. Smell is an intimate and direct way to interact with the molecules that make up the world. Smell arises from two tiny patches of sensitive skin placed out of sight in the front of our head, behind and a little below our eyes—the olfactory bulbs. From this location our world is fleshed out and given vivid textures, sensations, and meanings: the scent of galangal and kaffir lime leaves at your favorite Thai restaurant is much more than the scent of tom kha soup; it can be your last quarrel with your lover or a satisfying conversation with a dear friend. Scent is evocative, bringing strong images, memories, and feelings to mind.

Sacred Shape: Square

The square expresses the element of earth. It is the energy of fixed nature, matter, strong foundations, and order. In the physical domain it represents the static configuration of matter upholding the principle of volume in the physical world. The earthy square is associated with solidity, reliability, and sturdiness. You can rely on the square. To invoke and amplify the energy of earth and the root chakra, apply the oil(s) you are working with in a square shape on your lower back and/or the soles of your feet.

Plant Pairings: Using Scent and Sacred Shape to Invoke Earth Energy

A powerful way to access the earth element through all the bits of nature in this book is through the sense of smell. By inhaling the fragrance of a plant's oil, you tap into its gifts. It's that simple. You can do this by diffusing an essential oil or absolute blend, inhaling deeply and mindfully as you apply to your body, soak in the bath, or breathe it in directly from the container or a diffuser.

One of my favorite authors, Harold McGee, a James Beard Award winner, explores the world through scent:

> Smell is such a powerful and revealing sense because it detects actual little pieces of things in the world. Those little pieces are volatile molecules, so little that they're able to break away from their source and fly invisibly through the air to reach our nose. To begin to understand a thing's smell, then, is to identify the many volatile molecules it emits.

... When different things seem to echo each other with shared component smells, it's a sign those things have some volatile molecules in common.[2]

As scents echo one another due to shared molecules, we too, are made of the same elemental stuff. By taking in these sacred medicines through our nose, we awaken or actualize their energetic pattern or gift. In this way you can craft states of being by mindfully using fragrance. When engaging with your sense of smell, meditate on the gifts of the earth. With intention, you can access any aspect of the earth element's energy signature you wish to harness, as well as the unique plant signature you're working with.

Three plant oils come immediately to mind when I think of earth energy: Siberian fir absolute, brown boronia absolute, and virgin coconut oil.

The sublime scent of Siberian fir perfectly expresses the grounding energy of earth. The concept of *shinrin-yoku*, or "forest bathing," is a truly beautiful practice. It invites us to *earth* ourselves in nature, deeply connecting with the environment and allowing its energy to heal and restore. The forest offers a space to address our concerns and reflect on life's bigger questions; it acts as a mirror of our inner landscape, a kind of "school of life."

For those who can't physically visit a forest, diffusing Siberian fir absolute provides a satisfying alternative. With its grounding, supportive energy and scent, Siberian fir can evoke the same sense of balance and calm that comes from walking on the rich earth beneath a canopy of towering trees. Siberian fir guides you back to your roots, reconnecting you with your personal history, teaching valuable lessons about community, your place in the larger world, and navigating the complexities of daily life.

Siberian fir essential oil's key aromatic molecules are monoterpenes (alpha-pinene, camphene, limonene) and terpene esters like bornyl acetate. These phytochemicals give rise to a fresh, piney, sweet, woody aroma, with fruity-balsamic undertones.

Brown boronia absolute deepens your connection with your physical body to foster a more sensitive awareness of living in your flesh and bones. It invites a gentle dialogue with yourself, offering support if you have concerns about your relationship with whole foods, are feeling exhausted, or need help with an exercise routine. This oil supports all aspects of daily life. If you don't feel at home in your body or on Earth, this absolute nurtures and guides you, helping you feel more grounded and at peace in this physical world. It also amplifies the wonder and beauty of being alive, encouraging you to fully engage with and appreciate all five senses.

The aroma of boronia absolute is primarily shaped by constituents derived from carotenoids, but it also contains several linalool-related compounds, including linalool, linalyl acetate, and a series of 8-hydroxylinalool esters. The result is a complex, richly layered, tenaciously earthy floral scent reminiscent of champaca, with fresh, green, fruity, tealike notes. Subtle nuances of soft cinnamon, tobacco, and a warm, woody undertone add depth and warmth to its fragrance.

Virgin coconut oil, a very earthy oil, is solid at room temperature. To use, place a dollop in the palm of your hands and allow the warmth of your body to gently melt it, releasing its buttery, sweet coconut aroma. Once melted, apply it to your lower back and the soles of your feet; after saturated, trace the shape of a square to further amplify the energy signature. Take a moment to absorb the sensation of solidity and strength, then meditate on the following:

This oil supports endurance and perseverance, helping you stay focused and committed to completing tasks. It provides steady, sustained energy, enabling you to "put your shoulder to the wheel," empowering you to manifest your full potential while navigating obstacles with strength and determination.

Coconut oil is a triglyceride composed of glycerol and medium-chain fatty acids (MCFAs), with approximately 90 percent of its fatty acids being MCFAs. Lauric acid accounts for about 50 percent of this content, followed by other fatty acids. These constituents allow the scent of coconut oil to unfold in layers, starting with top notes of nutty and sweet, followed by the fresh coconut fragrance in the middle. The bottom notes are creamy milk, creating a rich, comforting aroma that is both grounding and soothing for the body and senses.

Water: The Soul Medium

The element of water is the other part of the food body, or Annamaya kosha. Nature loves the principle of cohesion, and very rarely do the elements act alone, as most often they work in combination. In this case a good example is the interplay between water and earth. This combination is the basic energy that sustains everything; it is the building blocks of existence. This combination is sensual and procreative. The energy of the water element corresponds to the pelvic bowl, which cradles our creative energy and holds the body's wisdom.

Water is responsible for giving food its flavor; it holds the energies of attraction and fascination; it is feminine and lunar in nature; it is procreative and teaches the universal cycles of life. The water element imparts grace, calm, and sensuality.

Physical Gate: Taste

The element of water rules the sense of taste. We lavish our tongues and taste buds with flavors and sensations that not only feed our body, but also our mind, heart, and soul with taste. A favorite example of mine is one of the earliest recorded recipes for ice cream, *Neige de fleurs d'orange*, "Snow of Orange Flowers," a recipe taken from an antique 1682 book titled *Nouveau confiturier* that I found in my grandmother's collection of cookbooks:

> You must take sweet cream, and put thereto two handfuls of powdered sugar, and take petals of orange flowers and mince them small, and put them in your cream . . . and put all into a pot, and put your pot in

a wine cooler; and you must take ice, crush it well and put a bed of it with a handful of salt at the bottom of the cooler before putting in the pot. . . . And you must continue putting a layer of ice and a handful of salt until the cooler is full and the pot covered, and you must put it in the coolest place you can find, and you must shake it from time to time for fear it will freeze into a solid lump of ice. It will take about two hours.

This is not just a recipe—it's a love letter to nature, an invitation to awaken your gentle nature. Orange flowers, known as *neroli* (see the entry in chapter 2), bring the energy of refinement, beauty, and light. This delectable dessert is a frozen cloud on your tongue that spreads joy throughout your body and soul.

Sacred Shape: Crescent Moon

The word *crescent* is from the Latin word *crescere*, "to increase." The Sanskrit word for water, *apas*, which, interestingly, also translates as "sacred act," is derived from the root *aap*, which means to "to pervade." The moon and water are mirror energies of each other. One energy hangs in the sky in eternal motion, starting with a crescent shape that waxes and then eventually wanes back into a crescent shape. The other is the pregnant, watery womb of the oceans here on Earth, which rise and recede with a gentle push from her celestial sister. Both deeply influence humankind's rhythms, thoughts, and behaviors, as noted by Rumi:

> *A new moon teaches gradualness*
> *and deliberation and how one gives birth*
> *to oneself slowly. Patience with small details*
> *makes perfect a large work, like the universe.*
>
> FROM "NEW MOON, HILAL,"
> TRANSLATED BY COLEMAN BARKS

The Vedas say that water is the most creative element, as it is vital for birthing new environments. As well, we humans gestate in water. It is said that the physical universe arranged itself in the water element before its emergence, thus the term *pregnant waters*, alluding to the idea of the universe contained within the great womb that is *apas*, water.

"Apas" or water is derived from the root "aap," which means "to pervade." Apas tattwa can be described as a vast quantity of intensely active matter which has begun to emerge out of agni tattwa. It is matter that has not yet been broken up into cohesive and separate bodies, because the atoms and molecules reverberating within this tattwa are still in a state of chaos. It is said that the physical universe is arranging itself in apas tattwa before its emergence. Hence the term "pregnant waters," alluding to the idea of the universe contained within the womb of apas.[3]

Water and her governing body, the moon, open a portal to the soul, the divine feminine, and the collective unconscious. Dreams are the primary way this element communicates to humankind. To invoke the energy of water and the sacral chakra with the oil(s) of your choice, apply in the shape of a recumbent crescent moon on your pelvic bowl area—the lower stomach and sacrum.

Plant Pairings: Using Taste and Sacred Shape to Invoke Water Energy

The line, "Restaurants are to people in the '80s what theaters were to people in the '60s," from the 1989 romantic comedy *When Harry Met Sally*, highlights the fun, fascination, and drama that can occur in the mouth! The sentiment "eat to live, not live to eat" is often interpreted as meaning that food should be consumed primarily as a necessity to sustain life, not as the primary focus or pleasure in one's life. By no means am I suggesting gluttony, but I would like to recast the idea of food as only fuel to be rigidly counted out in calories and nutritional data. Treat the act of tasting as the miraculous, informative gift it is, and be blessed.

In ayurveda, the subtle elements that are the objects of the five senses are known as the *tanmatras*, from the root words, tan, meaning "subtle," and matra, meaning "element." The water element in ayurveda originates from the tanmatra of taste, known as *rasa*; this is the primordial energy that enables the experience of taste. While rasa itself is not taste, it is the subtle energetic quality that provides the potential for it to manifest, and the tongue is the sense organ through which the rasa tanmatra manifests. Since taste relies on the water element, any imbalance in water can disrupt the ability to taste. Taste buds only function when water or saliva is present—without water, there is no taste. This underscores the essential role of the water element in our sensory experience.

In many ways, taste is a living representation of experience: the substances we take in and our body's response to them. Ayurveda teaches us to fully appreciate and savor the variety of flavors we encounter each day. By doing so, we can harness taste's power to create specific states of being. As taste has a special affinity for the water element—when you taste the following recipes, feel into that unique connection and allow flavor to connect you with the water element.

A beautiful and very simple way to take in the energy of water is to anoint yourself with fixed peach oil. A ripe peach, glowing in the vibrant hues of the second chakra and the water element, offers feminine gifts both sensual and life-giving. Peach oil resonates with the energy of the muses, inspiring creativity and artistic expression. The peach's gift is to awaken the muse within your pelvic region, unlocking a flow of joyous, creative energy. To amplify this, apply the oil in a recumbent crescent moon shape on your lower stomach and across your sacrum, enhancing this creative flow.

🌿 Moon in My Mouth Pulling Blend

½ cup coconut oil
6 drops magnolia absolute

Mix the coconut oil, which is antimicrobial, with magnolia absolute in a dark bottle or mason jar. Give the jar a good shake. Place a tablespoon of the formula in your mouth and swish for fifteen to twenty minutes, breathing through your nose. If that's difficult, start with five to ten minutes and gradually increase the time. Once done, spit the oil out, do not swallow it. Most experts recommend brushing your teeth immediately afterward.

The milky blooms of magnolia offers the energy of the full moon, suggesting the White Queen from *Alice in Wonderland*, offering a perspective on creativity and time out of time, all the while guiding you toward soulful fulfillment. One way to incorporate this energy is through your sense of taste. Magnolia flowers have a sweet flavor with hints of spice reminiscent of ginger, jasmine, and vanilla. This flower can also support oral health, helping with mild forms of gum disease like gingivitis by reducing swelling and bleeding of the gums.

🌿 Sweet Dreams are Made of This Salad Dressing

1 small shallot, minced (about 2 tablespoons)
1 small clove garlic, minced (about 1/2 teaspoon)
2 teaspoons Dijon mustard
3 tablespoons white wine vinegar
1 tablespoon water
6 tablespoons grapeseed fixed oil (*vibrates to the soul*)
6 tablespoons black currant seed fixed oil (*opens a doorway to the collective unconscious and your dream state*)
Sel gris salt to taste (*connecting with the in-between places*)
Black pepper to taste
Drizzle of honey (*the sweetness in life*)

Combine the shallot, garlic, mustard, vinegar, honey, and water in a large bowl and whisk to combine. Slowly drizzle in the combined oils while whisking constantly until emulsified. Alternatively, place all ingredients in a tightly sealed jar and shake vigorously until emulsified. Season to taste with salt and freshly ground black pepper. This vinaigrette will keep in the refrigerator for up to two weeks.

Try adding this dressing to a salad of rocket, goat cheese, and apple. Any apple is delightful, but pink lady is my favorite. Apple's gifts unlock the secrets of the realm of water, connecting you to the divine feminine and the collective unconscious. This dressing will help you understand water and its mirror, the moon, as living energies within your body; you create portals to your soul with each bite. Through this, dreams become the primary messenger of this element's wisdom, amplifying your ability to have and work with numinous dreams.

Black currants have a rich, complex flavor, blending tartness, sweetness, earthiness, and a subtle astringency. This unique combination makes them both refreshing and deep, with a bold, vibrant taste.

Fire: Awakening

The burning flame within provides the energy to *make conscious*. Said another way, this element is the energy of awakening, in which all the rich, fertile information within is mined and brought to the surface for the intellect to use. The element of fire corresponds to the solar plexus, the body's own "sun center," which rules the fire of digestion and the ability to act in the world. People with strong fire energy are usually farsighted and have no trouble with night vision. If this sense is developed, one can have etheric or even astral vision, a paranormal attribute.

An easy way to take this out of the abstract is to show with an example. The following is a dream that was a precursor to this book. I always had the information within me to write this book; the complexity lay in bringing this information to the mental level to be expressed in words. Fire rules comprehension.

I dreamed I was in a classroom with a small group of people, and the Human Design* analyst Cathy Kinnaird was instructing. A younger woman with long, curly hair started out by addressing the group with announcements, one being that the group dance following class had been canceled because someone had stolen the golden sun from the last dance, and until it was returned there could not be another dance. She started handing out bound booklets with plant profiles done in a very unique way.

Cathy came to the back row where I was sitting and told me she knew it had been hard for me to get there but she was happy I had come. She then flipped open my book and asked me if I had seen anything like the information in it. The plant signatures had all the information you would expect. Two notable exceptions that I can remember upon awakening are: First, if one is using a specific plant, it lists words you should not say, as these words lessened the power of the plant. Second, it had shapes that represented the plant with its corresponding color. She asked me if I had ever seen anything like this before. I answered, "I would call these yantras." She said, "Not exactly," then asked me to look closer, and it was a Fibonacci sequence. As this pattern spiraled on the page, it diagramed what colors and shapes correspond to what plants. She asked me to stare at the images, and I knew that would help me on a personal level with my well-being, and so I did. She then disappeared, and her curly-haired assistant came and took the book from me and said that was enough.

I cannot completely remember what was on the page, but I was allowed to bring with me dark blue squares with smaller squares taken out, laid out on a page showing me a progression in sequence. The other diagram she had me study was in black ink and parchment, a very detailed spiral going in, and in, and in, with small illuminations at specific places with other images I needed to see.

---

*Human Design is a "revealed" (in 1987) esoteric system that synthesizes the ancient systems of astrology, the I Ching, the chakra system, and the Kabbalistic Tree of Life tradition with the contemporary disciplines of quantum physics, astronomy, genetics, and biochemistry.

This was nature speaking to me; the act of making conscious information and using images that stimulated sight, in part, to do so—to help me remember, awakening in me first so that it could ultimately awaken in others something that has been deep in the recesses of our collective consciousness. It's time for this knowledge to come forward. This is how awakening works over time as we each remember and share. At this point I have already harvested a teaspoon of information, and as time goes by I eagerly await the action of fire to help me refine and further understand, to the point when I can distill and share yet another layer of information. As new information emerges from an unconscious level to a conscious level, the act of writing helps me further understand what is being communicated to me. Even then it is just a glimpse; in a year or two when I reread this book it will be striking to discover how much I still did not understand.

I cannot say this enough: this type of learning is slow and infuses all of the self, so be patient and stay in the conversation. Find your personal way of refining information in the fire of the mind.

Physical Gate: Sight

The element of fire depends on light; it is behind the creation of great works of art that are cherished by others, which feed the sense of sight. We build architectural wonders filled with light and create sublime shapes by which to worship and feel closer to God. We learn about ourselves, others, and the world through works of art. René Magritte, in his famous self-portrait *The Son of Man* (1946), paints his question concerning form and reality. As quoted in the introduction, about this painting he said, "Everything we see hides another thing, we always want to see what is hidden by what we see. There is an interest in that which is hidden and which the visible does not show us."[4] Is this not in part what we are seeking to understand in this book?

Sacred Shape: Triangle

At its base, each angle of a triangle represents a part of who we are. The mind, the physical body, and the subtle body as represented by the triangle is a reminder that all beings need to be cared for and are equally important in our lives. The triangle encourages us to cultivate harmony, wisdom, and understanding. To invoke and amplify the energy of fire and the third chakra in your life, anoint your solar plexus with the oil(s) of your choice in the shape of a triangle.

Plant Pairings: Using Sight and Sacred Shape to Invoke Fire Energy

Trataka, yogic visual concentration, involves focusing intensely on a candle flame without blinking, holding your gaze until tears are produced. This practice is believed to improve eye health and helps combat mental sluggishness. Scientific studies have explored its impact on cognition and vision, revealing that trataka can enhance cognitive performance, improve attention, and promote autonomic relaxation. The practice brings mental clarity and offers a calming effect, making it a valuable tool for balancing both cognitive and emotional states, especially in times of heightened, hot emotions.

Apply sunflower seed oil to your solar plexus in the shape of a triangle to balance your internal fire energy. Sit comfortably in a quiet space with a candle about three feet in front of you. Focus on the flame without blinking, keeping your gaze steady. When your eyes start to water or feel tired, close them and focus on the afterimage of the flame. Continue for five to ten minutes, then sit quietly for a moment, breathing deeply and allowing the sensation of a balanced fire element to wash over you.

From the Ashes Oil Blend

½ cup chia seed oil
7 drops myrrh absolute
1 drop cinnamon leaf essential oil

One of fire's main gifts is its ability to consume in order to renew. Apply this oil blend to your solar plexus in the shape of a triangle to release what no longer serves you. Allow fire's energy to burn away the old, uncovering hidden treasures within the ashes. Through this process you are reborn with new knowledge and fresh eyes to see the world anew.

Chia means "strength" in the Mayan language, and this plant truly embodies its name, resonating with the element of fire. This resilient desert plant is drought-tolerant and is a "fire-following" plant, one of the first to emerge after a wildfire. Consider the phrase "fire-following" through mythic eyes. What life circumstances call for something to rise from the ashes, scorched, yet destined to grow again? Chia is the energy of rebirth and resilience, reminding us that even after destruction, new life can emerge, stronger and more determined.

Myrrh absolute holds the energy of the fabled phoenix, mirroring the mythical bird's cycle. The phoenix, said to live for five hundred years, flies to the City of the Sun when its time has come. There it builds a nest of myrrh, cinnamon twigs, and spices. Ignited by the sun, the phoenix dies in flames, only to rise again, reborn. Myrrh invites transformation, encouraging you to embrace the sacred process of death and rebirth.

Cinnamon essential oil pulls you out of the depths of defeat and self-pity. It shifts the energy of negative self-fulfilling prophecies to empower you to overcome self-destructive patterns. Cinnamon promotes warmth, strength, and the courage to care for yourself.

৩ Caught in a Maze of Confusion Blend

When clarity feels just out of reach, connect with the element of fire. This fire blend ignites inspired action, filling body, mind, and spirit with enthusiasm, bliss, and the joy of waking experiences.

12 drops labdanum absolute
5 drops petitgrain essential oil
½ cup safflower fixed oil

Apply to your solar plexus in a triangle in a clockwise motion. Labdanum absolute helps organize your thoughts, while petitgrain essential oil cultivates discernment. Blended in safflower fixed oil, this combination supports the development of knowledge, consciousness, and willpower. It warms the mind, helping you tap into your inner resources to bring information from your water element and the collective unconscious to the surface. This blend helps you recognize your strengths, using them as stepping stones for growth, allowing you to build trust in your own path.

Next, sit or lie in the sunlight, either outdoors or through a window, and let its warmth ripen your thoughts. As they incubate, allow them to become clearer and clearer. Soften your gaze, focusing on the diffused light on the horizon. Feel the combined energy of fire from the oils, the sun's heat, and the nourishing light feeding your vision. Allow this radiant energy to stoke your inner fire, clearing your mind and bringing clarity to your thoughts.

If doing this practice outdoors, make sure stomach is covered.

Air: Dream Container of the Self

The element of air is gaseous in form and has the nature of wind. Air represents kinetic energy in all its forms—electric, chemical, vital, and so on. Air is the breath of life. It is the prana that allows us to be animated and vital. It expresses movement through contraction and expansion. It also creates instability and restlessness, so it is not helpful for material gain. The air element is responsible for unanticipated insights, making it an auspicious element to invoke when creating original work. Air's corresponding location in the body is the center of the sternum, a crucial point in the body that according to Taoist teachings can accumulate negative energy such as when people shout at us or when people are angry at us. The remedy is to invoke balanced air, and this can be supported by the use of plants that correspond to this element.

Invoking air facilitates positive change and stimulates the intuition. Air promotes curiosity, learning, and flexibility on all levels, allowing the mind to receive new insights and fresh perspectives. This element stimulates abstract understanding and daydreaming, as air is the element of active dreamers and supports visualizing what could be. Air promotes freedom from attachments and supports shifting consciousness and swiftness in all its forms. It bridges the mundane and the Divine to foster love, forgiveness, and compassion.

There are silences and there are silences. In the context of air it is not the lack of something being expressed, but rather the deep silence in which the Divine can be heard. All sacred traditions understand that this kind of inner spaciousness—the quality of airiness—is required for profound mysteries to reveal themselves to us. It is here that strength and inspiration are found. It is not a negative to seek self-empowerment in silence and inactivity, because it is from here you can be filled with dreams and inspirations without the intrusion of the mundane, which can dull the mind and tax the spirit. If you allow yourself to be replenished from this place of quietude, profound knowledge can emerge.

A teaching dream once spoke to me of this. Silence is sometimes hard for me, as I like sensations and often do not even realize that I'm not listening:

> *I dreamed I was speaking to a Jungian analyst over the phone, and I was telling her about my air dream, and there was a hollow sensation at the end of the phone, like space without form. It was a feeling beyond words, but I felt it in my being. So I told her, "I do not find this satisfying," and she hung up on me. The sensation of nothingness then intensified. When my mind reengaged, I tried to decide if I should call her back, as I still had questions about my dream while still in my dream, but it did not feel like a dynamic exchange. Air showed me how she felt, as opposed to words and language, which are more of the mind.*

The aspect of my dream that I was trying to understand involves my mind. I have never actually noticed what space without form feels like. Even though I am surrounded by air at all times, within space my senses are always filled with sights, sounds, and scents. In this dream the Divine was kind enough to show me how air presents itself. My gut reaction was to want more: more sensation, more understanding, more information. I was not quiet. I was not listening. I was not melting into the teaching silence. I'm sure if I had rung air back in my dream she would not have answered, as having a conversation was not my lesson—silence was. People often ask what is the difference between meditation and prayer? I would say one aspect of meditation is that you are not asking for anything; you are listening with your whole being to discover if the Divine has anything to say to you. Try sitting in quiet curiosity, without an agenda.

Physical Gate: Touch

We feel movement and have sensations when there is movement. This sense can be developed so that psychometric skills can manifest. Some people know the entire history of an antique object by who handled the object in the past. Some people know how to read gemstones or plants simply through touch. Our sense of touch goes far beyond the simple electrical impulses triggered in the skin—it is interwoven with our emotions, memories, and sense of self and sense of others; it creates richly textured stories and lets us know if something is pleasing or not, thereby helping us form opinions.

My sisters texted me from New Orleans while at dinner as I was writing this; they wrote, "The *amuse-bouche* is worth mentioning, this bite-sized hors d'oeuvres arrived in a chicken egg." They sent a picture (very pretty), and when I asked about the taste, they replied, "It was tomato-based and served cold. We remember the texture and not the taste." For them, the big takeaway was the mouth feeling, not the flavor. Many of my food preferences are texture-based and not based only on flavor. I personally like my fruit underripe, meaning hard, and my asparagus cooked just a tick longer than most, meaning soft. This has caused many a donnybrook in my kitchen, and someone once told me that my love of firm fruit was a sign of a personality deficit, although I am sure my dinner guest's love of mushy, overripe fruit is equally as telling (wink). There is no right or wrong, only sensory preferences. It is interesting to note how opinionated people frequently are about the texture of food and the strong reactions that are produced.

Touch is why mouth sensations are important, why being enveloped in strong arms feels so comforting, why babies like to be swaddled, and why the warmth of the sun on your face warms your soul. Touch alerts us as to whether a surface is too hot or cold; it allows us to know if our pillow is comfortable and our thread count satisfying. We rely on touch to walk properly, to feel the subtleties and irregularities of the earth beneath our feet, to know where our bodies are in space and how the position of one hand relates to another while buttoning up our shirt, to know how to hold and maneuver chopsticks. Touch grants the ability to place your hand in your purse and fish out the exact item you want without looking.

Language reflects how much touch informs how we process information: it is perfectly clear what we mean when we say someone is soft-hearted, hard-headed, a pain in the neck, or their disposition is either hot, warm, or cold. Touch links us in an intimate way with the world and people around us, allowing us to experience passion, ecstasy, arousal, comfort, and discomfort. Skin can be soft as petals, lips lush as a peach, abs rock-hard, and a chin like sandpaper. The human soul breathes in contentment at the lushness of a pashmina shawl against bare shoulders, the cool brush of a silk dress in the summer, the comfort of a thick woolen sweater in the winter—all these wonders are due to touch.

Sacred Shape: Circle

I always know when I have a new and substantial understanding being served up because I will dream of a circle in a significant way. With my first book the circle showed me how to release the aggregate of holding on to deep pain and not forgiving. This led the way to authentically letting go to let love in and let understanding pervade my relationships. With my second book, the circle alerted me to the fact that I was not letting a new way of thinking in and was shutting out inspiration.

The circle is the shape of unity, integrity, the true self, fulfilment, sanctity, blessing, chance and omens, friendship and intimacy, time and eternity. The functions associated with it are protection and guarding, self-knowledge, that which is indestructible, and divine epiphany. To invoke and amplify the energy of the circle, the element of air, and the heart chakra, apply the oil(s) of your choice to your spiritual heart, midline between the nipples, both front and back.

Plant Pairings: Using Touch and Sacred Shape to Invoke Air Energy

As you apply the following blends to your body, focus on the sensations that arise from touch. Notice the satisfying "scratch" of the salt scrub and the smooth glide of the oils as they slip between your hands, then slide over your skin. Revel in the tactile experience, allowing the sensations to connect you ever deeper to the air element.

ༀ If You Cannot Behave Blend

The element of air is centered in the sternum, an area that according to Taoist teachings can accumulate negative energy, such as when others direct unkind energy toward you. To safeguard and heal this center, apply the following oils in equal proportions to your energetic heart in a counterclockwise circular motion, releasing any hurtful energy.

1 part raspberry seed oil
1 part blackberry seed oil

Raspberry seed oil offers protection for the emotions and actions of others. It creates a protective boundary around your aura, allowing you to detach from others' behaviors and engage only in the interactions you choose. Blackberry seed oil helps heal the tendency to sacrifice yourself to meet others' expectations. It provides strong support against gossip and "helpful meddling," those actions by others who claim to benefit you but actually cause harm. It shields you from these negative influences and supports self-preservation.

ༀ Entering the Silence Body Scrub

⅓ cup Kilauea onyx sea salt
12 drops white rose absolute
½ cup Epsom salts (neutral energy)
Fractionated coconut oil (enough to saturate salt)

Mix the salt, white rose absolute, and Epsom salts in a jar with a lid. Fill with fixed fractionated coconut oil until completely saturated. Cap and shake to blend. Use this as a full-body scrub to awaken the benefits of introspection, silence, and listening. In this sacred silence where the Divine speaks, profound insights emerge. This is not inactivity, but the productive, quiet space where new insights, inspiration, and freshness are found. Through air, inspirations flow, unburdened by the mundane.

Kilauea onyx sea salt invites you into the quiet of the self, a gateway to daydreaming. In this silence and introspection, you enter a sacred space where you can listen to the Divine. In this space, inspiration can emerge. White rose absolute expresses the alchemical quality of sub-rosa ("under the rose") psychic transformation that occurs in self-contained silence. This silence is necessary to enter into the matrix of the self, the "rose" where the self is quietly conceived and transformed in secret. Fixed fractionated coconut oil supplies a neutral energy.

❧ Flexibility and Movement Massage Oil Blend
20 drops cardamom essential oil
1 cup cranberry seed oil

Blend the essential oil and the cranberry seed oil. For an extra layer of sensation, pour this oil blend into a metal measuring cup and place on an electric disk coffee warmer for five minutes, warming to the perfect temperature before applying. Tap into the power of symbolic anatomy by massaging this blend into the legs, our pillars of support. The legs are the foundation of movement, grace, and power, reflecting the stages of growth and evolution. This blend supports and balances the transitions of growth, offering flexibility, strength, and stability throughout life's journey.

Cardamom essential oil dissolves patterns of rigidity, encouraging a flexible mindset and freeing you from inflexible behaviors and thoughts. It opens the mind, allowing adaptability and flow. Cranberry seed oil promotes a balanced mix of flexibility and restraint, helping you find harmony between action and stillness.

Ether: The Cosmic Egg

The universe is an interplay between two fundamental principles: nature and supreme consciousness, or Source. In the body the mythic understanding of nature resides in the earth element, while supreme consciousness lies in the element of ether. They are two sides of the same coin. Supreme consciousness is the masculine principle that pervades all things; it is the sustainer. It is the ultimate, out of which mind and matter proceed. Nature is the feminine principle that in-*forms* this information; she is responsible for procreation, for birthing earthly existence. The juxtaposition of these two elements is the basis of all creation, the power of evolution. This is also referred to as Shiva-Shakti, yab-yum, yin-yang, Father Sky–Mother Earth—in essence, male and female energy combined, giving rise to experience.

Ether corresponds to the hollow of the throat, or in the chakra system, vishuddha, which relates to communication and self-expression. When ether is balanced in the body we're able to express our truth without worrying about what others think; when it's unbalanced we tend to overtalk and we don't listen very well.

Ether is the ethereal essence pervading the cosmos, the imperceptible force that holds the universe together. It is the nonlocal holographic field of consciousness that connects the human brain with the cosmos. Here, space and time are mixed, folded into a dimension of frequencies that is an implicit hidden order within space-time. In this field of frequencies, dimensional fluctuations occur as well as more intense undulations such as the holographic patterns that build the space-time dimension. This explicit order is our manifest universe.

In the implicate order, everything is folded into everything. This is the premise of the holographic universe theory: the universe is enfolded in each discrete part, as reflected in the esoteric maxim "As above, so below"—and as expressed by elemi essential oil. Each part may unfold in different degrees and ways, revealing and giving rise to different aspects of human experience and consciousness.

Physical Gate: Sound

Sound is the sensation associated with ether. Our ears drink in sound, the natural music of nature as well as that which is created by humankind listening to an internal melody. *The Four Seasons* is a suite of four violin concertos composed by Vivaldi based on four poems he wrote, each of which he expressed in music. "Spring" is freshness and beauty and includes birdsong and a spring storm, a shepherd who sleeps with his faithful dog by his side, and a lively spring dance. "Summer" sounds like that season's intense heat as slowly the lazy heat begins to be replaced by a cool and refreshing breeze, while dramatic undertones warn us that this breeze could turn into a storm. "Autumn" is communal; it is the sound of comradery, a country dance at a harvest festival. The sound is crisp and carefree, and you can hear the gaiety, as "full of Bacchus's liquor," Vivaldi writes, "they finish their celebration with sleep." With the sound of gently arching strings, you can hear the cooler air of autumn arrive, the crackling of dried leaves beneath the hooves of the horses and the sound of barking dogs as they dash across the autumnal landscape. In "Winter" we first hear the smooth and persistent rhythms of snow falling, which cause the teeth to chatter due to the intense cold. Next we hear the sound of being contentedly safe and snug indoors next to a fire, watching snowflakes falling rhythmically against the windowpanes. Vivaldi writes, "So it is the winter, but it also has great beauties."

Plants communicate through volatile chemical signals and a network of fungi connecting their roots. They also produce sound waves at low frequencies (50–120 Hz) and emit ultrasonic vibrations (20–100 kHz) that can be detected by sensors attached to their bodies. These sounds are released from different plant organs at various growth stages and in response to different environmental factors. Using sensitive sound receivers, researchers have found that plants emit sounds from the xylem and produce faint ultrasounds when under stress. They can even "hear" a caterpillar chewing and activate defense mechanisms in response. Plants can also detect pollinators and respond within minutes by instantly sweetening their nectar.

An exciting development in plant communication is a device called PlantWave, which converts the electrical conductivity changes in plants into audio, allowing them to "sing." As plants undergo electrochemical reactions in response to their environment, these fluctuations are translated into musical patterns. Pairing plant music with plant oils allows you to delve into a deeper relationship with a plant. Once you've chosen your plants, apply your choice of oils or absolutes, diluted in fractionated coconut oil, to your entire body, focusing especially on the throat and ears. Then lie back, relax, and listen to the plant's unique melody (either listening to online recordings or using your own device), allowing yourself to connect with its energy and vibrations.

Sacred Shape: Oval, or the Cosmic Egg

The cosmic egg represents all that is possible. It is full of the promise of new life, expressing the rebirth of nature and the fruitfulness of the Earth and all of creation. In many traditions the egg is a symbol for the whole universe, the cosmic egg. The golden orb of the yolk represents the divine masculine, which is enfolded by the divine feminine, the egg white, with both in perfect balance.

Plant Pairings: Using Sound and Sacred Shape to Invoke Ether Energy

The ethereal force, present within you, mirrors the cosmic essence that connects the universe, forming a nonlocal holographic field of consciousness, linking your mind to the cosmos. In this realm, space and time merge, revealing a hidden order within the fabric of existence. Feel the energy of ether flow as this blend connects you to the vast cosmos.

The microbiome is a diverse collection of bacteria and other microorganisms that live inside the human body, playing essential roles in digestion, immunity, and overall health, even effecting the mind. Each person's microbiome is unique, and maintaining its balance is vital for one's well-being. Next time you want to nurture your microbiome, try playing music after anointing yourself with one of the following blends. While we can't directly observe how sound affects our inner world, it's a fun way to imagine how it might influence the delicate balance of your microbial community.

In a fascinating study, Swiss cheesemaker Beat Wampfler and researchers from the Bern Academy of Arts explored how music affects cheese. Nine 22-pound wheels of Emmental cheese were placed in wooden crates and exposed to a continuous twenty-four-hour loop of a single song for six months. The result? Cheese that "listened" to hip-hop developed a funky flavor, while those exposed to Led Zeppelin or Mozart had milder, subtler tastes. It seems music can influence the fermentation process due to bacteria behavior, much like it might influence the bacteria in our own microbiome.

Cosmic Egg Blend

½ cup blueberry seed oil
8 drops hyacinth absolute
2 drops juhi absolute
1 drop elemi essential oil
1 drop frankincense absolute

Blend all ingredients and apply to the hollow of your throat in the shape of an oval (the cosmic egg), and if you wish, lightly anoint your scalp in a uniform pattern. As you do, tune into the living essence within you, birthed from the ether.

The Sound of Music Blend

½ cup fractionated coconut oil
¼ cup borage oil
1 tablespoon macerated daisy oil
8 drops blue chamomile essential oil
1 drop spinach absolute

Apply this blend to your stomach and throat in an oval and ear shape, put on your favorite music, lie back, and listen. Then listen deeper. Can you feel your microbiome responding? Let the vibrations of the music and the oils guide you into a deeper connection with your body's inner rhythms and the gift of sound.

6

The Chakras

The Seven Centers of Spiritual Power

There was neither non-existence nor existence then; there was neither the realm of space nor the sky which is beyond. What stirred? Where? In whose protection? Was there water, bottomlessly deep?

RIG VEDA, 10.129

Nature is the original storyteller: crafting tales in the curve of a river, the grace of your hips, the age rings of a tree, the history held in your bones, the migration of birds, your evolution of thought. Each chakra weaves its own narrative into your flesh, a language older than words, where seasons mark chapters, cycles are characters, and landscapes are living plots. Nature tells stories of resilience in the deep roots of a desert plant; we find these stories in jojoba oil. Cyclamen absolute reflects transformation in the wings of a butterfly. And Siberian fir absolute tells the story of harmony in the interdependence of forest life. These stories are not only etched in the contours of mountains and riding the ebb and flow of tides, they are within you as well. Nature doesn't rush to conclusions; instead, she invites us to witness the unfolding, to listen and *remember our place* within her infinite plotlines. Our internal archetypes.

The chakra system can be understood as a series of energy centers, each embodying distinct states of being, much like deep pools in the body's subtle energy landscape. Through the *nadis*, or energy channels, a flow of vitality moves throughout the physical and energetic bodies, harmonizing and awakening these pools. The Sanskrit word *nadi*, meaning "stream," aptly captures this dynamic, as the nadis act as the body's sacred rivers, carrying and delivering the subtle energy currents that sustain each chakra. The nadis support the energy centers in this dance, as they purify, guide, and feed them with the energetic nutrients they need to evolve, ultimately facilitating the rise of kundalini. Just as rivers nourish the land, these channels uphold the inner terrain of consciousness, attuning it to the wisdom of both earth and sky—the ever-present flow of "as above, so below." Here, nature reflects in our very bodies, as we are in constant exchange with the world around us, and through this ancient, yogic circuitry, the life force within moves toward deeper clarity and unity.

As you move through each absolute and oil profile in this book, think of it as an invitation to uncover the story of your hidden self. With each scent, each chakra, you're piecing together layers of your journey, connecting to those parts of yourself that hold grounding, compassion, insight, or power. This journey is one of self-discovery, a gradual unveiling of who you are on a deeper level, and each individual is unique. It tells the story of you. Each oil's essence can awaken memories, stir emotions, and open pathways within you. This practice is more than sensing the fragrance of the oils—it's about connecting to their energetic imprints within yourself, reflecting back to you where you've been, where you are, and where you're headed. In honoring the subtle yet profound support these oils provide, you are also honoring your own unique story—one of growth, transformation, and ever-deepening understanding.

As you connect with each oil, ask yourself: *How does this apply to me? Where do you feel its energy calling in your own body or life?* Let these reflections reveal insights into the current state of your energy centers. In this soft, inward approach, you may uncover new layers of understanding, feeling into the support each oil can bring to your unique journey.

The chakras are often depicted as spinning wheels or lotus flowers. Each lotus has a specific number of petals, which is determined by the number and position of the nadis that maintain each chakra. The number of petals for each chakra is noted in each of the chakra descriptions, along with the chakra's location and associated element. As well, in this exploration we find that each chakra embodies an element of nature, grounding us to the world around us and aligning our inner landscape with the natural forces that shape all life. Plants that are known to vibrate to the frequency of each chakra are provided, and some of these plants vibrate to all seven chakras. Reflect on how each plant frequency supports the chakra it is paired with, sensing its qualities intuitively. For example, how does a certain oil's grounding energy align with the root chakra's stability? Or how does a heart-opening fragrance cultivate and expand the heart center?

Opening the Chakras Using Plant Allies

Certain absolutes, essential oils, and fixed oils in this book resonate with specific chakras, as indicated in each chakra description below. In addition, there are certain plant allies that resonate with all seven chakras, making them good partners to work with as you begin your exploration of the entire chakra system. These include:

- **Absolutes:** benzoin resin
- **Essential oils:** lavender, red spikenard
- **Fixed oils:** apple seed, apricot seed, buriti, cantaloupe seed, jojoba, onion, passion fruit seed

Whether you're focusing on the entire chakra system or a specific chakra, an easy way to do this is to anoint the chakra center(s) you would like to focus on with your choice of plant oils. Alternately you can mist your full body, setting the intention to work with a specific center as you visualize it. A third option is to diffuse your choice of plant aromas throughout your environment while setting your intention.

For example, as I am mostly a water incarnation—based on my dosha type and astrology as well as my strengths and water-centric inclinations—my preferred method of working with the chakras begins with the Mindfulness Bath described in the appendix. I start every day with a twenty-minute bath where I clarify my intentions, set goals, and ask for direction, using the botanicals that support what I need by matching those to the energy center or centers that I wish to work with. With the information I receive, and while still moist from the bath, I follow up with a full-body application of one of the fixed oils, often adding the absolute or essential oil (at a 2 percent dilution) that corresponds to the chakra(s) I'm focusing on.

The Root Chakra: Muladhara

I saw that the divine beauty in each heart
is the root of all time
and space.

RABIA, FROM "JEALOUS OF A POND,"
TRANSLATED BY DANIEL LADINSKY

Location: base of the spine, coccyx
Number of petals: 4
Element: earth
Plant frequencies: *absolutes*: brown boronia, lilac, spinach, sweetgrass; *essential oils*: oakmoss, pink pepper seed, vetiver; *fixed oils*: chia seed, coconut, corn, oat, red cabbage seed, wheat germ; *macerated oils*: saffron

The root chakra, muladhara, is the foundation of our connection to earth's solid ground. Like the roots of a tree, this chakra draws strength from the soil and symbolizes survival, security, and your primal connection to your ancestral roots. This center resonates to the number 4, which is about strength, stability, dependability, and practicality.

In the beginning, your beginning, the cosmic seed or essence of you germinated, sending out an exploratory root, the primary root that anchors you in this earthly realm. Your root pushed down into the soil, searching the darkness for nutrients and a foothold in viable ground. From this base root, other roots grew and spread, extending further to absorb water and dissolve minerals from the inorganic realm to feed and aerate the living stem that is your physical self.

Your root system gives you solidity and the ability to survive. It sustains your sense of self, creates and maintains community, nurtures your family unit, and feeds your understanding of your ancestral, cultural, ethnic, and geographic roots, which comprise the psychic and material matrix that produced you. Your roots allow you to thrive and generate new growth. This in turn allows you to grow a multifaceted, safe, abundant life and plant with discretion the garden of you. Once your root system has taken hold, you have a stable base for creating the internal and external life you want.

If you have found yourself in shallow, unfertile ground, experiencing a sense of ungrounded rootlessness, it's likely your root chakra is blocked. You'll feel you are drifting without a clear direction, cut off from life's ability to give succor, afraid and alone, with no sense of you who you are or your life's purpose. Relationships do not feed you, and an abundant life filled with life's pleasures seems elusive.

The Sacral Chakra: Svadhishthana

It is just
that your soul is so vast
ST. CATHERINE OF SIENA,
FROM "HIS LIPS UPON THE VEIL,"
TRANSLATED BY DANIEL LADINSKY

Location: sacrum, pelvic bowl (beneath the belly button)
Number of petals: 6
Element: water
Plant frequencies: *absolutes*: black currant, carnation, cyclamen, lilac, magnolia, myrrh, Siberian fir, Spanish broom; *essential oils*: blood orange, clary sage, jasmine, kumquat, mandarin orange, marjoram, neroli, oakmoss, patchouli, peppermint, pink pepper seed, tangerine, vanilla, white birch; *fixed oils*: date, grape, mango kernel, oat, papaya seed, peach kernel, pumpkin seed; *macerated oils*: saffron, orchid; *other*: babassu butter, all salts

Flowing and adaptive, the sacral chakra aligns with water, the source of life and creativity. It mirrors the fluidity of rivers, lakes, and oceans, embracing change, sensuality, emotional expression, and the inner child. It is your gateway to the collective unconscious. It is expressed by the number 6, the frequency of compassion and empathy.

Svadhishthana, "the dwelling place of the self," is the sacred ocean within, cradling the deep, primal layers of our human psyche. This ocean, revered as the Mother of Mothers, symbolizes the origin of life, the vast womb from which all beings emerged. Though humanity has evolved beyond these waters, an indelible part of us remains tethered to this deep wellspring, echoing an oceanic memory that mirrors the hidden depths of our minds. Here, the visible ocean and the invisible psyche unite, two manifestations of the same profound reality.

In this oceanic realm, otherworldly and concealed elements swirl together much like the impenetrable depths of the sea that teem with ancient life forms and living fossils that have existed unchanged for eons. Similarly, our psyche holds archetypal energies, archaic forces that have withstood the test of time, silently shaping our thoughts and actions. These dark, untouched depths resemble underwater ecosystems flourishing beneath the surface, influencing our lives in ways we often remain unaware of. This energy center resonates deeply with Carl Jung's concept of the collective unconscious and the shadow aspect of the individual personality that conflicts with the ego's idea of who we are, causing us to project that shadow onto other people and situations. Svadhishthana serves as a gateway to the shared potentials and archetypes that subtly guide our behaviors and decisions. Yet accessing these oceanic depths is not a matter of mere will or intellect; it requires that we gently surrender to being open, like knocking softly on this portal and waiting patiently for entry into its sacred domain.

In this realm, dreams become the primary language of communication, imparting cryptic messages that reveal the mysteries of our inner world. People with an unprocessed shadow side sometimes describe this energy as overwhelming, cold, and impersonal, a daunting landscape that holds the archetypal power of the collective unconscious. However, within the second chakra this oceanic depth embodies emotions, creativity, sensuality, the divine feminine, and the child within, serving as both a source of illumination and a realm of challenge.

Here we learn that true self-knowledge is a journey that requires humility and patience. The self reveals itself gradually, often through feelings, dreams, and symbols rather than through mental or intellectual effort. In embracing this fluid, soulful energy, we dive into the depths of our being, reconnecting with our primal essence and unlocking the treasures hidden within. As we navigate this vast inner sea, we discover the beauty of our interconnectedness, the power of our creativity, and the wisdom that flows from embracing the full spectrum of our humanity.

The Solar Plexus Chakra: Manipura

So when earth, after the flood, still muddy, took the heat, felt the warm fire of sunlight, she conceived.
          OVID, *METAMORPHOSES*, BOOK 1

Location: at the solar plexus, between the navel and the bottom of the rib cage
Number of petals: 10

Element: fire

Plant frequencies: *absolutes:* cyclamen, labdanum, narcissus, oak wood; *essential oils:* bergamot, black pepper, cardamom, cinnamon leaf, common orange, grapefruit, lemon, peppermint, white birch; *fixed oils:* almond, broccoli seed, cashew nut, cherry kernel, chia seed, coconut, Arctic cranberry seed (*Oxycoccus palustris*), cranberry seed (*Vaccinium macrocarpon*), olive, safflower, sunflower; *other:* kokum butter

The solar plexus, manipura, burns with the energy of fire, fueling our confidence, purpose, and inner power. Like the sun, with which it resonates, it radiates warmth and life, driving our personal growth, passion, and willpower. It resonates to the frequency of the number 10, which signifies cosmic harmony and luck, strength, optimism, and effortless flow.

Manipura, "the abode of glittering gems," is produced by the element of fire and embodies the vibrant qualities of solar power and the dynamic masculine principle. When we connect with this radiant center we become, adopted children of the Sun gods, embracing a noble purpose that calls us to act with integrity. In this space we are inspired to shine our inner light brightly, serving not only our immediate circle but also the bigger world around us.

This chakra embodies the sovereign aspect of the psyche that is akin to the sun, a potent, life-giving force that comforts, sustains, and reassures those in need, particularly those facing challenges beyond their control. It is the foundation of vigor and abundance, fostering a well-ordered life rooted in leadership, lofty ideals, and disciplined, consistent actions.

The energy of manipura stimulates intellectual growth, illuminating our minds with brilliance and clarity, which drives personal and societal progress. Here we cultivate a profound understanding of systems and a passion for exploring the inner workings of all things. This aspect of the psyche encompasses personal power, intellect, and an ever-deepening sense of self. It is here that ego or the sense of an "I" comes into being. Manipura sharpens our focus on the ego, consciousness, and logical thought, nurturing the will, courage, and self-worth necessary for effective leadership and purposeful action.

In essence, the solar center radiates the luminous qualities of confidence, structure, and the strength to uplift others. It illuminates our path forward, guiding us with clarity and purpose as we navigate life's challenges. As we embody the energy of manipura, we become beacons of light, inspiring those around us to embrace their own potential and step boldly into their roles as co-creators in the grand tapestry of existence. In this sacred dance of power and service, we recognize that the light we share amplifies the brilliance of the whole, igniting a collective awakening that benefits all.

The Heart Chakra: Anahata

> *Because of your love*
> *I have lost my sobriety*
> *I am intoxicated*
> *by the madness of love*
>
> RUMI, FROM "INTOXICATED BY LOVE,"
> TRANSLATED BY CHOPRA AND KIA

Location: the level of the energetic heart, the center of breast bone
Number of petals: 12
Element: air
Plant frequencies: *absolutes*: aglaia, pink damask rose, spinach, sweetgrass, violet leaf; *essential oils:* kumquat, neroli, pine, sweet basil, vanilla; *fixed oils*: avocado, guava seed, mango kernel, papaya seed, pistachio nut, tomato seed; *other*: macadamia butter

The heart chakra, anahata, the essence of air, is expansive, offering love, compassion, and interconnectedness. Just as the air moves freely and supports all life, this chakra connects us with others and brings harmony to the mind, body, and spirit. It resonates to the frequency of the number 12, which represents growth from the physical to the spiritual realm and vice versa, as well as creativity and patience.

The Sanskrit word *anahata* means "heart lotus," the perfect description of the boundless space of love and compassion that can be found within your heart center. Like a celestial sphere, anahata resembles a cosmic snow globe where the sky arches above, cradling the sun, moon, and stars while we remain firmly rooted in the earthly realm. This chakra is the final frontier before the vast expanse of outer space, where the familiar begins to dissolve into the infinite. It is here that the atmosphere nurtures life, filtering sunlight, balancing temperatures, and providing the breath that sustains us—a harmonious blend of prana, the life force that animates all living things.

In yogic philosophy, the sky embodies wonder, containing the vast potential of uncontainable air. Air flows freely, the medium that expresses the mind's swift, kinetic movement—fleeting thoughts and sensations breeze by like whispers on the wind. This essence of prana is expressed through each inhalation and exhalation, a rhythmic dance of expansion and contraction. Through pranayama, the sacred art of breath control, we forge a connection to this vital energy, harmonizing body and mind, expanding awareness, and moving toward spiritual balance.

Air, ever restless and dynamic, invites us to embrace change, welcoming flashes of insight and fostering imagination. It is an auspicious energy for those seeking a shift in consciousness or new perspectives, igniting the imagination and offering the joy of exploring what could be. Through the heart chakra, this energy supports us in transcending the limitations of the ego, nurturing the qualities of compassion, forgiveness, and love.

This is the prana of unconditional love—unifying, expansive, and divine. Anahata holds the capacity for all forms of love: from romantic devotion to sacred veneration, grace, and surrender. It is the center that transforms conflict into understanding and the mundane into the divine, filling us with a sense of boundless compassion. In this sacred space we are encouraged to soften, to open, to surrender in trust, and to let love flow freely, fostering unity within and with all beings.

As we deepen our connection to our heart center, we awaken the power of love that resides there, allowing it to radiate outward, touching every life we encounter. In this harmonious embrace of air and love we find solace, healing, and a profound sense of belonging, reminding us that we are part of a greater whole, a divine tapestry woven with threads of compassion and understanding. Here, in the heart's embrace, we celebrate the joy of connection, the beauty of vulnerability, and the limitless potential of love to transform our world.

The Throat Chakra: Vishuddha

We come spinning out of nothingness, scattering stars like dust.

RUMI

Location: base of the throat
Number of petals: 16
Element: ether
Plant frequencies: *absolute*: hyacinth; *essential oils*: blue chamomile, pomelo; *fixed oils*: blueberry seed, kiwi seed

The throat chakra, vishuddha, resonates with ether, the vast, open space that contains all sound and vibration. It invites us to communicate truthfully and express ourselves, recognizing the power of voice to bridge inner experience with the outer world. It resonates with the frequency of the number 16, a number of introspection that reflects wisdom and intuition, and also a karmic number that can bring karmic lessons, sometimes challenging ones.

Vishuddha, meaning "pure," embodies the natural law of cause and effect—a dance of interdependence woven into the fabric of existence. Within this sacred center you awaken to the power of truth and authentic expression, allowing the voice of your innermost self to flow freely into the world. This is the realm of the inner muse, where your deepest thoughts find form.

In this psychic space of communication you connect with your true essence, aligning with your core beliefs and purpose. Each word becomes a brushstroke on the canvas of your life, shaping reality through intention and sound. Ether is synonymous with the Akashic Record, a vast repository of all the wisdom of the past, present, or future. This is where your intuitive gifts bloom, guiding you on your journey.

As a beacon of truth, the fifth chakra illuminates the path of self-discovery and expression, with each utterance resonating with your higher Self and crafting the reality you are here to experience.

The Third Eye: Ajna

It's not what you look at that matters, it's what you see.
HENRY DAVID THOREAU

Location: centered between the eyebrows
Number of petals: 2
Element: all of the elements combined/light
Plant frequencies: *absolutes*: gardenia, orris root, elderflower, frankincense, magnolia; *essential oils*: citron (Buddha's hand), frankincense, jasmine, petitgrain; *fixed oils*: blueberry seed, borage, cashew nut, fig seed

The third eye chakra, ajna, connects to light. Just as light reveals hidden forms, this chakra illuminates inner wisdom and clarity, guiding us to see beyond surface perceptions. It resonates to the frequency of the number 2, representing the supreme feminine force, the power of grace, and cooperation and peace.

Ajna, meaning "to command," is the center of intuition and insight, a vast realm of consciousness beyond the physical eyes. This chakra helps to create your reality on every level, mental, emotional, psychic, and physical, allowing you to access the interconnected threads of the past, present, and future within a single, unified awareness.

In this expansive inner space you cultivate individuality and self-expression, forming meaningful connections that bring clarity and purpose to your path. The ajna chakra empowers you to explore different dimensions of yourself, gaining insights that span all times. Here, thoughts crystallize, emotions communicate profound truths, and you access the flow of cosmic wisdom.

As the third eye opens, you gain the ability to see beyond everyday perception, recognizing your oneness with the universe. Each insight becomes a guiding light on your journey of self-discovery and authentic expression, ultimately bringing you closer to the essence of your true self.

The Crown Chakra: Sahasrara

Enlightenment is the key to everything.
MARIANNE WILLIAMSON

Location: top and center of the head
Number of petals: 1,000
Element: beyond the elements
Plant frequencies: *absolutes*: frankincense, juhi, orris root, white rose; *essential oils*: cedar (Eastern white), citron/Buddha's hand, lime, sandalwood, white lotus; *fixed oils*: cloudberry seed, goji berry seed, papaya seed, poppy seed; *macerated oils*: saffron; *other*: yak's milk

Beyond the elements, the crown chakra embodies pure cosmic energy, linking us to the infinite. It is the gateway to universal consciousness, transcending individual identity and dissolving us into the boundless energy that unites all existence. It is represented by the number 1,000, as in the thousand-petaled lotus, signifying our vast, unlimited potential and connection with the Divine and the higher Self.

Sahasrara, "the dwelling place without support," resides in the sacred expanse beyond the elements and physical senses, embodying the pure void, an infinite space where the mind's activity ceases and all distinctions dissolve. Here, the illusion of an individual self melts away, revealing the essence of your true self in a profound state of enlightenment. As this energy swirls around the crown of your head, it connects to the radiant channels of light flowing gracefully through your being, grounding itself through your feet. This sacred energy bridges you with the Source, the oneness of consciousness that encompasses cosmic awareness.

In this divine space, you merge with the universe, uncovering your unique purpose in this lifetime, your divine blueprint. Sahasrara reflects the intricate patterns of every cell in your body, a testament to your interconnectedness with all that exists. As this luminous energy fills you, it invites you to remember the times when you were pure light beyond form. This energy envelops your being, reminding you of your innate connection to the universe and guiding your life toward divine perfection. In this sacred union you awaken to the truth of your existence, embracing the cosmic dance of creation. Here, you find ultimate freedom and the boundless joy of simply being, where the universe flows through you, and you become one with all that is.

7

Symbolic Anatomy

The Body as Story

The body is called the Field, because a man sows seeds of action in it, and reaps their fruits. Wise men say that the Knower of the Field is he who watches what takes place within this body.

BHADGAVAD GITA

This chapter is about looking at the ensouled body through mythic eyes so we can better explore the interconnectedness between the natural world and our authentic selves, using plants to better understand how these mythic stories apply to our spiritual journey. We'll begin at the top, with the head, all the way down to the toes.

Of course we all know what a human body is according to secular materialism: the physical structure of a person, including the bones, flesh, and organs. Psychotherapist and bestselling author Thomas Moore believes that we are much more than our physical selves, however, which is the subject of his book *Care of the Soul*:

The human body in fifteenth-century Florence was an entirely different body from the one you see in the New York of, say, the 1990's.

The modern body is an efficient machine that needs to be kept in shape so that its organs will function smoothly and for as long as possible. If something goes wrong with any part, it can be replaced with a mechanical substitute, because that is the way we picture the body—as a machine.

In the Florentine view, the human body was a manifestation of the soul. It was possible to entertain a soulless notion of the body, but that was considered an aberration. Such a body was unnaturally split off from soul. We might call it schizoid—lifeless, meaningless and without poetics. But an ensouled body takes its life from the world's body, as [fifteenth-century Italian humanist philosopher Marsilio] Ficino said, "The world lives and breathes, and we can draw its spirit into us." What we do to the world's body, we do to our own. We are not masters of this world, we participate in its life.[1]

The doctrine of signatures appears in many wisdom traditions. As mentioned earlier, it is the belief that the physical traits of a plant, such as its shape, color, or texture, reveal its potential behavior. In effect, nature "signs" plants to show how they can aid in our healing, an idea rooted in the belief that God or Universal Intelligence designed nature with these clues. For example, the color of a plant can be linked to the chakra it vibrates to, giving insight into its properties. Language often describes behaviors through body parts, reflecting a visceral understanding of the stories within us. This chapter aims to encourage you to listen to those stories and explore how specific oils, when applied to specific body areas, can amplify and highlight certain traits in your personality and life.

Hair

The slender filaments that crown our head hold our stories: hair follicles contain nucleic acid DNA, and the hair shaft contains mitochondrial DNA, both of which reveal our ancestral inheritance and individuality.

Assessing hair structure from the cells at the roots of the hair can be a way of finding out if people are related or to discover other aspects of a person's reality. For example, forensic hair analysis can help identify whether a person has been present at a crime scene. Hair analysis can also reveal drug use habits, genetic diseases, heavy-metal poisoning, and overall nutritional health.

How a person wears their hair speaks volumes to those around us and about society in general. Voluminous long hair signals extraordinary potency: in men, a warrior who is brave, virile, and strong, and in women, fertility, sexuality, and beauty. In times past, because the angels were said to be attracted to the gorgeous hair of human women, it was required that they cover their heads: "For if a wife will not cover her head, then she should cut her hair short. But since it is disgraceful for a wife to cut off her hair or shave her head, let her cover her head. For a man ought not to cover his head, since he is the image and glory of God, but woman is the glory of man" (1 Corinthians 11:2–16). Most traditional Catholics still believe the head covering of a nun is an act of modesty and a visual reminder that she belongs to God and is not for herself alone.

The same voices that instructed Joan of Arc to put on men's clothing and eject the English from France also told her to crop her long hair to disguise her feminine beauty. Most accounts say that she wore her hair in the pageboy style common among knights of her era until soldiers shaved her head shortly before her execution.

The German fairy tale heroine Rapunzel, who was locked away in a tower by a sorceress, was famous for her long golden braid. The tower had no steps or doors, so she could not leave, and so when the sorceress wanted to get to her she had to call out: "Rapunzel, Rapunzel, let down your hair that I may climb your golden stair." Rapunzel would then let down her hair. When a handsome prince who'd fallen in love with Rapunzel learned the secret of how to reach her, he climbed the "golden stair," and the love story ensues. In this classic fairy tale, which is a form of myth, hair symbolizes desire. Rapunzel's birth mother desired a leafy green vegetable known as *rapunzel* (*Campanula rapunculus*), also known as rampion bellflower, after which she named her daughter.* The sorceress desired Rapunzel, so later in life she locked her away in a tower. And the handsome prince also desired Rapunzel, so he found a way to get to her and make her his wife.

One can identify the male members of the U.S. armed forces by their short, militaristic hairstyle, characterized by the back and sides of the head being shaved almost to the skin and the option for the top to be blended or faded into slightly longer hair.

A popular fictional image shows a librarian shaking loose her bun, held in place with a pencil, to show the transition from being very proper to being a lioness.

Historically, the bob hairstyle for women, which came in with the suffragette movement of the early twentieth century, represented independence and breaking out of society's norms.

In the fantasy novel series *A Song of Ice and Fire* (which was turned into the television series *Game of Thrones*), the character Cersei Lannister, who was of noble birth, had her head shorn as punishment and to shame her publicly as a symbol of her fall from grace. After she regains her royal status, she keeps her hair short, a gesture that shows her defiance and increasingly aggressive and warlike behavior.

It's instinctive to cut your hair while grieving the death of an immediate family member or to signify a traumatic event or a major life change. Cutting one's hair at these key times represents the end of something, just as it can represent a new beginning. I cut my waist-length hair in seventh grade when my first major love broke up with me, without my understanding the grief behind this gesture at the time.

---

*This plant is not commonly grown in the United States. If you cannot find it at your local nursery, you can order seeds from StrictlyMedicinalSeeds.com and follow the instructions on page 150 for making your own macerated oil blend, using the whole flowers and fractionated coconut oil.

Plant Resonances

To perform a pre-shampoo oil treatment, start with dry hair and section it for even oil distribution. Choose an oil (or oils) that suits your desire or hair type—see list below—and apply it from the roots to the ends. Gently massage the oil in, focusing on the scalp and the ends, which tend to be drier. For deeper penetration, wrap your hair in a warm towel or use a heat cap. Leave the oil on for thirty minutes to overnight, depending on your preference, then shampoo and condition as usual. You can also add a few drops of any essential oil or absolute to your brush before styling your hair to infuse it with fragrance and invoke the matching energic gift. You are not limited to the following list; you can use any fixed oil for a pre-shampoo treatment to cultivate specific states of being.

- **Curly, dry, or frizzy hair:** Daikon radish oil provides smoothness and hydration without artificial silicones. Macerated banana oil hydrates and strengthens curls without adding weight.
- **Dandruff:** Use macerated banana oil or a blend of lavender and bergamot essential oils in fractionated coconut oil to soothe and hydrate the scalp and keep an overgrowth of a yeastlike fungus called *Malassezia globosa*, the source of dandruff, at bay.
- **Hair growth/hair loss:** Stimulate circulation and encourage regrowth with macerated banana oil, pine essential oil, or rosemary essential oil in fractionated coconut oil or onion fixed oil.
- **Damaged hair:** Strengthen and restore hair structure with cucumber seed oil, rich in silica.
- **Fine hair:** Watermelon seed oil nourishes thin, fine hair, adding volume without weight.
- **Oily hair:** Balance oil production with clary sage and petitgrain essential oils in fixed borage oil. Borage oil's astringent properties clarify the scalp with a dry finish.

❦ I Grieve Blend

> 6 drops narcissus absolute
> 13 drops myrrh absolute
> 22 drops lavender essential oil
> 2 teaspoons fractionated coconut oil

This blend creates a sacred space to honor loss, allowing you to feel all your feelings as you process them before moving into acceptance and healing. Narcissus absolute invites the acceptance of sorrow, of lamenting and letting your emotions flow, as expressed in the myth of Narcissus, where the nymphs mourned his passing by letting down their hair—an enduring symbol of vulnerability, surrender, and loss. Myrrh absolute resonates deeply with themes of death, mourning, and resurrection. Myrrh supports emotional healing, offering stability and clarity to navigate loss and grief so you can embrace the mourning process. Lavender essential oil soothes a broken heart and agitated mind. Mix with fractionated coconut oil, a neutral oil, massage into moist hair and scalp, and focus your intention before shampooing out.

❦ Personal Magnetism Blend

> ¼ cup macerated orchid oil
> 2 drops jasmine essential oil
> 3 drops vanilla essential oil
> 6 drops pink pepper seed essential oil

Macerated orchid oil embodies the energy of sexual magnetism—cultivating a natural allure born of confidence, authenticity, and a deep connection to one's unique beauty, radiating an irresistible energy that effortlessly draws others in. Mix with jasmine, vanilla, and/or pink pepper seed essential oil to amplify the above energy signature. Massage into moist hair and scalp and focus your intention before shampooing out.

❦ I'm Gonna Wash That Man Right Outta My Hair

> 6 drops white birch essential oil
> 1 tablespoon fractionated coconut oil

Blend the essential oil with the coconut oil. Wet your hair completely and massage this "break-up" blend into your scalp, visualizing all the things you want to leave behind. Wash and condition your hair as usual and immediately get out of the water. As the remnants of the blend wash down the drain, so does the energy and situations you want to leave behind.

Skin

Skin tells the story of our lives. Dewy-fresh and without blemish at birth, it is a blank page on which we write the story of our life. The skin holds the scars of childhood—falling from a tree, scraped knees on sidewalks, operations, and sometimes abuse. For some it reveals the stretch marks of motherhood as a belly swells with growing life. As we go through life, the skin is carved with lines that have recorded all of our smiles, frowns, and worries. Eventually it sags with age as gravity takes hold and grows thin and delicate as paper.

Your skin is your outer armor against the world. We say, "Don't let him get under your skin," and "You need to develop a thick skin if you are going to make it in this world." Skin is the physical barrier that serves as one of the body's first lines of defense against harmful microbes, with dedicated immune cells in the skin tissue that fight against harmful invasive organisms and keep you safe.

An average adult has approximately 21 square feet of skin, 300 million skin cells, and about 11 miles of blood vessels, which account for 15 percent of a person's body weight. Three layers of tissue make up the skin: the epidermis, the top layer; the dermis, the middle layer; and the hypodermis, the bottom fatty layer.

Writing on skin with permeant ink is common in most cultures, with different degrees of thoughtfulness. Māori tattoos are not merely decoration, but a carefully constructed language. In the United States, tattoos can range from a cartoon character, the name of someone you love, to something to regret, to an affiliation with a specific group. Some religious groups take issue with tattooing based on Leviticus 19:28: "Ye shall not make any cuttings in your flesh for the dead, nor print any marks upon you."

To "have skin in the game" is to have a personal investment in an organization or undertaking, and therefore a vested interest in its success. "Beauty is only skin-deep" means that while someone may appear beautiful, their character, their inner self, may not be.

Self-help author Louise Hay says skin problems stem from anxiety and fear and old, buried emotions.

Plant Resonances

Percutaneous (from the Latin *per*, meaning "through," and *cutis*, meaning "skin") is the medical term to refer to something that penetrates the skin. *Percutaneous absorption* is just a fancy way of saying your body rapidly metabolizes absolutes and essential oils and their components, transporting phytochemicals from the outer surface of the skin into the skin and from there into the blood. Essential oil molecules are so tiny that when they are applied to the skin they pass right through the stratum corneum, the outer layer of the epidermis. From there the oil molecules pass through the dermis, into the capillaries and into the bloodstream, entering the general circulation. The oils featured in this book have the ability to affect change on multiple levels—physical, emotional, mental, soul, and spirit.

The skin absorbs the benefits of each aspect of nature featured in this book, supporting a variety of needs—from soothing shingles with fixed onion oil, to calming acne with fixed tomato seed oil, to promoting collagen growth with fixed quinoa oil. White birch essential oil acts as a counterirritant, creating temporary hot and cold sensations that interrupt pain signals, offering relief. Petitgrain essential oil helps balance excessive perspiration, while neroli essential oil supports the reduction of stretch marks.

You can also match the energetic qualities of any of the plant oils featured in this book to corresponding body parts. When working with the air element or the heart chakra, apply spinach absolute or lime essential oil with fixed guava oil to the tender tissue of the breastbone. To ground and feel strong, apply oak wood absolute, vetiver, or patchouli essential oil to the feet and legs. To invoke the energy of ether or the throat chakra, apply fixed blueberry oil, lavender essential oil, or hyacinth absolute to your décolletage, derived from the French verb meaning "to expose the neck," referring to the delicate tissue from the neck to the top of the breasts. Every inch of your skin holds your personal stories written within. Brown boronia absolute allows you to access these memories, helping you remember what resides deep within.

Your skin will also benefit from the collective wisdom shared in each unique plant profile offered in chapters 1 through 4. For example, if you want to work with the Hera archetype, use white lily absolute; to invoke the goddess Athena, use olive oil; to ask for Venus's blessing, turn to pink damask rose absolute. Experiencing all-consuming sorrow? Go to myrrh essential oil. To foster contentment in the present moment, try fixed cherry oil. To contemplate the navel of creation, turn to juhi absolute. When time is not on your side, find relief in fixed wheat germ oil. As you apply and connect with each oil, you awaken the narratives held in each layer of your being.

❧ Not Under My Skin Blend
1 part raspberry seed oil
1 part cucumber seed oil

Fixed raspberry seed oil provides a nurturing shield, offering protection from absorbing the intense emotions and energetic states of others. It creates strong energetic boundaries, allowing you to engage only in the exchanges you choose, fostering a sense of being safe and comforted. Blend in equal proportions with fixed cucumber seed oil, a combination that offers broad-spectrum relief for challenging emotional states. Cucumber seed oil acts as a form of the Bach Flower Remedy known as Rescue Remedy, renewing and refreshing the whole self, particularly during times of exhaustion, illness, or emotional shock that can often render one especially vulnerable. This blend deeply supports the revitalization of your life force and inner vitality, helping you reengage fully in life.

🌿 More than Skin-Deep Blend
1 tablespoon sweet almond oil
1 tablespoon papaya seed oil
6 drops narcissus absolute

Sweet almond oil supports the release of fears surrounding aging, transforming the passage of time into a sacred journey beyond the physical body. It invites a deeper connection with the complex beauty of the self, including personality and the expression of talents and good works, reminding us that true beauty lies not on the surface, but is shown in a life well-lived. Narcissus absolute supports the journey of releasing attachment to the outer material world, guiding one away from deriving self-esteem and identity solely from one's physical looks. Papaya seed oil spiritualizes and refines sexual energy, transforming this raw vitality into a sophisticated inner radiance that uplifts and shines from the inside out, reflected in your poise and how you conduct yourself.

This blend promotes releasing fears of aging, guiding you to a deeper connection with the sacred journey of time beyond the physical. It helps you release attachments to an external self-image, allowing you to nurture a self-esteem rooted in inner beauty. It transforms the desire to be "frozen in time" in a youthful expression of beauty to stepping into a new expression that allows you to age with grace.

Brain and Head

The Brain is wider than the Sky—
For—put them side by side—
The one the other will contain
With ease—and You—beside

The Brain is deeper than the sea—
For—hold them—Blue to Blue—
The one the other will absorb—
As Sponges—Buckets—do

> *The Brain is just the weight of God—*
> *For—heft them—Pound for Pound—*
> *And they will differ—if they do—*
> *As Syllable from Sound—*
>
> EMILY DICKINSON

The brain is a soft, jellylike mass of billions of cells and their connections, weighing about two and a quarter pounds. As a generator of electrochemical energy it regulates conscious and unconscious sensations, perceptions, and behavior, as well as the sympathetic and automatic activities of the internal organs. In the brain stem and limbic system we experience our commonality with our animal and human ancestors.

As the physical base of the crown chakra, the brain houses the ability to visualize the higher universal mind as an internal representation of reality. The human mind reveals collective patterns of behavior called *archetypes*, such that the laws of nature are simply archetypes of the universal mind. Reality can be independent of the human mind, but our descent into matter requires identifying the outside with the inside to create a totality in which consciousness and matter and all other things are indissoluble and whole. In short, everything interpenetrates and is interpenetrated by everything else.

When wisdom traditions say that the universe is *maya*, the illusory appearance that is the phenomenal world, many people interpret this to mean that reality exists in our minds. Quite the opposite is the case: if all reality is cerebral, then the head and body, as parts of reality, exist first in the mind. This may sound shocking at first, but it is entirely consistent with everyday experience. There is nothing to the body but our felt perception of it.

In the language of symbols, the uppermost part of our body, the head, houses the elements of awareness, inspiration, and expression. Our eyes, ears, nose, mouth, and brain allow us to take in the world around us, while sight, sound, scent, and taste are the means by which to interpret this information. We form opinions, make judgment calls, and organize our experiences into categories that form the basis of our behaviors based on our awareness of reality.

Michael Talbot, in his book *The Holographic Universe*, offers insight into what is known as nonlocal consciousness, one of the central tenets of quantum physics, which says that human consciousness is not confined to specific points in space and time. This phenomenon is commonly behind most spiritual experiences:

> Our brains mathematically construct objective reality by interpreting frequencies that are ultimately projections from another dimension, a deeper order of existence that is beyond both space and time: The brain is a hologram enfolded in a holographic universe . . . The objective world does not exist, at least not in the way we are accustomed to believing. What is "out there" is a vast ocean of waves and frequencies, and reality looks concrete to us only because our brains are able to take this holographic blur and convert it into . . . the familiar objects that make up our world.[2]

This sheds light on the idea that we ourselves are but composite vibrations existing in a primordial soup until we manifest in the flesh. The brain is the vehicle by which we explore our reality. Most wisdom traditions teach that our thought processes are not neutral, and in general humankind cannot interpret what is occurring right in front of them. Instead, our present reality is in part defined by repeating calcified energy patterns that greatly limit what our awareness can perceive and absorb. Generally speaking, we can only know that which already exists within our realm of awareness, and we must use this small opening of awareness to scan the vast ocean of accumulated knowledge and information to begin the process of becoming more aware. This can be complicated because not only do we need to learn what we know as well as what we do not know, but also what we do not know what we do not know!

Symbolically, the essential spiritual nature of a person or a deity or any other being is located in the head. Blessings are given by the laying of hands on the head; Christ is the head of the church, and his followers are the body; monsters in myth, once killed, must have their head removed to sever them from their ability to reconnect to their life force and return. In the Greek myth of Perseus and the gorgon Medusa, the potent magic of Medusa's head was passed down to Athena, whose blood gave birth to the Muses. In Tibet, rounded human skulls are used in tantric rituals as drinking vessels, as the head is considered a vessel of transformation. Athena's birth from the head of Zeus symbolizes a turn of consciousness, making chthonic mystery teachings available for common use. The head often symbolizes oracular powers that continue after death, such as the myths of Osiris and Orpheus.

Only recently has humankind started to associate the brain with consciousness. For the ancients, the abode of thought and feeling was believed to be in the heart or the liver. Nonetheless, over time the brain has become a symbol of the procreative life force, as in the Delphic philosophical maxim "Know thyself" that was inscribed on the Temple of Apollo. Our culture is peppered with positive declarations concerning the head and mind, as in William James' famous statement, "If you can change your mind, you can change your life." This reminds us that our future is created from the choices we make moment to moment.

Plant Resonances

Aromatherapy using essential oils has been scientifically linked to improvements in cognitive function for people with dementia. For systemic effects, the active components in essential oils must be absorbed through the skin, where they then enter the circulation to cross the blood-brain barrier. Increasingly, plant-based substances like essential oils are being explored as complementary therapies to address Parkinson's disease and other neurodegenerative disorders. Linalool and geraniol, prominent compounds in lavender, are among those being extensively studied for their potential benefits in addressing a variety of neurological conditions.[3]

The central nervous system, including the brain and spinal cord, faces unique challenges and so is protected by the blood-brain barrier, which prevents harmful substances from entering while allowing necessary nutrients to pass through. However, systemic chronic inflammation and oxidative stress as seen in conditions like type 2 diabetes can destabilize the blood-brain barrier, leading to cerebral inflammation and cognitive decline. This highlights the importance of anti-inflammatory interventions to restore the integrity of the brain's microvasculature.

Terpenes and terpenoids, the primary constituents in marjoram and rosemary, are small, fat-soluble molecules that can penetrate the skin and nasal mucosa. Their lipophilic nature allows them to cross the blood-brain barrier, offering potential therapeutic effects in neurodegenerative conditions.

In cases of Parkinson's disease, to reduce inflammation of the brain, use frankincense essential oil (*Boswellia carterii*). For reducing tremors, a combination of the essential oils of basil, clary sage, frankincense (*Boswellia carterii*), lavender, marjoram, and vetiver is effective. To help with stiffness and rigidity, turn once again to frankincense (*Boswellia carterii*), as well as to basil, lavender, and sandalwood essential oils.

To address Alzheimer's, try lemon and rosemary essential oils in the morning, and lavender and orange essential oils in the evening. These can be diffused or added to macerated ginkgo oil.

The deeper structures within the brain include the pituitary gland, hypothalamus, amygdala, hippocampus, and pineal gland. The pituitary gland is known as the "master gland." It regulates the function of the other glands in the body by controlling the flow of hormones from the thyroid, adrenals, ovaries, and testicles. It receives chemical signals from the hypothalamus via its stalk and blood supply. It also regulates the third eye. Oils that help regulate the various hormonal systems include clary sage essential oil, date fixed oil, frankincense essential oil, lavender essential oil, peppermint essential oil, and rose otto absolute.

The hypothalamus is located above the pituitary gland, to which it sends chemical messages to control its function. It regulates body temperature, sleep patterns, hunger, thirst, and plays a role in memory and emotions. The hypothalamus is linked to the crown chakra. It works with the pituitary gland to regulate the endocrine system, influencing biological processes and hormone communication through the nervous system. The crown chakra corresponds with the cerebral cortex, governing consciousness, perception, and thought, similar to how the pituitary gland regulates the endocrine system through hormonal control. Essential oils that work with the hypothalamus include lavender and bergamot, which are rich in linalool and linalyl acetate and are renowned for their relaxing properties that promote restful sleep. Have a low appetite? Essential oils of grapefruit, lemon, and orange are best. Struggling with anorexia? Try brown boronia absolute and patchouli essential oil.

The amygdala is a small, almond-shaped structure located under both hemispheres of the brain. Part of the limbic system, the amygdala regulates emotions, memory, and is associated with the brain's reward system. It plays a crucial role in detecting potential threats and triggering the fight-or-flight response, which aligns with the root chakra's concern for basic survival needs. Essential oils that work with the amygdala, specifically the fight-or-flight response, include lavender, lime, mandarin orange, sandalwood, and tangerine as well as aglaia absolute and white rose otto absolute.

The hippocampus is a seahorse-shaped organ located on the underside of each temporal lobe. It supports memory, learning, navigation, and the perception of space. It interacts with the cerebral cortex and may play a role in Alzheimer's disease. The hippocampus plays a key role in forming and retrieving memories, thus aligning with the third eye chakra's association with insight and deep knowledge, inner vision, and the recall of past experiences. Our brains integrate scent with information about space and time to form episodic memories, allowing us to use any oil from this book to reconnect with past moments.

The pineal gland is found deep within the brain, attached to the top of the third ventricle by a stalk. It responds to light and darkness, secreting melatonin to regulate circadian rhythms and the sleep-wake cycle. The third eye chakra, also connected to the pineal gland, represents the vision that transcends physical sight—our inner vision, intuition, and clear perception, as well as the power to manifest through visualization. Many studies have shown that inhaling lavender essential oil can significantly boost melatonin levels and promote better sleep and body-clock regulation. Fixed almond oil and macerated banana oil contain magnesium and vitamin B_{12}, which also help balance the body-clock and circadian rhythms.

Ears

The human inner ear has an intricate spiral shape often compared to the shells of mollusks, particularly the nautilus. Sound waves enter the outer ear and travel through the narrow passageway that is the ear canal, which leads to the eardrum. The eardrum vibrates from the incoming sound waves and sends these vibrations to three tiny bones in the middle ear: the malleus, the incus, and the stapes.

Vibrational fields connect everything in existence, from the infinitesimal to the infinite. Everything vibrates to divine order. Your ear is a symbolic doorway, a portal that opens to new perceptions and the whispers of life. As artist and musician Laurie Anderson says, "I've always thought that one of the most serious defects of the human body was that you couldn't close your ears. You can't point them anywhere or close them, they just sort of hang there on the sides of your head. But an acupuncturist explained to me that the pressure points in the ears are very important, because the whole body is represented right there in the ear."[4]

In folklore, the left ear is connected to your inner voice and to divine intuition; if you hear a brief, clear ringing sound, it's letting you know you're on the right track. Mine is often accompanied by a momentary flash of pure white light. Hindu cosmology tells us that the primordial vibration of the sacred syllable OM is the sound of creation before the creation of form. Through profound introspection we can tune in to this vibration, which wakes us up to eternal truths.

Being heard is powerfully important; it means you have been understood, since your voicing something does not necessarily guarantee you are heard and understood.

The painter Vincent van Gogh famously cut off his left ear. As stories take on a life of their own, the following are all versions of why he did this: He got in a nasty row with Paul Gauguin. He heard phantom wedding bells after receiving a letter notifying him that his brother Theo was getting married. He was suffering from unrequited love with his widowed cousin. He gave it to a prostitute named Rachel as a token of affection that he neatly wrapped in newspaper. He wanted to show his favor to a farmer's daughter named Gabrielle.

The famous painting by Vermeer, *Girl with a Pearl Earring*, has long captured imaginations and has been featured in poems, novellas, and film. The painting is not a portrait of a living person, but what is known as a *tronie*, a painting that is intended to show a certain facial expression, in this case an imaginary figure—a girl in exotic dress, wearing an oriental turban and sporting an improbably large pearl in her ear. Only her face, a slight portion of her neck, and her ear are visible. The rest of her, including her hair, are covered. Her tender earlobe beguilingly slips from her turban and the radiant pearl seems to be suspended against the dark background. Pearls can suggest innocence, the loss of innocence, and femininity.

There are approximately 25,000 nerve endings in the ear, considered an erogenous zone. Stimulating the vagus nerve inside the ear can make the surrounding tissue swell just like it does in the genital region, bringing intense pleasure.

Aztec tradition believed that by stretching earlobes one could hear the gods and spirits more easily. In Buddhism, large earlobes signify wisdom and compassion (the Buddha has the ability to hear the cries of the world). Maasai men and women consider long, stretched earlobes to be a symbol of wisdom.

Plant Resonances

Continue your exploration of the ear with the following blends.

ꙮ Cries of the World Blend

2 teaspoons goji berry fixed oil
6 drops spinach absolute
3 drops white rose otto absolute
2 drops patchouli essential oil

The comination of goji berry fixed oil and spinach absolute helps you connect with the wisdom of the female buddha, Green Tara, who embodies enlightened activity, wisdom, and compassion in action, precisely attuned to the needs of each moment. Listen to her guidance for what is needed to facilitate liberation from any ensnaring situation, whether for yourself or a loved one. White rose absolute brings the energy of the diamond mind, illuminating the path to compassionate action, and patchouli summons every ounce of your being for good works.

Apply this blend to your ears and intone Green Tara's mantra: *Om Tare Tuttare Ture Soha*. Or simply apply any oil that vibrates to the sixth or seventh chakra (see chapter 6) to increase your wisdom.

ꙮ Swelling with Desire Blend

1 tablespoon macerated orchid oil
1 drop cardamom essential oil
1 drop patchouli essential oil
1 drop white rose otto absolute

Massage this blend gently onto your ears with a slow, firm, rhythmic motion to amplify the sensation of pleasure in yourself or for a loved one. If you're doing this for another person, to increase the pleasure have them nestle the back of their head in your crisscrossed legs, with a pillow in the gap, like a little nest; then turn off the lights and have them close their eyes before beginning.

❧ Earache Blend

1 tablespoon olive or coconut oil
1 drop basil essential oil
2 drops lavender essential oil

Do not apply essential oils directly into the ear canal! And avoid using essential oils if you have a ruptured eardrum. Always dilute essential oils in a cooling fixed oil such as olive oil or coconut oil before using. A few drops of the diluted oil can then be applied to a cotton swab or the fingertips and gently wiped around the outside of the ear. Basil and lavender essential oils offer various therapeutic benefits: basil oil is antibacterial and antiviral, while lavender oil is soothing and helps reduce pain and inflammation.

❧ I Am Listening Blend

1 tablespoon blueberry fixed oil
1 drop blue chamomile essential oil
1 drop elemi essential oil
1 drop gardenia absolute

Mix all ingredients together with your pinky finger (ruled by Mercury, the god of communication), then apply to your ears to amplify your ability to truly hear and comprehend. This blend also makes for a thoughtful gesture before a dinner party or salon. Pass it around for your guests to explore deeper connections and sensitivity with one another.

Beard

When hair first appears on a boy's face at puberty, it signifies he is leaving childhood and beginning his journey into manhood, his hero's journey and all that entails.

The beard can represent being capable, manly, brave, exploratory, and almost superhuman. Daring men come to mind, such as Joseph Walker, who served as a guide for men who forged our history, the explorers of the American West Benjamin Bonneville and John C. Frémont. While working for Bonneville in 1833, Walker led an expedition from Wyoming to California across the Sierra Nevada that was fraught with difficulties (including having to eat their horses to survive). After emerging from the mountains they became the first white men to experience the giant sequoia trees and other wonders of the Yosemite Valley. This so impressed Walker that he had the words "Camped at Yosemite" inscribed on his tombstone.

The legendary bearded folk hero Paul Bunyan was a giant lumberjack who represented ingenuity, strength, and endurance. His exploits, as told in the tall tales of his herculean labors, were told for decades around campfires from Maine to California, providing inspiration for men working in grinding and often impossible situations as they built the backbone of what eventually became our cites.

In Egypt, the beard was considered to be a divine attribute of the gods, and even after the fashion among Egyptian men was to be clean-shaven, figures such as Osiris and other divine entities were depicted with beards the color of lapis lazuli. In keeping with this religious principle, the pharaoh would express his status as a living god by wearing a blue-colored false beard. So widespread was this type of beard in formal royal portraiture that even Queen Hatshepsut is depicted wearing a false beard.

Beards can also symbolize the darker, more disquieting side of masculinity, as depicted in numerous fictional accounts. The folktale figure Bluebeard is a good example of the shadow aspect when his murders of his many wives is revealed in a shocking manner. The god Pan is depicted with a goatish beard that can symbolize animalistic impulses and excessive, unchecked sexuality. In the Grimm Brothers' fairytale *Rumpelstiltskin*, a mysterious, gnomelike man with a white beard spins straw into gold to aid a beautiful miller's daughter, but he does so in exchange for her future firstborn child. He is neither good nor bad, but instead represents the importance of telling the truth and being accountable for your mistakes, or the price might be heavier than you are willing to pay. Captain Ahab is another fictional character who symbolizes madness, an obsessive nature that leads to ruin, and being destructive and not in right relationship with nature.

As a man ages, his beard grays, then whitens; the white-bearded man suggests wisdom, knowledge, and one in possession of magical powers, as symbolized by figures such as the wizards Merlin and Gandalf the Grey (who later became Gandalf the White). The potency of the words and logic of philosophers such as Socrates, Plato, and Aristotle as they tugged and stroked their beards while puzzling out eternal truths and morality comes to mind.

Plant Resonances

The Greek word *pogonotrophos*, "man with a beard," is a synonym for a philosopher. The word *pogonotrophy* ends with the Greek *trophe*, "nourishment," so its literal sense is "beard feeding," though it may be understood as growing a beard or cultivating one. Don't forget to feed your beard with one or more of the fixed oils found in chapter 3.

The primary difference between beard hair and head hair lies in their texture and growth patterns. Beard hair is generally coarser, thicker, and curlier due to the unique structure of facial hair follicles, which produce thicker, more curved hair shafts. In contrast, head hair tends to be finer and straighter. Beard growth is also heavily influenced by androgens like testosterone (white rose otto absolute can stimulate growth), resulting in a distinct growth pattern compared to scalp hair. Any oil in this book can be used to feed your beard, nourishing it with care and intention. However, the following formulas are designed to evoke some of the more potent archetypal themes, adding depth and symbolism to your grooming ritual.

✤ Hero's Journey Blend

13 drops oak wood absolute
6 drops narcissus absolute
6 drops sandalwood essential oil
2 teaspoons safflower oil

Oak wood absolute carries the noble energy of Zeus, king of the gods on Mt. Olympus, as well as Jason's mythical quest for the Golden Fleece, a journey to seek spiritual wisdom that begins with masculine qualities but ultimately requires embracing feminine support to overcome deeper challenges. Narcissus absolute represents the inner marriage, harmonizing both poles of your existence. Sandalwood essential oil brings the warm glow of expansion through experience. Blended with safflower oil, this mixture softens the heart, broadens your perspective, and opens your awareness to the vast possibilities life offers so you can truly be all that you are.

❧ Overcoming the Shadow Blend

¼ cup guava seed oil
1 tablespoon macerated saffron oil
3 drops labdanum absolute
18 drops lavender essential oil

Guava seed oil cleanses and opens the heart, supporting the healing of distorted emotions. Adding macerated saffron oil balances overly lascivious second chakra energy, anchoring the soul in sacred sexuality. Labdanum absolute softens and redirects tendencies toward power-over and control into a protective, nurturing strength. Lavender essential oil encourages vulnerability and fosters genuine connections. This blend addresses the shadow side of masculinity, often expressed as dominance, aggression, emotional repression, or a fear of vulnerability. It works to transform these imbalances, fostering a harmonious integration of courage, protection, and connection, while transcending ego-driven pursuits to embrace authentic wisdom and unity.

❧ Mountain Man Blend

1 cup safflower oil
22 drops lemon essential oil
6 drops Siberian fir absolute
4 drops oakmoss essential oil
4 drops patchouli essential oil
4 drops vetiver essential oil

This blend cultivates rugged independence, grounded strength, and a deep connection to nature. Rooted like the mountains, it balances resilience, self-reliance, and courage with quiet reflection and the wild call of adventure, helping you embody life's raw beauty with humility and steadfastness. If you are making this beard blend for another person, offer it as a silent prayer for their growth and support.

Neck and Throat

The peach-dyed kimono
patterned with maple leaves
drifting across the silk,
falls from right to left
in a diagonal, revealing
the nape of her neck
and the curve of a shoulder
like the slope of a hill
set deep in snow in a country
of huge white solemn birds.
Her face appears in the mirror,
a reflection in a winter pond,
rising to meet itself.

CATHY SONG

This poem by Cathy Song, inspired by a woodblock print by the Japanese artist Kitagawa Utamaro, describes the elaborate work of a geisha who has painted lines on the back of her neck to make it appear longer and slimmer.

Most sensory inputs occur in the head. This makes limber neck movement vital to survival, as the neck serves as the conduit for the brain to communicate with the rest of the body. Motor and sensory information and nutrients from the body to the head and vice versa must all pass through the neck.

The river of life flows through the neck via the jugular veins, three veins in your neck: the interior, exterior, and anterior veins. This makes the throat highly vulnerable, as the veins there are close to the surface; it also makes the throat an excellent pulse point for the application of perfume, as every heartbeat releases a subtle layer of fragrance. Oxygen is whisked through the nose and mouth and into the lungs via the neck. If any of these processes are constricted or severed, serious or even fatal damage can occur.

The fifth chakra, vishuddha, meaning "pure," resides in the hollow of your neck. This energy center is produced by ether (*akasha* in Sanskrit), which suggests that the entire story of the creation is alive within you.

To say "make the hair stand up on the back of your neck" means to scare or horrify someone, a reaction that directly connects to our instinctual, animalistic nature. We say someone is "stiff-necked" if they are haughty or entrenched in their views despite the facts. A person is a "pain in the neck" if they are intentionally difficult.

The American artist Man Ray (né Emmanuel Radnitzky, 1890–1976) dabbled in cameraless photography and explored surrealism, a movement that "reveal[s] the uncanny coursing beneath familiar appearances in daily life." He proclaimed, "I have finally freed myself from the sticky medium of paint and am working directly with light itself." In his work *Anatomies*, "through framing and angled light, he transformed a woman's neck into an unfamiliar, phallic form"[5] that emphasizes the sensuousness of this swath of skin.

The larynx, located in the neck, is involved in swallowing, breathing, and voice production. Sound is produced when air passes through the vocal cords and causes them to vibrate, which creates sound waves in the pharynx, nose, and mouth. Words and sound are vital to being human, the primary way we communicate and exchange information, news, and ideas. We are islands within ourselves, born with our own predilections and karmic imprints, and we need to express what we see, feel, and know. Our words are messengers that carry all of this information. As our words arrive to the ears of others, they are colored in an overlay of our predilections and karmic imprints. In the Bible, John 1:1–3 proclaims the primacy of the spoken word: "In the beginning was the Word, and the Word was with God, and the Word was God. He was with God in the beginning. Through him all things were made; without him nothing was made that has been made. In him was life, and that life was the light of all mankind."

I recently had a discussion with a man who is dear to me, and I used the term *hardwired*, which to me suggests getting back to one's original blueprint or natural self before we are layered with the calcified energy patterns of learned behaviors. My saying that distressed him. As someone who was raised to not accept his emotions, he had only recently found that he wanted to become more aware of his emotional body, and so the term *hardwired* translated as "robotic" to him—the exact opposite of what he wanted for himself. I was trying to express exactly that to him, but the words I chose did not translate that to him, so I had to explain what I meant. We were fortunate in that we both care deeply about each other and want to communicate clearly, although it is incredibly easy to be misunderstood through one's choice of words. Let us only use our words to create and bring things into manifestation that are worthwhile, kind, and enriching.

Plant Resonances

Continue your exploration of the neck and throat with the following blends.

Bluer than Blue Expression Blend

2 teaspoons blueberry fixed oil
18 drops lavender essential oil
4 drops hyacinth absolute
3 drops blue chamomile fixed oil

Mix all ingredients and apply to the hollow of your neck and the external occipital protuberance, known as the "occipital knob" or "occipital bun," at the base of your skull. This blend taps into the frequency of the throat chakra, the seat of communication, as expressed by its vibrant blue color. It supports the expression of truth spoken in a way so as to heal, not hurt, and to overcome any difficulty in discerning truth or feeling confused in conversation. It enhances clarity, wit, and spontaneity, and aids in understanding the impact of words on reality.

❦ Geisha Blend

3 drops violet absolute
3 drops white rose otto absolute
2 tablespoons peach fixed oil
6 drops aglaia absolute

In Cathy Song's poem above, we can visualize the peach-dyed kimono flowing gracefully, falling from right to left in a diagonal, gently revealing the nape of the geisha's neck. This blend evokes the subtle sensuality of the poem—violet absolute for vulnerability and modesty, white rose for chaste intimacy, and peach fixed oil for elegance, beauty, and poise. Aglaia absolute embodies ethereal grace, the kind that's almost too delicate for this world. Apply this blend to pulse points on your neck, transforming this area into a focal point for releasing fragrance, subtle gestures, and nonverbal communication, thereby enhancing your allure.

❦ No Longer Garrulous Blend

7 drops narcissus absolute
6 drops benzoin absolute
¼ cup cantaloupe seed oil
¼ cup blackberry seed oil

A garrulous person tends to talk excessively without getting to the point, which can disrupt effective communication, causing exasperation. Narcissus absolute symbolizes the need to reflect on how words are used, as Echo lost her voice due to being overly talkative, a curse from Hera. Benzoin absolute helps correct this by guiding you to choose words with precision. Cantaloupe fixed oil supports self-acceptance and feeling comfortable enough that you do not need to fill all the empty spaces with sound, while blackberry seed oil ensures mindful speech, avoiding gossip and careless words.

Spine

You sit here for days saying, This is strange business.
You're the strange business.
You have the energy of the sun in you,
but you keep knotting it up at the base of your spine.

RUMI, FROM "STRANGE BUSINESS,"
TRANSLATED BY MOYNE AND BARKS

The Bhagavad Gita speaks of a fig tree, the giant Aswattha, "The Everlasting," a metaphysical tree rooted in heaven with its branches bending earthward. Each of its leaves is a song of creation, with the buds that come forth being the things of the senses. The Aswattha tree is a metaphor for the stories of humankind that come into creation and are recorded on the spine. It symbolizes the Tree of Life, also known as the Tree of Knowledge. In the Bhagavad Gita, Krishna describes it as a metaphysical entity representing the life force that transcends the physical realm. Derived from *aswa*, meaning "eternal," the tree's branches extend across both spiritual and material dimensions, while its deep roots signify karma's influence. This tree embodies the cycles of life, karma, and the path toward detachment and eventual enlightenment. Its roots are grounded in the Divine, with branches extending into the manifest universe, encompassing the struggles of birth, old age, grief, and death, as well as all the joys in life.

For human beings to be able to walk upright, the spine must be a pillar of stability that connects the feet, which are rooted firmly on the earth, and the head, held aloft in the sky. The *djed* is an ancient Egyptian symbol that is depicted as a pillar. The word means "enduring" and "stable" and is commonly understood as representing the spine. Chapter 155 of *The Egyptian Book of the Dead* illuminates the power of the djed, a representation of which was ceremonially placed on the throat of the deceased during funeral rites: "Raise yourself up, Osiris! You have your backbone once more, O weary-hearted One; you have your vertebrae!"[6]

Symbolically the spine represents the esoteric dictum "as above, so below," indicating what is within is without, that the human being is a microcosm of the macrocosm. The ancient Greeks and Romans viewed cerebrospinal fluid as the stuff of life. The word *sacrum*, the seat of the spinal column, means "sacred bone." Jung hypothesized that the collective unconscious is "localized anatomically in subcortical centers, the cerebellum and the spinal cord."[7]

Craniosacral therapy is a form of bodywork consisting of exceedingly light finger and hand pressure on the cranial bones and sacrum. It addresses the rhythmic system that lies at the core of our physiology: the craniosacral fluid that flows through the spine, between the head and the pelvic area, to provide the pulse of energy. "A pulse through the fluids proceeds through the entire craniosacral system, like a tidal wave, from the sutures in the skull to the spinal cord."[8] "The craniosacral wave isn't just a physical phenomenon," according to osteopath Hugh Milne. "It's also a field of information and intelligence. In the tiny movements of the system, and in the still points in between, is consciousness."[9]

The symbolic power of the Tree of Life is a profound teaching, a version of which is found in nearly every culture on earth. The teachings explore our divine nature that is often thought of as located in the spine. The archetypal image of a person hanging from the Tree of Life is a symbol of inviting the experience of change. Jesus hung on a metaphorical Tree of Life, the cross, to signify his descent into the land of the dead, his return to the land of the living, and then his movement beyond our reality into the realm of God.

The Sun Dance is a ceremony practiced by a number of Native American tribes, particularly the Plains culture, who consider this ceremony to be one of their most important rituals. Each tribe has its own distinct rituals and methods of performing the Sun Dance, but many of these ceremonies have certain features in common, including dancing, singing, praying, drumming, experiencing visions, and fasting. The ritual is conducted around a central pole, representing the Tree of Life or the spine, to which the dancer is attached by rawhide cords that pierce the chest or back of the dancer.

The Norse god Odin, who plays a hermetic role in pagan worship, uses the Tree of Life, called Yggdrasil (a giant ash tree), to travel between realms and receive wisdom. According to myth, he hung upside-down for nine nights to obtain the magical rune alphabet.

> When considering Odin's travels, it is that he can travel up and down the great tree at the center of the world, the axis of the world. Traveling up the tree leads him to the land of the gods; traveling down the tree leads him to the land of the dead. Like Greek Hermes, he mediates between the worlds. He is the energy that travels between realities, and he is the borderless reality in between. Mercury is what some cultures might refer to as a shape-shifter, one who has access to all worlds simultaneously just as he belongs to none. James Hillman writes: "For Hermetic consciousness, there is no upperworld versus underworld problem. Hermes inhabits the borderlines; his herms are erected there, and he makes possible an easy commerce between the familiar and the alien."[10]

The Kabbalah, a representation of the Tree of Life, offers direction for personal transformation and guidance for spiritual development. The tree is comprised of ten spheres or channels on the tree called *sefirot*, meaning "lights" or "emanations"; these depict the different aspects of humankind's spiritual nature. One of the most poetic aspects of the Tree of Life is that it illuminates how our bodies are a hologram of the matrix of creation:

1. **Kether:** Uppermost on the tree, the primordial energy out of which all things are created; the dimension of universal consciousness and how this interacts with physical manifestation
2. **Chokmah:** Next, the dimension of spiritual consciousness where one experiences a desire to understand the soul's purpose and the meaning

of life; the energy of wisdom and the connecting point between the eternal mind and human thought
3. **Binah:** The dimension of light consciousness and the value of wisdom emerges; primordial feminine energy that is cooling and nourishing; the celestial mother of the universe that receives energy from Source and gives rise to innumerable forms throughout the cosmos
4. **Chesed:** The dimensions of universal, spiritual, and light consciousness and the value of mercy as one experiences universal love
5. **Geburah:** The dimensions of universal consciousness, personality consciousness, and individual will emerging through strength in action; the energy of judgment, power, and punishment
6. **Tiphareth:** All dimensions of consciousness and the values of beauty, harmony, compassion, and balance; the energy of the trunk of the tree, or its spine
7. **Netzach:** The dimension of subjective consciousness and the value of unselfishness; the energy of the endurance of God
8. **Hod:** The dimension of objective consciousness where one experiences an expanded perception of reality, the splendor of existence, and truthfulness in action as a source of prophecy; the energy of the majesty of God
9. **Yesod:** The dimension of personality consciousness; the foundational energy where a sense of individuality emerges and the energy of self-realization; the energy of the procreative forces of God merging with physical form
10. **Malkuth:** The lower dimensions of consciousness; personality; the energy of the physical plane, where one experiences physical groundedness, where the ability to discern emerges.

Plant Resonances

The word *spine* comes from a botanical word meaning "thorn" or "prickle." Each individual vertebrae in the human backbone has a plantlike dorsal projection known as a *spinous process*. The trunk of a tree is its heartwood, the central, supporting pillar of the tree, its backbone, so to speak; another way to think of this composite of needlelike cellulose fibers is as a spine.

❧ Climbing Your Spine Oil Treatment
Fig seed fixed oil

The giant Aswattha tree, a fig tree, is described as everlasting and rooted in heaven, with its branches bending earthward. Each leaf is a song of creation, and its buds are its senses. From here we begin the climb back to our celestial roots, remembering as we go. Fixed fig seed oil opens higher channels of the mind, unlocking memories of your deepest origins to reveal the inner fruit and nectar stored within your soul. You become the alchemical vessel, accessing your deepest knowing and essence. Have your massage therapist (or if you can reach the entire length of your spine) apply fig seed oil with light, feathery strokes, starting at your coccyx and moving upward to the base of your skull. Meditate on the gifts of fig and recall your celestial roots.

❧ All of Creation

4 drops vetiver essential oil
6 drops labdanum absolute
12 drops lemon essential oil
4 drops narcissus absolute
7 drops Siberian fir absolute
¼ cup buriti oil
¼ cup fractionated coconut oil

The spine holds the potential for all of creation. As you read the oil profiles in this book, consider each of the sefirot in the Tree of Life. For example, Malkuth expresses groundedness (vetiver essential oil) and discernment (labdanum absolute and lemon essential oil). Yesod is where the sense of "I" occurs (narcissus absolute). Tiphareth encompasses all dimensions of consciousness (Siberian fir absolute). Try blending any or all of the above oils in fixed buriti oil, and note that in Portuguese *buriti* means "tree of life."

Arms

Arms complete *homo faber*, or "Man the maker," the concept that humans' ability to make and use tools allows us a degree of control over our environment. Arms link our erect spine with our capable hands and intelligent mind to do our bidding. We build things with our arms; we cradle babies with our arms; we find refuge in strong arms; and we can destroy things with our arms.

Images of the Tibetan buddha Chenrezig (aka Avalokitesvara) with four arms are said to represent the qualities of loving-kindness, joy, equanimity, and compassion. In storytelling and myth, arms explore concepts such as strength, support, and bringing a sense of unity, often helping those in need and letting us know how capable a person is.

During the Renaissance, a popular subject of artists was the dance of the Three Graces—Aglaia (personifying radiance), Euphrosyne (joy), and Thalia (flowering). The Renaissance artist, poet, and philosopher Leon Battista Alberti described the Three Graces as sisters: one gives, the other revives, and the third returns the benefit. Through this interaction one learns the dance of reciprocity. (See aglaia absolute in chapter 1 to further understand this energy.)

Conversely, being "up in arms" means you are angry or upset about something. A firearm by definition is a weapon, a tool that can take life.

A coat of arms is a symbol representing a specific family lineage. Initially appearing on shields and flags during the Crusades, coats of arms were a way of differentiating one knight from another on the battlefield.

The Cubist painting *Genie Out of the Bottle*, by contemporary artist Denise Marts, depicts one flesh-toned arm pulling itself out of a bottle against a background of blue, brick red, and white, alluding to the idea that once you put something in action, there will be unpredictable consequences that you might not be able to imagine at the time.

Rumi invites us to melt into love of a heavenly and earthy nature, safe in encompassing arms:

Lose yourself,
Lose yourself in this love.
When you lose yourself in this love,
you will find everything.

FROM "THE BLACK CLOUD,"
TRANSLATED BY JONATHAN STAR

Plant Resonances

Continue your exploration of the arms by embracing the following blends.

❧ The Dance of Reciprocity Blend

1 cup corn oil
6 drops aglaia absolute
6 drops gardenia absolute

This blend cultivates a harmonious exchange of energy between giving and receiving, the fluid balance of giving freely while remaining open to receiving in return. This dance allows for the flow of love, support, and abundance; it fosters deeper connections and a sense of interconnectedness with the world around you. Through this practice, you cultivate a space of mutual understanding and softness. To amplify these virtues, apply on your arms before hugging someone, or meditate on the aspects of each of the ingredients in this blend and how you can further deepen their activities.

❧ Lost in Love Blend

½ cup date fixed oil
1 tablespoon avocado fixed oil
1 tablespoon fractionated coconut oil
6 drops neroli essential oil
3 drops pine essential oil
3 drops basil essential oil
1 drop rose otto absolute

This blend embodies the feeling of a warm, reassuring hug. Date fixed oil opens your eyes to seeing and feeling life as a lover, the way ecstatic poets like Rumi did. Avocado fixed oil allows you to become more vulnerable to others without fear. Neroli essential oil embodies the energy of pure love and the sweetness that comes with it. Pine essential oil allows you to experience your emotions in real time versus playing out echoes from the past. Basil essential oil makes it easy to quickly forgive. Rose otto absolute encourages you to carefully tend the garden of your love, helping it grow until only love remains. Apply this blend to your arms to embody and amplify these gifts.

In My Arms

½ cup fig seed oil
3 drops labdanum absolute
4 drops orris root absolute
1 tablespoon fractionated coconut oil

The expression "up in arms" refers to being upset about something to the point of violence. Fig seed oil helps soften the energy of anger, tantrums, and being easily upset. A coat of arms is a symbol representing a specific family, used on shields and flags to distinguish knights in battle. Similarly, labdanum absolute serves as a protector for those who cannot help themselves—true knight energy. In Denise Marts's painting *Genie Out of the Bottle*, an arm emerges from a bottle, symbolizing how taking action often leads to unforeseen consequences. Orris root absolute guides you to explore and understand the energies within actions before taking action, to reveal potential outcomes. Blend the above in fractionated coconut oil to ensure your arms take right action.

Hands and Fingers

We use a raised palm to gesture *stop!* Our pointer finger curling toward us gestures *come here*. A raised middle finger shows extreme displeasure. A single finger over the lips signifies silence. We "pinky promise" by locking our small fingers with another person, a binding childhood oath. We hold hands for comfort and to show affection. You place a quiet, reassuring hand on a shoulder when words are not enough. You use your hands and fingers to excite your lover. "The hand is the visible part of the brain," asserted the philosopher Immanuel Kant. The palms contain a literal map of the body that alerts us to our strengths and weaknesses, the state of our emotions, and our changes over a lifetime. Only fingerprints do not change. Palm readers say that the state of our emotions is revealed in every part of the hand.[11]

If you are an artist, musician, builder, designer, healer, massage therapist, or craftsman, your hands and fingers are your primary tools by which you work with your materials; they allow you to birth ideas into material form. An entire language is spoken with fingers and hands, such as signing for the deaf. Hand gestures can serve as punctuation for words, adding depth of meaning in such expressive languages as Italian. In Hindu and Buddhist traditions, hand positions known as *mudras* encompass a complete symbolism used in sacred rituals.

The small, mysterious, prehistoric handprints found in the French cave of Pech Merle are a 20,000-year-old reminder of those who came before us, testaments to our ancestors' ingenuity, artistic talents, and connection to the Divine. These "negative hands" were created by blowing pigments, likely black manganese dioxide, through a tube onto a hand placed against the rock surface. Those remarkable hands also created paintings rendered in reds and earth tones, depicting a variety of animals, including horses, mammoths, bison, and bears alongside human figures, sparking curiosity about their relationship and suggesting a fluidity between the human, animal, and spirit realms. The red ochre used in these paintings comes from the mineral hematite, a word, like *hemoglobin*, that is derived from *haima*, Greek for "blood." Red is probably the oldest color in use. Our Paleolithic ancestors started painting using a red created from a mixture of ochre with saliva and/or blood to make prints of human hands on the walls of caves in Europe, India, Africa, and Asia. Thus humankind's first cave paintings, created with hands from a primal matrix of spit and blood, seem to proclaim, "We are here, I am alive, I am here!" We still say it requires "blood, sweat, and tears" to accomplish something difficult, something that requires *all* that we are.

Plant Resonances

Continue your exploration of the hands and fingers with the following blends.

STOP!
Prickly pear oil

A firmly upraised hand signals "stop" and is strong medicine for discontinuing negative habits or patterns, encouraging you to return to your ideals, regain a balanced spiritual path, and reconnect with your own divinity. Prickly pear oil helps you stay centered, promoting inner calm as you pause, breathe, and thoughtfully assess situations instead of reacting impulsively. Apply this oil to your palms to regain clarity and act mindfully—stop, breathe, assess, and act.

Lotus Mudra
10 drops white lotus essential oil
1 cup cloudberry oil

The lotus mudra, or padma mudra, represents the lotus flower, symbolizing the divine light within and the wisdom of the heart. It serves as a blessing for ease, comfort, and safety as we grow. Perform this mudra by pressing the palms together in front of the heart, with the palms, thumbs, and fingers touching. Gently spread the index, middle, and ring fingers, mimicking a lotus flower opening. Apply lotus essential oil (the path of awakening) blended with cloudberry oil (the indestructible purity of your soul) to your hands before performing this sacred mudra to support your path.

I Am Here Blend
5 drops brown boronia absolute
3 drops vetiver absolute
3 drops red spikenard essential oil

6 drops lemon essential oil
½ cup fractionated coconut oil
1 tablespoon cabbage seed oil
1 tablespoon puumpkin seed oil

This blend boldly declares: *I am alive, I am here!* Brown boronia absolute and vetiver absolute reflect grounding energies that anchor you in your body, calling forth your full strength. Red spikenard essential oil is a testament to grit, embodying the blood, sweat, and tears needed to overcome challenges. Lemon essential oil is the energy of steady, step-by-step progress needed to accomplish your goals. Fractionated coconut oil and fixed cabbage seed oil provide sustained vitality and energy. Fixed pumpkin seed oil echoes the essence of humanity's ancient wisdom and all before you.

Blend any or all of these oils to align with this powerful signature. Apply the mixture to your hands, to the soles of your feet, and to your lower back, to foster a deep connection to your first chakra and earth energy, to honor the wisdom of all those who came before you, and to embrace the knowledge they have passed down for your descendants to inherit.

Legs and Feet

I want to be where your bare foot walks,
Because maybe before you step you'll look at the ground.
I want that blessing.

RUMI

Legs and feet are sturdy pillars of support that allow flexibility of movement, grace, and power. The malevolent Sphinx tormented travelers by challenging them to answer this question: "What creature walks on four legs in the morning, two legs at noon, and three legs in the evening?" The answer, of course, is we humans. We crawl in youth, walk on two legs in our prime, and in our twilight years we lean on a cane.

We walk and dance for pleasure; the legs of prisoners are shackled to restrict their freedom of movement; we are metaphorically "hobbled" when we are not at our full power; to render someone powerless you "cut them off at the knees."

The story goes that Achilles' mother, Thetis, made him invulnerable by dipping him in the River Styx while he was still an infant. She held him by the heels, which were not wetted, thus creating his only vulnerability. To this day to have an Achilles' heel is to have a known weakness that can be exploited.

Legs inspire lust and desire. The "gams" of Hollywood golden era pinup girl Betty Grable were insured for one million dollars. ZZ Top sings, "She's got legs, she knows how to use them." To be a Rockette at Radio City Music Hall a dancer must be between 5'5" and 5'10½" tall, with perfectly formed legs. "Ladylike" behavior dictates that in public women must keep their legs and knees together, crossing at the ankles but never at the knees. In the poster for the movie *Flashdance*, leading actress Jennifer Beals is shown sitting with her knees wide open, alluding to her natural, free-flowing sexuality. A common theme in the book series *Game of Thrones* is to "bend the knee," meaning to submit to another.

Plant Resonances

Our feet root us into the ground, our most intimate connection to Mother Earth. At one time the native plants in any given area addressed every possible health condition. We evolved walking barefoot, our feet crushing plants that released their precious oils, which our feet then up-wicked to benefit our entire system, as we are created to be nourished by plants. The pores on the bottom of the feet are made to quickly pull essential oils from our plant allies into the bloodstream. Reflexology is a holistic art that says that every organ in the body is represented by a corresponding area on your feet; this form of massage allows you to work on organs tucked deep, deep inside, like your liver and kidneys, by applying pressure to these points. A reflexology session using essential oils and absolutes is an exceptionally dynamic way to tonify your entire body, inside and out. Walking barefoot on uneven and rocky surfaces is another way to give yourself a reflexology massage; if you feel unwell, disconnected, or adrift, simply remove your shoes and go for a walk and upwick the gifts of nature in the form of plants and minerals through the soles of your feet.

Bare Feet Blend

6 drops spinach absolute
3 drops white rose otto absolute
1 tablespoon grapeseed oil
½ cup strawberry seed oil

Spinach absolute evokes the feeling of soft grass under your feet. It is the miracle of green growth, soft as spring awakening a winter-worn world, pulling light, earth, and water together in a miraculous act of celebration. White rose otto absolute allows you to walk in tandem with love in harmony with the heart. Grapeseed oil offers softness toward the human experience, while strawberry oil invites adventure and joyful exploration.

Blend any or all of these oils and apply them to your feet, connecting to the earth with astonishment and embodying the spirit of wonder and adventure as you step through life. Anoint your beloved's and your own feet as a blessing of togetherness.

Reflexology Key

Next time you want to connect with your internal organs, keep reflexology in mind. If you don't have a reflexology book, *The Complete Illustrated Guide to Reflexology: Therapeutic Foot Massage for Health and Well-Being* by Inge Dougans, is a great resource to get started. If precision isn't a concern, simply apply the oils of your choice to the entire foot and massage with firm, even pressure. If an area is tender, linger there. Use a thick fixed oil such as avocado or virgin coconut as the base, as feet are usually dry. Add any absolutes or essential oils you desire, such as the following to support specific organs.

Liver: blue chamomile, juniper, lemon, peppermint, rosemary essential oils

Spleen: blue chamomile, cardamom, frankincense, lavender, lemon, patchouli essential oils

Gallbladder: grapefruit, lime essential oils

Lungs: bergamot, cinnamon, rosemary, thyme, white cedar essential oils

Heart: lavender, marjoram essential oils, white rose absolute, macerated saffron oil

---

Just Look at Those Gams!

To create a preshaving oil blend, combine any fixed oil from chapter 3 with a few drops of an essential oil or absolute for fragrance and a smooth shave. Slather the oil mixture onto your legs before shaving. Follow with your preferred shaving cream or soap and shave as usual. Rinse with warm water, and for added moisture and skin health, apply your chosen fixed oil and allow to air dry. Some suggestions:

- Apple seed oil for youthful plumpness
- Apricot seed oil for soothing and supporting the skin's protective barrier
- Avocado oil for increasing water-soluble collagen content in the dermis
- Blackberry seed oil for smoothing blotchy skin tone, wrinkles, and reducing large pores

- Blood orange essential oil for fighting cellulite and dull skin tone
- Cantaloupe seed oil for a significant visual reduction of cellulite on thighs
- Common orange and jasmine essential oils for dry skin
- Frankincense essential oil for keeping red shaving bumps at bay and tightening tissues
- Marjoram essential for encouraging healthy cell growth

Keep in mind that any oil in this book will support happy, healthy legs. Feel free to explore different fragrances, textures, stories, and the luxurious slip of oils to create a radiant, nourishing experience.

PART 3

The Blends

Recipes, Prompts, and Inspiration

8
Alchemical Creations
Blending Story, Art, and Sensations

Now that I am older and almost ready to face the world, I look back on my youth and wonder if I will ever be able to smell the world in the same way again.

WALTER HUBERT,
NAKED FLOWERS EXPOSED

When you first learn a new art or craft it is normal to at least initially study another person's work and style. I bought my first aromatherapy book when I was in junior high, Marcel Lavabre's *Aromatherapy Workbook*. My mother would take me shopping with her to the only health food store in my small town, and the moment I laid eyes on this book I knew I needed to have it. I was magnetized. I saved up and bought it with my allowance. I studied it like it was scripture, devouring every word, concept, and blending recipe until the ideas felt like my own. This was not me duplicating another person's thoughts. Lavabre's book gave me the tools and information I needed at the time, sending me down a fascinating and lifelong path of learning and exploring to find my own unique path. I am eternally grateful for this seminal book.

Once you've absorbed the basics of any subject, your unique approach emerges. This chapter is about finding your own unique approach to creating blends that stimulate, heal, and nourish. In this chapter we'll explore stories and art works to discover the sensations that connect us to our plant allies. To facilitate this, I offer some prompts that suggest certain possibilities, although it's important to understand that you can blend any story or feeling with your chosen plant allies by simply using your intuition.

Principles for Blending

The following are some guiding principles or creative focal points when making blended distillations based on stories, art, songs, or dreams:

Symbols: Symbols are generally suggestive rather than explicit in meaning. For example, a rose can suggest beauty, love, femininity, and transience, without being limited to any of these meanings in particular.

Allegory: An allegory is a story within a story. There is the surface story and another story below the surface. For example, the surface story might be about two boys playing sword-fighting with sticks, but the hidden story would be about war between countries. Unlike symbols, which broadly suggest, allegory is a narration or description usually restricted to a single meaning because its actions, events, characters, and setting represent specific abstractions or ideas. Allegories are not symbols because there is little or no room for broad speculation and exploration, as they are intended to teach a precise virtue.

Irony: This is when there is a contrast between expectations and reality, for example, the difference between what something appears to mean versus its literal meaning. Irony is associated with both tragedy and comedy.

Metaphor: This involves a comparison between two things without using the terms *like* or *as*; with metaphor, the subject *is* the object. Metaphors are more direct than similes, which can make them seem stronger or more surprising. For example, the remarkable Kate Bush sings, "A wonderful sunset / honeycomb / In a sea of honey / A sky of honey." This type of figurative language communicates the point in an intuitive, sensory way.

Simile: This is a way of comparing two things by saying they are "like" each other; with simile, the subject is *like* the object. Similes remind us that a comparison is being made, which sometimes makes them easier to understand and follow. For example, Laurie Anderson, in her captivating song "Let X = X" sings, "Oh yeah, P.S. / I, I feel, feel like, I am in a burning building, and I gotta go / Cause I, I feel, feel like, I am, in a burning building / And I gotta go."

Who Am I in This Moment?

This blending exercise requires that you suspend your logical brain that tells you things like "Grass is green" or "I am a fifty-year-old woman with curly hair" so you can step into the innate storyteller that you are. This aspect of you creates sometimes fantastical ideas and images such as "A bird and a whale get married," "I am a dust mote on a ray of sunshine," "I am the strength and flexibility of the willow," "I have the depth and wisdom of an inky night sky."

Forget yourself. Merge into everything around you—the birds singing, the warmth of sun through a windowpane, a cup of tea, the weight of a warm bathrobe on your bare skin. Allow your heart and mind to wander, to unwind, to weave in and out of thought strands. Then ask your inner oracle to describe to you in textured detail who you are in this moment.

Don't try to make a cohesive story with a sensible plot line. Don't worry—your logical mind might panic and try to stop you from considering what brings ecstasy. Allow that doubt to arise, observe it, and the panic will pass and ecstasy will come in its place. When you catch on to the feeling, sight, or the idea of a scent, the moment you are one with it you will have a sublime blend.

Write down all the images and sensations that arise. These might include colors, phantasmagorias, feelings, crystalized thoughts, snippets from music, a song, poems, and so on. Feel into each bit and find the correlation (this can be a literal match or a feeling match) from the plants profiled in this book. Take each sensation and write down which plant or plants express this. Once you've gathered all the materials you need, blend, letting intuition be your guide. Keep mixing and adjusting until the scent of your blend smells and feels like you in this very moment. Keep detailed notes—this allows you to revisit snapshots of yourself in time.

For example, my snapshot in time as I write this today: I am a gnarled swamp witch made of oak wood, using my roots to go down, down, down below the water to the silty bottom so I can drink up, up, up the information that supports my writing today.

❧ Galvanizing Blend

- 6 drops vetiver (*deep roots going down, grounding me, grounding in ideas*)
- 3 drops red spikenard (*shunting information from my upper chakras down to my root for practical use*)
- 1 drop white lotus (*seeing in the dark*)
- 6 drops elderflower (*asking nature as an oracle my questions, listening for her response*)
- 3 drops lemon (*burst of mental insight*)
- 1 drop oak wood (*asking questions and receiving answers*)
- ½ cup safflower fixed oil (*helping me see and make connections*)

I use this blend as a full-body application out of the bath, while still moist, when I want all aspects of myself working together.

Contributing to the Cosmic Library

A library is a place where knowledge is stored. Each book in the library is not necessarily the absolute truth, but rather a snapshot of the writer's understanding that gives us context for a specific point of view. Thousands of books are offered on the same topic, each presenting a bit more insight to add to the collective knowledge of that subject.

Our collective consciousness is like a cosmic library. We each supply our unique and specific knowledge in the cosmic library that is the quantum field, which is then available for anyone to access. We also have access to all the rich information that has been deposited in the cosmic library by countless others. For instance, the write-up on lilac (*Syringia vulgaris*) in chapter 1 is a collection of insights and memories about lilac that are not mine specifically but represent shared knowledge.

The following is my purest, most intimate experience of lilac:

When I was a child, my maternal grandmother had a magnificent pale violet lilac tree in a secluded spot in her backyard, where it bordered the edge of her lawn and the wild fields beyond. This tree felt like my own private world. Grandma would lay a quilt under the branches of the tree where dappled sunlight dripped through. The intense summer heat amplified the scent of the lilac flowers as she instructed me on how to pluck a single tiny bloom and suck the nectar from the hollow neck of the flower. On a small table low to the ground that she set up for me she would place a glass of water, small sandwiches, and her favorite books—everything a child needed to while away an afternoon. That moment in time was (and still is) pure love, a feeling of absolute contentment, a memory of wonder, safety, and the spaciousness of an endless summertime.

This memory is mine, I generated it, although it is forever intertwined with the energy of the lilac tree. It's the sensation of checking into the cosmic library. Those feelings of pure love, absolute contentment, wonder, safety, and the spaciousness of time are now available for everyone working with the energy of lilac, as I have fed the quantum energy field, the cosmic library, with my experience of lilac. Now that you have read this it will be easier for you to access the energy of this plant. And even if you had never read this you could still access all these sensations because they are a part of the cosmic energy field. Most likely you would not flash to my specific memory, but you may have access to the feelings I have about lilac.

Allow yourself to file through your favorite sense memories that are tied to a specific plant. Relive them in rich detail. Write them down, and as you do so imagine you are placing your "book" of sense memories in the cosmic library for everyone to enjoy. If you happen to choose a plant featured in this book, go to that chapter and write your insights and intuitions in the margins so that whoever inherits your book will be blessed with this knowledge.

The following blend is to assist you in tapping into your library of sense memories:

❦ Tucked in Time Blend

- 12 drops lilac absolute (*a suspended moment in time, pure love, feeling absolute contentment, wonder, safety, and the spaciousness of time*)
- 1 tablespoon watermelon oil (*seeing the beauty in my life and resting in that sweetness*)

Apply to the heart center, pulse points, behind the ears, neck, knees, and wrists.

The Scent of Childhood

The science behind how scent evokes vivid memories lies in the direct connection between the olfactory bulb (responsible for processing smells) and the limbic system, which includes the amygdala and hippocampus. These regions are deeply tied to emotions and memory storage, making familiar scents trigger strong, often emotional, memories—sometimes even long-forgotten ones. As we've learned, the earth element's physical gate is your sense of smell. The following blend focuses on the poetry of scent, memory, and emotion. It was created from a place of sensory memory, inspired by how my front yard literally smelled.

Think of your own childhood, and as you file through your sense memories, stop at one that feels vibrant and detailed, meaning you can clearly see and feel the environment. Once you have chosen the memory, feel into each detail that makes it alive and write it down. You can then use these sense memories to craft a plant blend that expresses all the feelings you associate with that memory. Suspend your mind and uncap the oils you are working with. Breathe them in deeply and see if the fragrance profile feels and smells like your recalled time and place.

My childhood home was on a gravel road across from an alfalfa field, and behind that, the mudflats of Utah Lake. Two houses down lived a woman named Annie who had a miraculous green thumb. She would plant over a half an acre of spectacularly scented flowers that perfumed the air. Her property gave way to a natural spring that fed into a small pond, which trickled down into an irrigation ditch. Along the edges of the ditch grew cattails, milkweed, and Russian olive trees. I can still vividly recall the intense smell of sun on earth and water, baking and warming, the decaying smell of the mudflats, the rich green notes of plant life, and the sweetness of the flowers. This was the scent of my front yard growing up.

My Front Yard in Summer

- 4 drops oakmoss essential oil (*warm, intense and damp earthy smell*)
- 6 drops magnolia absolute (*complex and evokes sweet, effervescent notes reminiscent of sparkling champagne or light on the water, combined with a bouquet of white flowers and creamy fleshed fruits*)
- 3 drops pink rose absolute (*spicy, green, and honeyed; powerful combination of floral and fruity elements, reminiscent of lychee fruit*)
- 3 drops carnation absolute (*rich, sweet honey-like aroma with bright spicy clove-like notes, deep floral undertones, and a subtle minty-herbaceous finish in a long dry down*)
- 3 drops sweetgrass absolute (*lightly sweet, earthy, and warm yellow-green scent, reminiscent of freshly cut alfalfa drying in the sun*)

- 3 drops spinach absolute (*bright green, slightly earthy, vegetal scent with a touch of sweetness*)
- 10 drops bergamot essential oil (*sunshine on a hot summer day*)
- Optional: 1 cup oat fixed oil (*embodies longing for home, evokes a deep sense of yearning for a place, time, or person that may no longer exist*)

This blend is based on *scent only*. I diffuse it when I'm feeling nostalgic and homesick for a place that no longer exists. The neighborhood has changed, and those elements are no longer there, but I can take myself back in time to that place of my childhood with the gift of scent and vibration, allowing my heart and soul to bask in those warm memories. Alternately, I blend the above in one cup oat fixed oil, which wraps my heart and soul in those childhood sensations, feeding and comforting those places of longing. I then use this as a full-body application immediately out of the bath or shower, while still wet, and then I air dry.

Blending Poetry

Poetry offers a doorway to our shared experiences, which combine our understanding about living, loving, dying, and the Divine. Poems welcome you in, revealing ideas that may not have been in the forefront of your mind. Poems have a magical quality even when it's impossible to articulate exactly what it is.

Poems speak to us in many ways, although their forms may not always be direct or narrative in style. Sometimes the essence of a poem comes closer to saying what cannot be said in other forms of writing to suggest an experience, idea, or feeling that you know but cannot entirely express in a literal way. The meaning of the words that comprise a poem go beyond the literal to convey an impression, an idea, a feeling, or an experience that you can't quite put into words but that you know is real.

This very much reflects the Divine as found in nature. For as long as written language has existed, poets have tried to distill the essence of the experience of seeing an impossibly beautiful sunrise or sunset, the perfection of a bud opening into a flower, grass golden in the late afternoon sun. In that precious moment of transcendence that is beyond the mind, one does not analyze the effects of sunlight when the sun is low on the horizon, or the fact that sunlight passes through more air at sunrise and sunset than during the day, when the sun is higher in the sky. One does not calculate that more atmosphere means more molecules to scatter the violet and blue light out of your line of sight to allow yellow, orange, and red to make their way to your eyes . . .

Aurora is the Roman goddess of the dawn, sunrise, and new beginnings. It is said that she rose out of the ocean and opened the gates of heaven so that her brother, the sun, could enter through them and illuminate the sky. Her energy provides a gateway to new ideas and being receptive to inspiration that is dormant, waiting for you to seek and express.

Saffron Musings

Saffron macerated oil offers a saturated glimpse of the poetry of a sunrise and a sunset. Choose one or two musings from the list below and *feel into* the energy of a sunset or sunrise and see what distillations come to mind that express that energy. Remember, there are no right or wrong answers—this is pure creativity expressing nature through you. For me, "The whisper of the dusk is night shedding its husk" feels like black currant bud absolute, orris root absolute, and cyclamen absolute in a base of strawberry fixed oil.

Dean Koontz: "The whisper of the dusk is night shedding its husk."
Jennifer Aquillo: "Sunset shows that life is too beautiful to hold on to the past, so move on to the present."
Mahatma Gandhi: "When I admire the wonder of a sunset or the beauty of the moon, my soul expands in worship of the Creator."
Jack Kerouac: "The sunsets are mad orange fools raging in the gloom."
Claude Debussy: "There is nothing more musical than a sunset."

The plant distillations featured in this book are your palette; you can think of the properties and attributes of each plant as the colors and shades of their personalities. Prompts are offered as suggestions to prime your creative process. As with art, there is no right or wrong way; similarly, blending is a soulful medium with no hard and fast rules. The following recipe is to help you get those creative juices flowing. You may want to start with a full-body application of kiwi and peach fixed oils (apply while still moist from the bath or shower and let yourself air dry while lying down), or submerge yourself in the vibration (water is endlessly creative) by using this blend in a bath:

ও Politely Invite Your Muses to Call

1 teaspoon kiwi fixed oil (*muse energy*)
1 teaspoon peach fixed oil (*muse energy*)
1 cup goat's milk (*to cultivate wild abandon*)
½ cup fleur de sel sea salt (*appreciating the arts*)

Fill your bath with warm to hot water and add the above under the running tap; stir in the shape of a figure 8 and ask infinity to come a calling—and see what flows.

Poetry is a deep expression that can be cathartic, happy, sad, or anything in-between. My mother is often moved by nature and has been known to jot down her thoughts on the nearest piece of paper with no intention of saving those scraps. The following poem, which she wrote when she was seventeen, was rescued by her sister, my auntie, which is the only reason why I can include it here. This poem beautifully illustrates the art of blending.

Outside My Window,
by Sandra Searle Peterson

From outside my window, warm rays of sun penetrate the glass.
(The sun reference feels soft and diffused to me, not sharp.
For me, saffron can feel like a lazy afternoon, a first inkling,
warm and supportive. Labdanum is also the energy of the sun
but feels sharper and more intense.)

The streaming rays appear like the long, silken strands of a spider's web. (This feels like time weaving and holding our stories, bringing to mind orris root.)

Light rays flounce into the room, exploding into the expectation of spring.

Stillness clutches at the soft surroundings as a trap would grasp a wild animal. (This feels like a realization of how on some level we are not autonomous creatures, bringing cyclamen to mind, as it helps one work with this energy.)

A gust of wind races through the colorless grass, (Her use of the word "wind" suggests I should apply this blend to the temples, suggesting the sky, and the center of the breastbone, suggesting the element of air.)

Lacing the long, dark locks of the girl's hair, (I would also apply this to the scalp and hair.)

The boys' kite dashes into the air like a gallant, chivalrous soldier off to war. (This explores positive male energy in its protector role; labdanum vibrates to this energy.)

Then, as suddenly as it came, the wind gave a last dying, soliloquy breath, leaving the children alone with their kites floating like an autumn leaf to the lifeless ground.

Then the clouds reach out, trusting the rays of sun into their cotton pockets. Stillness predominates again. (This feels like the energy of sub rosa to me, silence "under the rose," as being alone allows one's development to gestate. The energy of narcissus comes with the sun, the divine masculine, trusting its rays into the cotton pockets, her earthly feminine, starting the process of the alchemical marriage within.)

꧁ My Mom's Blend

Inspired by my mother at the age of seventeen:

- 1 cup cloudberry seed oil (*This fixed oil feels like pure light, a big theme in this poem.*)
- 6 drops macerated saffron oil (*diffused sunlight through the window*)
- 3 drops orris root absolute (*web of time weaving stories*)
- 6 drops cyclamen absolute (*like a trapped animal, not completely free*)
- 6 drops labdanum absolute (*male protector energy; a gallant, chivalrous soldier*)
- 3 drops white rose absolute (*stillness, sub-rosa*)
- 3 drops narcissus absolute (*the divine inner marriage required for maturation*)

Blend together in a clean dark glass container. Apply to the energetic heart and temples. You can also lavish it into moist hair for about four minutes before shampooing out. While still wet following a bath or shower, apply to your entire body, lie down, and let the active dreaming of the air element take you as your body air-dries.

Poems to Inspire Your Blend

I suggest that as you read any of the following poems (or you may wish to choose one of your own), stop at any point when a specific energy strikes you and then write down which distillation(s) holds that energy for you. After recording all your impressions, simply blend your ingredients together to express the whole. If you aren't sure about how many drops to use in a blend, start low and add to your chosen fixed oil base, and then smell or intuit until the number of drops feels right. Keep a notebook with all of your recipes and revelations. Remember, this is not a flat exercise—the ultimate goal is to wake up and work with the plant energies to alchemize your mythic self and to support the stories of your life as they unfold.

Who Has Seen the Wind?

Who has seen the wind?
Neither I nor you.
But when the leaves hang trembling,

The wind is passing through.
Who has seen the wind?
Neither you nor I.
But when the trees bow down their heads,
The wind is passing by.
                                  CHRISTINA ROSSETTI (1830–1894)

Prompt: This poem's energy is woven throughout this book, expressing ideas about the wonder, power, and beauty of nature and its ability to impact you. You can read "wind" as the element of air, giving further insight into where to anoint your body with this blend.

A Man Said to the Universe

A man said to the universe:
"Sir, I exist!"
"However," replied the universe,
"The fact has not created in me
A sense of obligation."
                                  STEPHEN CRANE (1871–1900)

Prompt: The discrepancy between what a character aspires to and what universal forces provide constitutes cosmic irony. You are invited to move beyond surface appearances and sentimental assumptions to see the complexity of experience. What emotions and thoughts arise when you read this poem?

Acquainted with the Night

I have been one acquainted with the night.
I have walked out in rain—and back in rain.
I have outwalked the furthest city light.
I have looked down the saddest city lane.
I have passed by the watchman on his beat
And dropped my eyes, unwilling to explain.

I have stood still and stopped the sound of feet
When far away an interrupted cry
Came over houses from another street,
But not to call me back or say good-bye;
And further still at an unearthly height,
One luminary clock against the sky
Proclaimed the time was neither wrong nor right.
I have been one acquainted with the night.
ROBERT FROST (1874–1963)

Prompt: When approaching this poem, try reading for literal meanings first, then follow with symbolic readings. How does the repetitive use of "I have" make you feel? Is this a "night" that is located in the soul and mind? What about walking to and from the city? Do you have a strong personal symbolism when it comes to night? If so, what are these traits? Conventional symbolism means something generally recognized by many people as representing certain ideas. For example, roses are associated with love and beauty. Laurels suggest fame and growth. The moon reflects magic and the uncanny. Conventional symbolism helps to convey tone and meaning. What comes to mind when reading this poem's night imagery? Insomnia, loneliness, isolation, coldness, death, fear, being alienated from community and perhaps even time? Could it mean adventure, questing, looking within, a place out of time, a search for meaning? Symbols are very personal in that we each have our own associations with night and darkness that we can bring to the poem. Many of the absolutes included in this book have been presented in a way to make it is easy to identify their conventional symbols when creating a blend.

Under Cherry Trees

Under cherry trees
Soup, the salad, fish and all . . .
Seasoned with petals.
MATSUO BASHO (1644–1694)

Prompt: You might try blending this poem as a way to present a bright emotion or vivid image of nature that leads to a spiritual insight. The blend could be as simple as using fixed cherry kernel oil with your favorite florals blended in.

The Frog

What a wonderful bird the frog are!
When he stand he sit almost;
When he hop he fly almost.
He ain't got no sense hardly;
He ain't got no tail hardly either.
When he sit, he sit on what he ain't got almost.

ANONYMOUS (DATE UNKNOWN)

Prompt: Try reading and blending the above poem through the eyes of whimsy and give your inner child the reins. To get you started, tangerine and mandarin orange essential oils stimulate your inner child. Dragon fruit fixed oil brings a sense of whimsy, while pineapple fixed oil adds a playful, light-hearted silliness.

From "Looking for Your Face"

I am bewildered by the magnificence
of your beauty
and wish to see you
with a hundred eyes.

RUMI, TRANSLATED BY CHOPRA AND KIA

Prompt: Take a moment to close your eyes and feel into the energy of being so captivated by something or someone that you long to experience it from every possible angle. Then blend from the perspective of having the overwhelming desire to truly see, understand, or be close to that beauty, even if it means expanding your own limits to do so.

The Road Not Taken

Two roads diverged in a yellow wood,
And sorry I could not travel both
And be one traveler, long I stood
And looked down one as far as I could
To where it bent in the undergrowth;

Then took the other, as just as fair
And having perhaps the better claim,
Because it was grassy and wanted wear;
Though as for that, the passing there
Had worn them really about the same,

And both that morning equally lay
In leaves no step had trodden black
Oh, I kept the first for another day!
Yet knowing how way leads on to way,
I doubted if I should ever come back.

I shall be telling this with a sigh
Somewhere ages and ages hence:
Two roads diverged in a wood, and I,
I took the one less traveled by,
And that has made all the difference.

ROBERT FROST (1874–1963)

Prompt: This is a great poem for understanding dependent arising, a key Buddhist doctrine that basically says that everything depends on everything else, which is the basis of our interconnectedness. This awakens one to the truth: you cannot have it all; each choice is a stone in your foundation. Though "sorry," this traveler could "not travel both," so he made a choice after careful consideration. Choosing "the road less traveled" has affected his entire life and "that has made all the difference." Explore a time when you had to make a difficult choice between two paths, reflecting on how you navigated that crossroads and the impact it had on your life's journey. Or imagine looking back on a decision you made and wonder how your life might have unfolded differently if you had taken the "other road." Or consider how a single choice has shaped the course of your entire life, or how choosing involves the natural law of cause and effect to gain further insight into how your choices have impacted you. Then try blending this poem by selecting oils that resonate with its themes and even with the landscape described by the poet. Apply the finished blend to your throat chakra. You can further this exercise by crafting a blend to support your next steps.

Song

Lovely, dark, and lonely one,
Bare your bosom to the sun,
Do not be afraid of light
You who are a child of night.

Open wide your arms to life,
Whirl in the wind of pain and strife,
Face the wall with the dark closed gate,
Beat with bare, brown fists
And wait.

LANGSTON HUGHES (1901–1967)

Prompt: Try blending by opening your mind and emotions to this person's impulses, hopes, aspirations, ideas, impressions, and perceptions to come via free association. Once this story is painted in your mind's eye, find the oil(s) that match those sensations.

Troublemakers

Since no one really knows anything about God,
those who think they do are just
troublemakers.

RABIA AL BASRI (717–801)

Prompt: Try blending this poem as an initiation or feeling into the themes of certainty, belief, and personal growth, each offering a unique angle for reflection.

- **Exploration of certainty:** Consider moments when you encountered those who claimed to have all the answers. How did their confidence influence your perspective?
- **Doubt and faith:** Reflect on a time when you struggled with your beliefs or understanding of something as abstract as the concept of God. How did you navigate the uncertainty?
- **Questioning authority:** Contemplate how those who assert they have the absolute truth can be perceived as troublemakers. How do we manage situations where certainty overrides open dialogue?
- **Seeking understanding:** Explore the importance of humility in seeking knowledge, rather than assuming to know everything. How does this pursuit shape personal growth and relationships?

I dwell in Possibility—

I dwell in Possibility—
A fairer House than Prose—
More numerous of Windows—
Superior—for Doors—
Of Chambers as the Cedars—
Impregnable of Eye—
And for an Everlasting Roof
The Gambrels of the Sky—

> *Of Visitors—the fairest—*
> *For Occupation—This—*
> *The spreading wide my narrow Hands*
> *To gather Paradise—*
>
> EMILY DICKINSON (1830–1886)

Prompt: Try blending this poem with your choice of oils, then consider the following when creating your blend:

- **Windows and doors:** Reflect on a moment when opening a new "window" as a result of a new experience, relationship, or idea led to deeper understanding and a change of fortune.
- **Gambrels of the sky:** Explore the metaphor of seeking an "everlasting roof" in life's ever-changing landscape. How do you navigate uncertainty while striving for stability?
- **Paradise within reach:** How would you blend the energy of small, deliberate acts that contribute to your sense of fulfillment. How do these moments shape your view of happiness and contentment?

Suggestion: try blending white cedar essential oil (sense of interconnectedness and wholeness) in blueberry fixed oil (the vastness of the sky). Consider anointing your hands (the "spreading wide my narrow hands") to further connect with and undersand this energy, and apply as well to the heart chakra.

Water is taught by thirst

> *Water is taught by thirst;*
> *Land—by the Oceans passed;*
> *Transport—by throe;*
> *Peace—by its battles told;*
> *Love—by Memorial Mold;*
> *Birds, by the snow.*
>
> EMILY DICKINSON (1830–1886)

Prompt: Try creating a bath blend that reflects how hardships and struggles have shaped your appreciation for something in your life. How has longing taught you to value what you hold dear? Explore paradoxical relationships using imagery from nature, such as snow teaching birds, or land defined by oceans. How does nature reflect human experiences through contrast? Or consider how a personal battle that ultimately brought you peace or clarity. How has adversity acted as a powerful teacher in your life?

Suggestion: benzoin and orris root absolutes explore the creative friction that comes from holding contrasting ideas and feelings until something new emerges. After you've made your choices, add this blend to your bath and/or anoint your second chakra to explore the complexity of how contrasts enable us to grow.

Blending Art

Vedic philosophy teaches that sight is related to the third chakra, manipura (see chapter 6), which is ruled by fire and governs analytical thinking. The sense of sight that is associated with this chakra seeks understanding though imagery and context. Seeing is literally the act of becoming awake. This reminds me of a Rorschach test in which a person's perceptions of inkblots are recorded and then psychologically analyzed. Of course, nature is more fluid and interesting in the way she engages us, but this is a good reminder that even modern science uses images reminiscent of nature to suss out our deepest knowledge.

Let's explore what some amazing people have had to say concerning this. One of my favorites is Carl Jung. Language is tricky, but what I understand him saying is: I am that. You are that. And that is us.

> All the mythological process of nature, such as summer and winter, the phases of the moon, the rainy seasons, and so forth, are in no sense allegories of these objective occurrences; rather they are symbolic expressions of the inner, unconscious drama of the psyche which becomes

accessible to man's consciousness by way of projection—that is mirrored in the events of nature.¹

The heart of my own spiritual path lies in Vedic thought: *I Am That. Thatness.* The Sanskrit word *tattva*, meaning "truth" or "reality," expresses this idea. I love this word, it is so succinct. It reminds us that all things are interconnected and that we contain everything. A part of what makes this so joyful for me is figuring out which plants hold stories containing information for us, and what is awakened as a result.

The visual language of art is a powerful tool of creative perception, as poet-philosopher William Blake observed: "The Eye, altering, alters all." Sit with that. Your perceptions filter the universe. Each of us will see a painting differently based on our background and karma. How you process your perception of a work of art depends on what you need in the moment.

Art and story allow us to open a gateway beyond the thin membrane of consciousness. This is where you will find deep deposits of the imaginal world, the teeming terrain of myth and archetype. Here you encounter the sacred and the profane, wise women and holy men, camels who live indoors, stone turtles who rain from the sky, plants that speak volumes silently, circular rooms, death and rebirth—all part of nature's rich and complex language, a language that provides a powerful way of discovering who we are, for myth is encoded in the DNA of the human psyche just as it is in nature.

Here we are blessed to live many different stories: we are the handless maiden of the Grimm Brothers' fairy tale, restored to wholeness. We are the green fields made verdant by Osiris, the green-skinned god who rules the cycles of nature. We are the essence of spinach, bringing abundance, love, and growth. We live out the love match of Venus and Mars. The meaning of these stories deepens as we blend them into our bodies and souls via nature's gift to us, the plants. Integrating these archetypes is an easy way to become larger than life.

Growth *anisotropy* describes the condition when growth rates are not equal in all directions. In contrast, when growth rates are equal in all directions, the growth is said to be *isotropic*. Anisotropy is a hallmark of plant growth. Almost without exception, a plant's cells grow faster in one direction than in another. I think this is such a perfect way to understand how the soul grows. The soul's nature is not uniform; it often stretches and pulls us in unexpected directions, leading to surprising and profound growth. Cardamom essential oil opens doors to unexplored aspects of the self, inviting fresh perspectives and unexpected twists and turns.

• •

Blending Tip — Working with the energy of anisotropy, this blend taps into the truth that things change depending on the direction you look. Try adding 1 cup apple kombucha, 1 drop cardamom essential oil, and 1 tablespoon fig base oil to a warm bath and meditate on the larger mythic cycle you are currently in, then within that, the unique growth pattern that is all yours. The meeting of two qualities within you, whether an element of a story or the energy of a plant, is like blending two chemical substances: if there is a reaction when they are blended, both are transformed.

• •

The painter Gustav Klimt (1862–1918) is famous for considering the viewer's participation in art as being critical to the artwork itself. This line of thought addresses one of the paradoxes of art: "Artists through the ages have aroused the same emotions in their viewers, yet people never tire of art. Why do we not become sated? Why do we continue to seek out and respond to new forms of art?" Klimt and his generation of artists "taught new truths about the unconscious instinctual urges that lay beneath the surface of their lives."[2]

The reader is encouraged to look at the following paintings online while reading the blending prompts.

Saturn Devouring His Son

I think a striking example of unconscious urges expressed visually can be found in the painting *Saturn Devouring His Son* by Spanish artist Francisco Goya (1746–1828). According to a prophecy, Saturn was destined to be overthrown by one of his children. To forestall this, he ate them as soon as they were born. He swallowed Vesta (Hestia), Ceres (Demeter), Juno (Hera), Pluto (Hades), and Neptune (Poseidon). Their mother, Rhea, heartbroken and unable to stop him, came up with a clever ruse: she presented Saturn with a rock swaddled as you would a baby to swallow instead of her newborn, the baby Zeus. Her deception worked. She then hid Zeus in Crete, keeping him safe until he grew to adulthood. Once he was of age, Zeus challenged his father's rule and saved his siblings by giving Saturn an emetic given to him by Gaia, which forced Saturn to disgorge the contents of his stomach in reverse order. In Goya's painting you see a sad and ghostlike Saturn illustrating this myth. Beyond the obvious, this painting explores deeper themes—God's wrath, the conflict between age and youth, and Saturn in his role as Father Time, devouring all things.

Notably, Goya lived in uneasy civic and religious times. The French Revolution shattered the relative peace of the eighteenth century and led directly to a series of Continental catastrophes, including the Peninsular War (1807–1814), when Napoleon's armies overran Spain. Meanwhile, Spain itself was ruled by an absolute monarch whose will was reinforced by an absolutely medieval Catholic Church, darkened by the Inquisition. These elements are reflected in the gloomy heaviness of Goya's subject.

Prompt: What oils come to mind when you meditate on Saturn? Wheat fixed oil vibrates to this myth. What about the other characters who populate Saturn's story? What emotions come up for you as you consider blending to this myth? Fear? Sadness? Being overthrown or replaced? Being consumed by circumstances? Lack of choice? Rebirth? Redemption? Perhaps a specific aspect of life represented by the swallowed gods and goddesses being stymied or revitalized? This is an opportunity to tap into and hear what your deep self has to say. What is your unique response?

❧ Saturn Blend

9 drops benzoin absolute
½ cup black currant oil
⅓ cup fractionated coconut oil

Blends do not have to be complicated to be profound. This simple yet powerful blend aligns with another character in Saturn's story, the Greek god Hades, the later name bestowed on Pluto, who is synonymous with the underworld, transformation, introspection, and the unseen realms. He represents the deep unconscious and shadow work. As the ruler of the underworld, Pluto governs the mysteries of life after death, the hidden forces within, and the treasures buried in the depths of the soul, the mind, and the emotions. Benzoin absolute captures the essence of descent into and emergence from the underworld, one of the most challenging of human journeys. The underworld is often depicted as a fiery hell or a realm ruled by ancient, forgotten forces. Yet within those depths lie unparalleled riches: pristine waters, as well as treasures of gold, silver, diamonds, rubies, coal, oil, and their symbolic meanings. To be a plutocrat—one who gains wealth from what lies beneath the earth—is to evoke Pluto's domain. This can be understood as the mining of one's interior psyche, soul, and subconscious, where untold treasures await those willing to delve deep. Black currant oil reflects the untangling of the composite self and the ethos you've carefully crafted over the years. It embodies the night journey to your primordial essence—not the false self that fades in the face of judgment, but your original self, the self of unlimited possibilities, your greater, deeper being. This oil serves as a guide as you explore your greatest potential.

Apply this blend to your second chakra, where dreams emerge as the primary language of communication, offering cryptic messages that unveil the mysteries of the inner world. This energy is often described as overwhelming, cold, and impersonal—a vast and daunting landscape that holds the archetypal power of the collective unconscious. Within the oceanic depths of the second chakra we encounter emotions, creativity, sensuality, the divine feminine, and the inner child. It is a realm where profound illumination resides as well as our greatest challenges, inviting us to explore and embrace the full spectrum of our being.

Mars and Venus United by Love

Let's consider this painting by Italian Renaissance artist Paolo Veronese (1528–1588), famous for his grandiose mythological and devotional subjects, as described in the Metropolitan Museum's online catalog:

> The love between Mars, the god of war, and Venus, the goddess of love, is encouraged by a meddlesome pair of cupids. One ties the couple together, while his co-conspirator restrains Mars's warhorse. The painting celebrates the civilizing and nurturing effects of love, as milk flows from Venus's breast and Mars is disarmed. A brilliant colorist, Veronese amplifies the sensuality of the subject through his lush palette. Works such as this had an enduring impact on later artists including Velázquez and Giambattista Tiepolo. Possibly commissioned by Emperor Maximilian II, the painting was owned by Emperor Rudolf II in Prague by 1621, along with other mythological works by the artist.[3]

❦ Mars-Venus Blend

- 1 cup fixed oils, half guava and half cloudberry (*These balance the emotions and clear the heart from any tensions and anger; they promote love and beauty in expressions and actions.*)
- 12 drops lily absolute (*In ancient Greece, lily was sacred to Hera, Queen of Heaven, and was said to have arisen from the drops of her breast milk as they fell to Earth during the creation of the Milky Way.*)
- 6 drops aglaia absolute (*The Greek goddess Aglaia, one of the Three Graces and a daughter of Zeus, brings the principles of beauty, refinement, peace, and cooperation into our everyday lives, which binds the god of war. She is known as one of Venus's favored companions and a reflection of her traits.*)

- 2 drops pink rose absolute (*Pink rose expresses the essence of Venus—deep, passionate, personal love rooted in another, profound love, romantic love, seeing divinity in your beloved, and beautiful femininity and all that it entails.*)
- 8 drops labdanum (*This is the essence of the divine masculine, expressing warrior energy, and quintessential maleness that is magnetizing, attractive, and powerful.*)
- 1 drop white rose absolute (*White rose is a flower sacred to Venus that expresses the energy of a higher spiritual love that refines.*)
- 4 drops spinach absolute (*Spinach is a joining force that cools and connects with the heart, bringing about the desire to build together in harmony. It brings a civilizing and nurturing effect.*)
- 2 drops narcissus absolute (*Narcissus represents the sacred or alchemical marriage.*)

Blend together and decant into a dark glass bottle. Apply to the heart and solar plexus or mix into a full-body massage oil.

Veteran in a New Field

Winslow Homer (1836–1910) is a celebrated landscape painter widely regarded as one of the greatest American artists of the nineteenth century. His paintings related to "the Great War" reflect Americans' changing attitudes toward war at that time, as described in the Metropolitan Museum's online catalog:

> Completed in 1865 following the surrender of General Robert E. Lee and the assassination of President Abraham Lincoln, this deeply symbolic painting embodies the tension between grief and hope after the Civil War. A discarded Union Army jacket and canteen in the lower right corner identify the farmer as a veteran, and the "new field" of the title reminds us of his old one, the battlefield. This return to productive, peaceful pursuits echoes the biblical passage from Isaiah 2:4, "They shall beat their swords into plowshares."
>
> While the bountiful Northern harvest signifies renewal and recovery, the single-bladed scythe evokes the Grim Reaper. Pigment that has become transparent over time reveals that Homer originally painted a

more elaborate scythe that he later simplified, intensifying its association with death.[4]

Prompt: How would you blend the energy of the scythe's single blade, which is reminiscent of the scythe held by the Grim Reaper, the harbinger of death, which emphasizes the veteran's past as a soldier and the connection between war and death? Do you personally know any veterans, and do you have any insight about this dynamic? How could you make a supportive transition blend for a returning veteran who is dealing with complex emotions? Alternatively, how can this painting be seen in relation to Isaiah 2:4: "They shall beat their swords into plowshares"? Consider blending the idea of the scythe as a tool for cultivating an abundant life that can only come from peace and stability. This blend is not necessarily just for a solider, it is also for anyone whose life has been disrupted by personal violence, whether emotional, mental, or physical. What oil(s) vibrate to cultivating a peaceful, safe life and growing a new environment to support it?

Broken Eggs

Jean-Baptiste Greuze (1725–1805) is noted for his sentimental and melodramatic genre scenes. His work was praised as "morality in paint" by his contemporary, the philosopher Denis Diderot. As described in the Metropolitan Museum's online catalog:

> In moralizing genre subjects such as this, Greuze bypassed the arcane subject matter of history painting to appeal to a broad public. At the Salon of 1757, a critic even declared that the pose of this young servant girl, whose loss of virginity is symbolized by the broken eggs, was worthy of a history painter. Greuze struck upon such subjects, based in part on seventeenth-century Dutch painting, while still a student in Rome, though he would spend the next decades stubbornly pursuing the official title of history painter.[5]

Prompt: Reflect on the concept of art serving as a moral tale, in which symbolism conveys deeper messages that are being expressed in the collective. Consider the implied judgment of the young woman and the symbolism of the broken eggs that basically say that once innocence is lost, it cannot be restored. What about the idea of a woman's worth and virtue being judged on her being virginal? Or feel into the expressions on the faces of the people in the room with her. How do they reflect societal views of morality and the complexities of human sexuality, especially for women? Do you feel those attitudes from 1700 to 1800 still persist today? If so, what feelings arise? Consider making a blend for addressing sublimated sexuality due to social views that often create guilt or stymie natural impulses. Or, as in *The Scarlet Letter* by Nathaniel Hawthorne, the heroine Hester Prynne wears a scarlet letter *A* on her dress as a public sign of shame for her adultery. How would you blend the energy of not living in shame in contrast with being branded for life due to expressing your natural sexuality?

The Strange Thing Little Kiosai Saw in the River

American artist John La Farge (1835–1910) was an Impressionist artist who worked in stained glass as well as being a painter and muralist. He was an inveterate traveler who explored Asia and in particular was greatly inspired by the formality of Japanese art.

> This small watercolor by John La Farge is striking for both its serenity and its graphic subject matter. Sharing his contemporaries' interest in Japanese woodcuts and drawings, *The Strange Thing Little Kiosai Saw in the River* is a scene from the life of a famous Japanese painter, who had found a human head floating down the river, most likely a political killing. Kiosai took it, made drawings of it, and then wrapped it in paper laden with prayers for the dead and gave it a proper river burial. La Farge's watercolor shows the head floating serenely on top of the river's surface, its hair floating in the moving water. He adds a pink

flower and casts dark brushstrokes to indicate the deep, coursing body of water. Though a scene of grisly decapitation, La Farge only gives hint of the violence by the slight discoloration of the water around the severed head as well as the slight drop of blood underneath its nose.[6]

Prompt: Consider blending the emotional and ethical complexities of La Farge's subject depicting the decapitated head. How does the serene depiction contrast with the gruesome nature of the subject? How would you blend this painting's deeper themes—mortality, respect for the dead, and seeing a wrong (you are not responsible for), but taking action to make right?

The Dream of the Shepherd

Ferdinand Hodler (1853–1918) was a Swiss symbolist painter whose landscapes and portraits portray the unity of nature and the mystery of human life. As described in the Metropolitan Museum's online catalog:

> In the lower, terrestrial portion of this composition, the shepherd kneels in an Alpine landscape, while in the upper, celestial portion, a vision unfolds of eight nude women. In contrast to the shepherd's muscular, naturalistically depicted body, their pale, ethereal forms indicate that they are apparitions. The women may symbolize enlightenment, harmony with nature, and erotic desire. Their frieze-like arrangement and stylized, rhythmic gestures recall the work of Puvis de Chavannes, which Hodler greatly admired. This ambitious composition, first exhibited in Geneva in 1896, was one of the paintings that earned the Swiss artist notoriety for his exploration of sexuality, mortality, and the unconscious.[7]

Prompt: *The Dream of the Shepherd* invites exploration of contrasting realms—terrestrial and celestial, reality and visionary. The shepherd kneels in an Alpine landscape, grounding the composition with the energy of spinach absolute, representing verdant green hills and earth energy. In contrast, the celestial portion reveals a vision of eight nude women, each embodying divine attributes beyond earthly bounds. This is captured by aglaia absolute, which symbolizes transcendent beauty of an ethereal nature. White lotus essential oil represents their heavenly essence and expression of wisdom. The women can also symbolize harmony with nature as represented by gardenia absolute, and erotic desire as embodied by macerated orchid oil. The shepherd's muscular, naturalistic form is paired with myrrh absolute, evoking the energy of Adonis, the impossibly handsome, supremely masculine and very much of this world mortal lover of the goddesses Aphrodite and Persephone. This blend offers a rich interplay of earthly depth and celestial mysticism, with a touch of awe. Blend any or all of these oils in fractionated coconut oil.

Diana and Actaeon (Diana Surprised in Her Bath)

French artist Jean-Baptiste-Camille Corot (1796–1875) is primarily known for his landscapes that featured mythological creatures and renditions of flora and fauna, the two often mixed together. As described in the Metropolitan Museum's online catalog:

> From its imposing size to its refined execution, this painting is elegant testimony to Corot's ingenuity: the landscape appears surprisingly natural, yet it is painstakingly composed. The narrative, from Ovid's Metamorphoses, recounts the fate of a young hunter Actaeon as he encounters the naked figure of the goddess Diana and her nymphs enjoying a woodland bath. Diana, in a fit of embarrassed fury, splashes water on the unwitting hunter, transforming him into a deer.
>
> There is a marked difference between the general tight handling of paint and tonal contrasts, and the background on the left, which is sketchy and silvery in tone, typical of Corot's late style. A year before the artist died, he was asked to repaint this passage as a courtesy to the picture's new owner.[8]

Prompt: The myth of Actaeon tells the story of a hunter who comes across the goddess Diana (the Roman counterpart of the goddess the

Greeks called Artemis) and her nymphs bathing in a secluded forest pool. Actaeon, drawn by the sight of their beauty, watches them from some distance. Diana, however, is angered and humiliated by his intrusion and punishes him by splashing water on him, transforming him into a stag. As a stag, Actaeon is hunted and torn apart by his own hounds, unable to escape his fate. Could this painting serve as a cautionary tale about respect for the divine feminine and the consequences of invading sacred spaces? If not, what comes to mind? What oils speak to this? To get you started, carnation absolute vibrates to Diana. Once you identify what themes you want to work with, what oils express what? Or consider which oils represent changing from one form to another, and why is that significant?

Watson and the Shark

John Singleton Copley (1738–1815) was a colonial American painter of primarily historical subjects in which he brought together subjects and the objects associated with their daily lives in lively compositions. As described in the Metropolitan Museum's online catalog:

> Copley painted this rapid study for "Watson and the Shark" from his first rendering of the iconic work—now in the National Gallery of Art, Washington—in preparation for successive versions, found in the collections of the Detroit Institute of Arts and the Museum of Fine Arts, Boston. It depicts the future Lord Mayor of London, Brook Watson, who, as a teenager, lost his leg to a shark while swimming in Havana harbor in 1749. A Black sailor forms the apex of the composition, holding a rope for the victim who later famously defended the slave trade in the West Indies. Copley's dramatic depiction of an ordinary man in the midst of an extraordinary event of unresolved peril in the Atlantic World revolutionized British-American history painting.[9]

Prompt: The shark symbolizes danger, the shadow aspects of an individual or a society, and primal forces in general. It also represents survival, resilience, and the fierce challenges that push people to confront their limitations and emerge stronger. The shark can also reflect fear, aggression, and the hidden depths of the human psyche. Which oils address these themes? What areas of the body can you anoint to further amplify and work with these energies?

Blending Folk Tales

Folk tales are stories that come from the oral tradition. They may seem odd at times, having elements that may stand out and even seem out of place, such as a fruit, vegetable, or tree; a number, a body part, or a mythic being. These random-seeming story elements are artifacts that have remained in the collective unconscious from the original telling of the story, so they hold deep, significant, and usually very personal meanings.

The Handless Maiden

Jacob Grimm (1785–1863) and his brother Wilhelm (1786–1859) were German philologists who transcribed stories and fairy tales told to them by common villagers. This story is also known as *The Girl Without Hands* and *The Helpless Maiden*. I've highlighted some aspects of this story (with the change to roman font) and provided prompts. These are only suggestions, so feel into what is vibrant for you in this story and what plant distillations resonate, and then make a list for your personal blend, or use my suggested blend at the end of the story as a starting point for your own custom blend.

> *Once there was a miller who had fallen into poverty. His mill was broken, so he had to go to the forest to chop wood. One day when he was* hacking at a tree stump, *an old man appeared and said,* "I'll make you rich if you give me what stands behind your mill."

Prompt: What is the energy of hacking? Explore your concept of riches and what makes for abundance.

The miller assumed the old man was talking about the apple tree out back, so he agreed to the deal, dollar signs flashing in his eyes. The old man told the miller he would return in three years to take what was his, and then he vanished.

Prompt: What is the symbolism of the apple? What do you associate with the number 3?

The miller returned home, and his wife asked about their newfound wealth. The house was filled with expensive furniture and their clothes were new and clean! Better than that, the mill was working again, faster and more efficiently. The miller, grinning from ear to ear, explained about the old man and the apple tree. But the miller's wife was horrified: "You stupid old duffer," she cried, "our daughter was standing behind the mill, and that old man was the devil. Our daughter was traded, not the apple tree!"

Prompt: What does the devil represents to you? What does the traded daughter mean for you?

Indeed, the miller's daughter was hanging out beside the apple tree, beautiful, pious, and oblivious to her fate. At last the dreadful day arrived when the devil would come to claim his payment: the maiden. That morning, the girl washed herself and drew a circle around herself with chalk. The devil appeared but couldn't come near her. Furious, he demanded she must not wash herself again, and then he left.

Prompt: What does a cleansing rite mean? What does the circle evoke?

When the devil returned the next day, the maiden wept and wept, and her tears ran down her arms to her hands, washing her clean. So the devil still couldn't touch her. Enraged, he ordered the girl's father to cut off her hands so she couldn't weep on them.

Prompt: What is the significance of losing her hands?

The miller was shocked and tried to refuse, but the devil threatened to kill him, his wife, and everything around the mill. Quaking in his boots, the miller approached his daughter and begged her forgiveness. She replied, "I am your daughter, do with me what you will." The miller took his sharpest axe and cut off both of her hands.

Prompt: How do you relate to the idea of a willing sacrifice?

The maiden wept and wept, and her tears ran down her arms and mingled with the blood that poured from her stumps. When the devil returned once more, he tried to claim his prize but still couldn't touch the maiden due to the cleansing waters that had washed her stumps clean. Muttering darkly to himself, the devil slunk off back into the forest.

Prompt: How do you relate to tears—water and salt with the ability to protect and purify? What is the symbology of life blood to you?

The devil retreated to the forest, and the maiden's parents did their best to care for their daughter. Her father begged her to stay, promising to provide everything she could ever want or need, but she refused. She had her bloody stumps cleaned and bound in fresh white gauze, and then set out toward the forest. The maiden wandered this way and that, not knowing where she was going. She walked all day and stopped at nightfall. She had arrived at a royal garden, and in the moonlight she could see trees covered with fruit. She was so hungry she could barely stand, but she couldn't enter the garden because it was surrounded by a moat.

Prompt: Water in a new context! Instead of purifying, it became a barrier. What comes to mind? What is the larger significance of leaving the forest and finding a garden but not yet being able to enter?

She fell to her knees, famished. Suddenly an angel appeared, a beautiful spirit in white *who made a dam in the water. After a short while the moat dried up and the maiden was able to walk across and enter the garden.* There she saw *lines of* trees heavy with ripe pears, but she couldn't reach them with her stumps.

Prompt: What is your relationship with the idea of divine intervention and angels? The maiden was granted passage but still needed help—can you relate this to your own life journey?

One of the trees, perceiving her need, *bent down to feed her a pear. And so, using only her mouth, she was able to eat a* pear, the juice running down her chin. The angel stood watch as the maiden ate.

Prompt: Nature, in the form of a tree, aided the maiden in her time of need. What do you think is the meaning of pear and tree in this context?

Across the garden, hiding behind a tree, stood the gardener. He watched the maiden and the spirit by her side, but he didn't interfere. He knew magic when he saw it and let the maiden be. Finally, after eating just one pear, *the maiden retreated across the* drained moat *and disappeared into the forest.*

Prompt: Bearing witness to the miraculous, ponder the highlighted words in this context.

The next day, the king was walking in his garden counting his pears, for he knew exactly how many were on each tree, when he realized that one was missing. He called the gardener and questioned him. The gardener explained to the king what he had witnessed the night before. A spirit without hands had been led into the garden by an angel and had eaten one of the pears. The king was curious and so that night he decided to watch the garden, and he took his magician with him. He waited until the moon was high in the sky before he saw a strange sight. Out of the forest came the maiden without hands, accompanied by an angel who led her across the dry moat and into the garden. Once there, the maiden began to eat a pear, just as the gardener had described. The magician approached the maiden and asked, "Are you of this world or not of this world?" The maiden replied, "I was once of the world, and yet I am not of this world." The magician returned to the king, who was eager to know, "Is she human or spirit?" The magician replied, "She is both human and spirit."

Prompt: "*I was once of the world, and yet I am not of this world.*" What does this mean to you?

The king rushed to the maiden and promised not to forsake her and took her to his castle. He loved the maiden with all his heart and had a pair of silver hands made for her, and then took her as his wife. And so the maiden became a queen with beautiful silver hands.

Prompt: What does silver signify to you?

The queen stayed in the castle and the king lavished her with love and care. But in time he had to leave to wage war in a distant land. Before he left, the king asked his mother to take care of the queen, for she was expecting his child. She must send a letter as soon as the child is born, he instructed. Some months later, the queen gave birth to a beautiful son, and the king's mother immediately sent a letter with the good news. But the messenger fell asleep by a river along the way. While he was dozing, the devil, who was still brooding over his humiliation in losing the maiden, exchanged the real letter for another. The devil's message informed the king that the queen had given birth to a monster. When the king received the letter, he was shocked but sent a reply asking his mother to take care of his wife at this terrible time. But once again, the messenger fell asleep on his journey. While he dozed beside the river, the devil exchanged the message once more and ordered, "Kill my wife and child." The king's mother couldn't believe her eyes when she received the letter, so she sent another message to the king, asking for *clarification. But the devil played the same trick again and switched the messages, there and back. Finally, the king's mother received a letter that ordered her to save the queen's eyes and tongue to prove to the king that she had been killed.*

By now, the king's mother believed her son had gone quite mad what with the war and everything, and she had no intention of killing the queen. Instead, she killed a deer, removed its tongue and eyes, and saved them. The king's mother then told the queen that she and her baby son were no longer safe in the castle. The queen must run and go far away, and never return. And so with the baby bound to her breast, the queen bid farewell to the king's mother. Weeping, she left the castle and returned to the forest. She wandered, not knowing where she should go or where she would be welcome. She prayed for guidance, and an angel appeared on the path. The angel led the queen to a cottage deep in the woods. Over the door was a sign that read, "Here all dwell free." A maiden dressed in white came to the door and greeted the queen. She welcomed the queen and the baby into her home and took care of their every need. The queen lived in the cottage in the woods for seven years.

Prompt: Royalty implies being divinely anointed by God, a step above mere mortals. Why is it significant that the handless maiden was taken in by the king and queen but ultimately not allowed to stay? Her first home was a castle. What does this symbolize? Power, sovereignty, a fortress, protection, sanctuary? Due to deception by the devil she is forced to leave and wander the forest until an angel once again intervenes and leads her to a cottage. Cottages are often depicted as being located at the forest's edge and can symbolize belonging and a space of love and warmth. Why do you think this change was required in her heroine's journey? What do you think is the significance of the sign above its door, "Here all dwell free"? Other significant themes include the eyes and tongue. Why these? What do they represent to you? Why do you think the archetype of the deer was chosen as a substitute sacrifice? The water of oblivion marks a pivotal change of course here. What is the significance?

One day as the queen bent over a stream to drink, the child fell from her arms into the water. Frantic, she called for help and an angel appeared. The angel wanted to know why the queen did not rescue her child. "Because I have no hands," she replied. The angel smiled and said, "Try." As the queen plunged her arms into the water and reached for her child, her hands regenerated, and the child was saved.

Prompt: Water once again plays a prominent role in this narrative. What is the significance of the child being submerged in water and water serving as the means by which the queen's hands are restored?

When the king returned from the war, he found that his queen and his child weren't there waiting for him. He asked his mother where they were. She was furious with him, and said, "How could you? I did as you ordered, you lunatic!" She showed him the eyes and the tongue, and the terrible letters he had sent. The king was shocked and heartbroken. He almost fell over in his grief. When his mother saw the anguish on her son's face, she realized the letters were not from him. She quickly explained that his wife and child were still alive and that she had sent them into the forest. The king vowed to find them and said, "I will not eat or drink until I find my wife and child."

Prompt: A grand deception is revealed, the truth comes to light, and the king starts his journey to right this wrong. He takes an oath not to eat or drink until his son and wife are found. What is the significance of not taking in physical sustenance on this quest?

The king left the castle and wandered for seven years. As he searched for his wife and child, his hands and face became blackened with dirt, and his beard grew wild until he looked more animal than man.

Prompt: What is the significance of the number 7 and the hands, face, and beard? White is most often used in this tale, why black now? What is the importance of looking more animal than man?

Finally, the king came to the cottage in the woods with a sign that read, "Here all dwell free." A maiden dressed in white invited the king inside. He was so exhausted from his search that he lay down and covered his face with a handkerchief.

Prompt: Why did the color white need to be mentioned again? Explore the archetype of the maiden. Considering that his face was animalistic a moment ago, what is the significance of the king covering his face with cloth?

The king slept deeply, and as he slept, the handkerchief slipped from his face. He awakened to find a beautiful woman and a small child gazing down at him. The woman smiled, for she recognized the man despite the filth of his wild beard. "I am your wife, and this is your son," she said. The king wanted to believe her but couldn't help noticing her hands. She explained, "With grace, my hands have grown back." The maiden in white retrieved the queen's silver hands from a trunk and showed them to the king.

Prompt: Ponder the concept of grace and what can come from this gift. How are the silver hands different now?

The king was overjoyed and embraced his long-lost queen and greeted his son warmly. All three returned to the king's mother, who helped to arrange a second wedding. In time, they had many more children and lived happily ever after.

Prompt: What is the significance of the number 3 and the father, son, and mother? And, of course—why can they live happily ever after?

Blending Exercise

Gather a notebook and pen and get cozy before you re-read your notes. You might want to diffuse gardenia, as she helps you see connections. Look for the following:

1. What overall themes of the human condition present themselves in this story? What oils vibrate to those aspects?
2. What actual plants are featured in the story?
3. What are interesting elements that stand out for you in this story? You do not need to immediately know their meaning, you can do some research or just let the energy marinate and reveal itself in time.
4. Write down all the numbers and body parts featured in the story. You may want to base the number of drops used in your blend on the numbers in the story. As well, you may want to apply to the body parts highlighted in the story to tap into their energy (review chapter 7, "Symbolic Anatomy").
5. Write down any and all information that comes to mind, no matter how small or significant.
6. How do you want to use your blend? As a cleansing bath? In a diffuser? As a body oil? As a body butter?

The following blend reflects my interpretation of this folk tale:

❧ Handless Maiden Bath Blend

1 cup camel's milk (*your inner king and queen, being developed, on your journey*)

1 tablespoon apple seed oil (*change in a state of being, divine intervention leading the way, a guiding star*)

1 drop benzoin absolute (*a difficult but important journey—symbolically, taken without the benefit of food or water*)

1 drop saffron oil (*in its aspect of submitting to the divine and asking for help*)

1 drop aglaia absolute (*the gift of grace*)

1 drop magnolia absolute (*magic, moon, the color white, and the energy of silver*)

½ cup apple kombucha (*The energy of fermentation provides anti-inflammatory properties, which can help calm and soothe irritated skin. Its high levels of organic acids make apple kombucha an effective natural exfoliant, helping to slough away dead skin cells*

and reveal a brighter, more even complexion. Invokes the energy of a cycle completed—a journey's end and the gifts received.)
1 pear cut into thin slices, to float three of them on top of bathwater, to impart the energy of pear. From my book *Vibrational Nutrition*: "Pear empowers you to bring the highest spiritual energy into the material realm and teaches you how to use this energy to find practical solutions to problems. It increases the awareness and effective use of personal power."[10]

Rapunzel

As you read through the classic story of Rapunzel, take note of all the words and phrases that pop out or strike you in a meaningful way. Write those down, along with whatever interpretations of those words come to mind as you free-associate while recording your impressions.

> There was once a man and a woman who had long wished for a child. At length the woman implored God to grant her desire. These people had a little window at the back of their house from which a splendid garden could be seen, which was full of the most beautiful flowers and herbs. It was, however, surrounded by a high wall, and no one dared to go into it because it belonged to an enchantress who had great powers and was dreaded by all the world. One day the woman was standing by this window looking down into the garden when she saw a flower bed planted with the most beautiful rampion (also known as rapunzel).* It looked so fresh and green that she longed for it. In fact, she pined for it so much that after a while she began to look pale and miserable.

Prompt: To blend this story, see chapter 7, page 220, "Hair." Meditate on the energy of hair and see what rises for you. Rampion, a plant with deep historical and cultural significance, is mentioned in various literary works dating back to the sixteenth century. Sir John Falstaff, a character in three of Shakespeare's plays, refers to rampion, indicating its signifance

---

*As noted in chapter 7, this plant is not commonly grown in the United States, hence its exclusion from the part 1 profiles.

at the time. The seventeenth-century English poet Michael Drayton also references rampion as a staple of the kitchen garden in his epic poem *Poly-Olbion*. Its title, derived from the Greek words for "many" and "Britain," reflects the poet's celebration of Britain's diverse geography. Drayton vividly describes the country's landscapes, rivers, and towns, while incorporating local flora, fauna, folklore, and regional customs, offering a rich portrayal of the British landscape and heritage at this time. In Italy, an ancient Calabrian legend tells of a maiden who discovers a staircase to an underground palace by pulling up rampion. Meanwhile, in nineteenth-century Germany, the Brothers Grimm popularized the tale of Rapunzel, a story based on the theft of rampion from a magic garden, which not only names the plant but also the maiden at the center of the story.

> *Her husband became alarmed and asked, "What ails you, dear wife?" "Ah," she replied, "if I can't eat some of the rampion in the garden behind our house, I shall die." The man thought, Rather than let my wife die, I'll bring her some of the rampion myself, let it cost what it will. So at twilight he clambered over the wall into the garden of the enchantress, hastily clutched a handful of rampion, and took it to his wife. She at once made a salad of it and ate it greedily. It tasted so good to her, so very good, that the next day she longed for three times as much as she had eaten the day before.*

Prompt: Why do you think the wife craved the energy of rampion—to the point of "dying" if she could not have it? What is the meaning of three?

> *If he was to have any rest the husband decided he must once more descend into the garden. In the twilight of the evening he clambered over the wall but he became terribly afraid, for he saw the enchantress standing angrily before him. "How dare you descend into my garden and steal my rampion like a thief! You shall suffer for it!" "Ah," he answered, "let mercy take the place of justice. I only made up my mind to do it out of necessity. My wife saw your rampion from the window and felt such a longing for it that*

she would have died if she had not gotten some to eat." The enchantress's anger softened and she said to him, "If the case be as you say, I will allow you to take away with you as much rampion as you want, only I make one condition: you must give me the child that your wife will bring into the world. It shall be well-treated, and I will care for it like a mother." The man in his terror consented to everything. And when the wife gave birth, the enchantress appeared at once, gave the baby the name of Rapunzel, and took her away with her.

Prompt: What oils hold the energy of twilight? Why is that time important? What oils hold the energy of decent, and why is that important? What emotions arise for you around taking something that is not yours but that is desired so greatly it confuses your actions? It is a common theme in fairy tales to lose a child due to personal actions—what do you think is the deeper significance? Also, the role of stepmother comes into play—what energies are being expressed at a deeper level?

Rapunzel grew into the most beautiful child under the sun. *When she was twelve years old, the enchantress shut her into a* tower in a forest that had neither stairs nor door, but at the very top was a little window. *When the enchantress wanted to go in, she placed herself beneath it and cried out, "Rapunzel, Rapunzel, let down your hair to me." Rapunzel had* magnificent long hair, fine as spun gold, *and whenever she heard the voice of the enchantress she would unfasten her braided tresses, wind them around one of the hooks of the window above, and then* let her hair fall down so that the enchantress could climb up by it.

Prompt: The most beautiful child under the *sun*, with magnificent long hair, fine as spun *gold*. Here we see above-world energies versus the decent into the garden and twilight. Why do you think this shift is important? Why is hair so important in the story—both as a signifier of beauty and a means to gain access to something impregnable?

In time it came to pass that the king's son rode through the forest and passed by the tower. Hearing a charming song, he stopped to listen. This was Rapunzel, who in her solitude passed her time letting her sweet voice resound. The king's son wanted to climb up to her and looked for the door to the tower, but none was to be found. He rode home, but the singing had so deeply touched his heart that every day he went out into the forest and listened to it. Once when he was thus standing behind a tree to conceal himself he saw how the enchantress was able to scale the tower: "Rapunzel, Rapunzel, let down your hair to me." He observed how Rapunzel let down her hair, and the enchantress then was able to climb up to her. "If that is the ladder by which one mounts, I too will try my fortune," he said.

Prompt: Think about your oil profiles; which explore the concept of forest as solitude? Also, the theme of ascending continues: the prince must climb a golden ladder of hair. Why is this important? And consider the energies of singing, giving voice, and listening. Where could you anoint this blend?

So the next day when it began to grow dark, he went to the tower and cried, "Rapunzel, Rapunzel, let down your hair to me." Immediately the hair fell down, and the king's son climbed up. At first Rapunzel was terribly frightened when a man such as her eyes had never yet beheld came to her. But the king's son began to talk to her quite like a friend and told her that his heart had been so stirred that he had no rest and had to see her. Hearing this, Rapunzel lost her fear, and when the prince asked her if she would take him for her husband, and she saw that he was young and handsome, she thought, He will love me more than old Dame Gothel does. So she said yes and laid her hand in his. She said, "I will willingly go away with you, but I do not know how to get down. Bring with you a skein of silk every time you come, and I will weave a ladder with it, and when it is ready I will descend, and you will take me away on your horse." They agreed that until that time he should come to her every evening, for the enchantress came by day.

Prompt: What comes to mind about wanting to do something but not having the means to do so immediately? What feelings arise about doing something in secret but for your own good?

> *The enchantress* noticed none of this, *until one day Rapunzel said to her, "Tell me, Dame Gothel, how it happens that you are so much heavier for me to draw up than the young king's son—he is with me in a moment."*
>
> *"Ah! you wicked child," cried the enchantress. "What do I hear you say! I thought I had separated you from the entire world, and yet you have deceived me!" In her* anger *she clutched Rapunzel's beautiful tresses, wrapped them twice round her left hand, seized a pair of scissors with the right, and snip, snap, they were cut off, and the lovely braids lay on the ground. Moreover the enchantress was so pitiless that she took poor Rapunzel into a* desert, *where she had to live in great* grief *and* misery.

Prompt: Can you relate to saying something absentmindedly that has dire results? Also, consider being completely cut off from the world and the energy of punishment. In this context, why the desert?

> *On the same day that she* cast out *Rapunzel, however, the enchantress fastened the braids of hair, which she had cut off, to the hook of the window, and when the king's son came and cried, "Rapunzel, Rapunzel, let down your hair to me," she let the shorn tresses down. The king's son ascended, but instead of finding his dear Rapunzel he found the enchantress, who gazed at him with* wicked *and* venomous *looks. "Aha!" she cried mockingly, "you would fetch your dearest, but the beautiful bird sits no longer singing in the nest; the cat has got it and will scratch out your eyes as well. Rapunzel is* lost *to you; you will never see* her again."

Prompt: What oils would support you when hijacked in a situation that you did not intend to enter into, and dealing with the fallout?

At this the king's son was beside himself, and in his despair he leapt down from the tower. He escaped with his life, but the thorns into which he fell pierced his eyes and blinded him. After that he wandered about the forest and ate nothing but roots and berries, lamenting the loss of his dear Rapunzel.

Prompt: What oils could you turn to when losing perspective and not being able to see?

Thus he roamed about in misery for some years, and at length he came to the desert where Rapunzel and the twins to which she had given birth, a boy and a girl, his own children, were living in wretchedness. He heard a voice that seemed so familiar to him that he went toward it, and when he approached, Rapunzel knew him and fell on his neck and wept. Two of her tears wetted his eyes, and they grew clear again, and he could see with them as before. He led her back to his kingdom, where he was joyfully received, and they lived for a long time afterward, happy and contented.

Prompt: Ponder the significance of twin children, both a boy and a girl. Consider water in the form of tears being able to heal and restore, finishing the journey, and living in joy and contentment.

❧ Freedom and Imprisonment Hair Rinse

- 1 tablespoon macerated daisy oil (*to clarify perspective, self-awareness, and growing into adulthood*)
- 2 drops lavender essential oil (*for emotional healing, when life is difficult, allowing you to come full circle, leaving limited stages of being behind*)
- 1 drop spikenard (*for courage and perseverance, making those difficult choices*)
- 1 drop violet leaf absolute (*for daring to be happy*)

Blend all ingredients and apply to wet scalp and hair and lie back in the bath and meditate on the following:

At the heart of Rapunzel lies the stark contrast between the physical confinement of Rapunzel in the tower and her deep, unspoken desire for freedom. The tower symbolizes both a prison and a sanctuary, keeping her safe yet isolated from the world. Despite the witch's control, Rapunzel's spirit yearns for independence, as seen in her secret longing for the outside world. Her confinement is not just physical, but emotional as well, representing the tension between security and the human need for exploration, connection, and self-determination. Her eventual escape with the prince marks a powerful triumph of personal freedom over the forces that seek to limit her.

When you feel ready, wash and condition hair as normal and visualize what you want to release going down the drain. Also, dream up what you want to plant in your life.

9

Butter, Scrub, and Oil Recipes

Waking Up Archetypal Stories Within

Deep in their roots, all flowers keep the light.
THEODORE ROETHKE

The recipes in this chapter express specific vibrations that amplify one's inner archetypes and create a state of balance and well-being. When you apply these blends, their inherent energies become enlivened and move to the forefront of your personality and life, shaping your behavior and attitudes.

When creating a blend, focus on the kind of energy you would like to expand in your life. When a particular distillation stands out, read its signature for a deeper understanding. I like a broad template, and some of the ingredients in these formulas may be unfamiliar to you. If you have a personality that likes exploration, wonderful—add to your apothecary with wild abandon. If you prefer a smaller toolbox, you can use the following recipes as inspiration for what you do have in stock. Simply look up the items you have on hand and see what theme(s) emerge and create from there. You may substitute most honeys, essential oils, absolutes, and fixed oils, and the recipes will still turn out. If runny, add more wax or plant butters. If too dry, add more fixed oils and hydrosols. You can play with a batch as much as you need to as you iron out the kinks. Simply reheat, stir, and adjust from there.

Most importantly, these are just ideas to guide you in how to blend; they are not set in stone. Use your intuition and adjust as needed to have each theme fit you perfectly.

What Is a Hydrosol?

Hydrosols are the aromatic water byproducts of plants used in the distillation process when creating essential oils. With the same properties as essential oils, these aromatic waters are much less concentrated, with aromas that are similar but often softer compared to their essential oil counterpart, with a greener note that comes from the water-soluble constituents in the plant material that are not present in the essential oil.

Poetic Lip Butters

Lips are imbued with profound spiritual meanings and ancient wisdom. They are the gateway for words and thoughts to be transformed from internal feelings to external expressions. They are associated with sharing wisdom, voicing feelings, and expressing emotions, and as such they hold the key to our voice, our truth, and our self-expression. They also hold profound spiritual significance as symbols of sensuality and intimacy, in which the act of kissing can be seen as a profound spiritual ritual.

Ecstatic poetry is the perfect avenue for exploring sensual pleasure, human connections, the nature of longing and desire, and most especially our relation to the Divine (often described as "the beloved" in the language of ecstatic poets). The lip butters in this chapter are inspired by the words of notable ecstatic poets.

❦ Lip Butter Preparation Guide

The following instructions apply to all the lip butter recipes in this chapter, with variations based on which recipe you are using.

- ½ cup fixed oil of your choice
- 2 tablespoons avocado oil
- 5 tablespoons beeswax
- ½ tablespoon honey
- 5 tablespoons plant butter
- 2 teaspoons lecithin powder
- 1 tablespoon hydrosol
- ½ teaspoon vitamin E oil
- 5 drops of essential oils and/or absolutes chosen from chapters 1 and 2

In a two-cup Pyrex measuring cup add base oils, wax, honey, and plant butter. Take a medium-sized pot and fill halfway with water and bring to a simmer. Once this is achieved, place the Pyrex measuring cup inside the pot. Stir continuously and keep an eye on the pot so it does not boil. Once all the ingredients have melted, add the lecithin and blend well. Remove from heat, add hydrosol, vitamin E, absolutes and essential oils, and mix well. Place in a large bowl filled with ice, making sure the Pyrex cup is secure and won't tip. Stir intermittently for about five minutes. Now place the bowl and measuring cup in the freezer for about ten minutes; take out and stir again, then put back in the freezer for about twenty more minutes, then remove. At this point the butter should be starting to harden—stir in earnest. Once it is smooth and firmed up, scoop into small jars with lids. This butter has a shelf life two to six months, depending on the environment; keep out of direct sunlight and intense heat.

Longing

In the orchard and rose garden
I long to see your face.
In the taste of Sweetness
I long to kiss your lips.
In the shadows of passion
I long for your love.

RUMI, FROM "THE AGONY AND
ECSTASY OF DIVINE DISCONTENT,"
TRANSLATED BY CHOPRA AND KIA

❧ Longing Lip Butter

- ½ cup apple seed oil (*desire, the allure of what lies beyond established boundaries, the human longing for the unknown*)
- 2 tablespoons avocado oil (*making the lips sensitive, using touch to express emotions*)
- 5 tablespoons beeswax
- ½ tablespoon tupelo honey
- 5 tablespoons shea butter (*aligning impulses with wholesomeness*)
- 2 teaspoons lecithin powder
- 1 tablespoon cucumber hydrosol
- ½ teaspoon vitamin E oil
- 2 drops pink rose absolute (*the heart aching in longing, for sweetness*)
- 2 drops lilac absolute (*yearning*)
- 1 drop pink pepper seed essential oil (*passion*)

Embrace of Beauty

And this brought me understanding, the audience with love,
and the way beauty can let us hold her
in mind and
arms.

MEISTER ECKHART,
FROM "THE PASSION IN HER WHISPER,"
TRANSLATED BY DANIEL LADINSKY

ꕤ Embrace of Beauty Recipe

½ cup date seed oil (*experiencing life as lover*)
2 tablespoons avocado oil (*using touch to express emotions*)
5 tablespoons beeswax
½ tablespoon orange blossom honey
5 tablespoons shea butter
2 teaspoons lecithin powder
1 tablespoon vanilla hydrosol (*savoring life's intensity*)
½ teaspoon vitamin E oil
2 drops clary sage essential oil (*aroused by life's richness*)
2 drops common orange essential oil (*the coppery glow of desire*)
1 drop jasmine seed essential oil (*fusing sensation with experience*)

Being Kissed by Spirit

There is some kiss we want
with our whole lives;
the touch of Spirit on the body
        RUMI, "THERE IS SOME KISS WE WANT,"
        TRANSLATED BY COLEMAN BARKS

ꕤ Kissed by Spirit Recipe

½ cup borage seed oil (*touching the divine, kissing spirit, being kissed in return*)
2 tablespoons avocado oil (*touch as a form of communication*)
5 tablespoons beeswax
½ tablespoon purple star thistle honey (*asking the divine in*)
5 tablespoon shea butter
2 teaspoon lecithin powder
1 tablespoon lavender hydrosol (*gentleness of the heavens*)
½ teaspoon vitamin E oil
2 drops lily absolute (*ambrosic drops from heaven*)
2 drops lavender essential oil (*tenderness incarnate*)
1 drop white rose essential oil (*feels like blessings, rare and sublime*)

Soul's Ecstasy

My soul is screaming in ecstasy
Every fiber of my being
is in love with you

RUMI, FROM "LOOKING FOR YOUR FACE,"
TRANSLATED BY CHOPRA AND KIA

My First Love Story Recipe

½ cup guava seed oil (*true love, original love, seeded in heart*)
2 tablespoons avocado oil (*touch as a form of communication*)
5 tablespoons beeswax
½ tablespoon wildflower honey
5 tablespoons mango butter (*intent to build a shared journey*)
2 teaspoons lecithin powder
1 tablespoon rose hydrosol (*desire to connect deeply*)
½ teaspoon vitamin E oil
2 drops blood orange essential oil (*cherishing your beloved's distinctiveness*)
2 drops neroli essential oil (*a pure love, a fated love, a timeless love*)
1 drop patchouli essential oil (*deeply felt sensations*)

Lost in You

I've disappeared from myself
and my attributes.
I am present only for you.

RUMI, FROM "DO YOU LOVE ME?,"
TRANSLATED BY CHOPRA AND KIA

We Two as One Recipe

½ cup papaya seed oil (*deepening connection of souls*)
2 tablespoons avocado oil (*sacred touch*)
5 tablespoons beeswax
½ tablespoon clover honey
5 tablespoons mango butter (*bonds of longing that fuels unity*)
2 teaspoons lecithin powder
1 tablespoon rose hydrosol (*flames of passion, intensity of the heart, intertwining spirits*)
½ teaspoon vitamin E oil

- 2 drops frankincense absolute (*understanding how to react in the moment, light by your beloved's inner glow*)
- 2 drops marjoram essential oil (*warms the soul, comfort of the heart*)
- 1 drop spikenard essential oil (*complete devotion, complete offering of self*)

Unfold Your Own Myth

*But don't be satisfied with stories, how things
have gone with others. Unfold
your own myth.*

RUMI, FROM "UNFOLD YOUR OWN MYTH,"
TRANSLATED BY COLEMAN BARKS

ᏉᏅ My Myth Revealed Recipe

- ½ cup kiwi seed oil (*unleashing your boldest, most imaginative self*)
- 2 tablespoons avocado oil (*touch as a form of communication*)
- 5 tablespoons beeswax
- ½ tablespoon safflower honey (*recognizing and working with your best qualities*)
- 5 tablespoons mango butter (*accessing your second chakra, what stories are ready to come to life?*)
- 2 teaspoons lecithin powder
- 1 tablespoon rose hydrosol (*the creation of self, the birthing of self*)
- ½ teaspoon vitamin E oil
- 2 drops brown boronia absolute (*tapping into your raw, natural talents*)
- 2 drops lemon essential oil (*boldness of self-expression, living without fear or regret*)
- 1 drop mandarin essential oil (*tenderness to your experience, as your myth unfolds*)

Heartquake

*What a cruel act to be untruthful.
Earthquakes happen in the heart that hears sounds
that are amiss.*

MEISTER ECKHART, "A PLAGUE,"
TRANSLATED BY DANIEL LADINSKY

ꕥ Heartquake Recipe

½ cup blueberry seed oil (*all actions and words—holding the essence of truth*)

2 tablespoons avocado oil (*touch as expression*)

5 tablespoons beeswax

½ tablespoon wildflower honey (*Natura, holding the heart during a shock*)

5 tablespoons mango butter

2 teaspoons lecithin powder

1 tablespoon rose hydrosol (*softness incarnate*)

½ teaspoon vitamin E oil

2 drops blue chamomile essential oil (*gentleness of speech, sensitivity*)

2 drops lavender essential oil (*tenderness as a means of expression, what is scorched can heal*)

1 drop white rose absolute (*using light to restore what felt lost, redemption*)

Innocent Follies

Be kind to yourself, dear—to our innocent follies.
Forget any sounds or touch you knew that did not help you dance.
You will come to see that all evolves us.

RUMI, FROM "THAT LIVES IN US,"
TRANSLATED BY DANIEL LADINSKY

ꕥ Resilience Recipe

½ cup strawberry seed oil (*dawn is coming, sweetness returns*)

2 tablespoons avocado oil (*using touch to communicate*)

5 tablespoons beeswax

½ tablespoon fireweed honey (*emerging after a dark night of the soul*)

5 tablespoons mango butter (*the coral fingers of dawn, arising, the flush of life back in your cheeks, wonder*)

2 teaspoons lecithin powder

1 tablespoon rose hydrosol (*keeping your own counsel until you can unfurl again*)

½ teaspoon vitamin E oil

2 drops black currant absolute (*darkness as a teacher, the silence within, integration of life lessons*)

2 drops macerated saffron oil (*melting of the emotions, the warmth of self-forgiveness and recognizing the wonder of you*)
1 drop labdanum absolute (*insights that set free, the diamond heart*)

For When We Wake Up Frightened

There are hundreds of ways to kneel and kiss the ground.
                RUMI, TRANSLATED BY COLEMAN BARKS

❧ Choosing Love Recipe

½ cup buriti oil (*ear to the ground, perceptions altered, what is nature saying?*)
2 tablespoons avocado oil (*communication with touch*)
5 tablespoons beeswax
½ tablespoon pumpkin honey (*new ways to pray, connecting with the echoes of the past*)
5 tablespoons shea butter
2 teaspoons lecithin powder
1 tablespoon rose hydrosol (*keeping the heart safe*)
½ teaspoon vitamin E oil
2 drops spinach absolute (*connecting to the earth, kissing the ground*)
2 drops vetiver essential oil (*protection and serenity*)
1 drop cardamom essential oil (*moving beyond the veil of fear, finding the path*)

Becoming Jezebel

When Jezebel heard about it
she painted her eyes, arranged her hair
and looked out of a window.
                2 KINGS 9:30

❧ Wild Woman Recipe

½ cup cherry seed oil (*let your hair down for a change of pace*)
2 tablespoons avocado oil (*touch as sensual expression*)
5 tablespoons beeswax (*lips as sweet as honey, kisses sweet as honey*)

½ tablespoon maple honey or tupelo honey (*hot-blooded*)
5 tablespoons mango butter (*exuding sensuality*)
1 teaspoon lecithin powder
2 tablespoons powdered beet (*passionate love*)
1 tablespoon vanilla hydrosol (*sexual magnetism*)
½ teaspoon vitamin E oil
2 drops vanilla essential oil (*bewitching*)
2 drops myrrh absolute* (*redemption, death, mourning, resurrection, veneration, reverence*)
1 drop pink pepper seed essential oil (*expressiveness, rapturous nature, loving to be in your body*)

Body Butters

Most likely you have heard these stories or something similar in childhood. All cultures have used morality tales to teach the simple points of good behavior to children and to instill base values. The moral of such a story is a lesson in how to behave in the world. Note that the word *moral* comes from the Latin *mores*, "habits."

❦ Body Butter Preparation Guide

This basic recipe applies to all the following body butter recipes, with variations based on which blend you are using.

½ cup fixed oil of your choice
½ cup different fixed oil
1 cup fractionated coconut oil (for texture)
1 cup plant butter
½–1 cup different plant butter
2–6 tablespoons beeswax
2–3 tablespoons lecithin powder
1 tablespoon arrowroot powder
1 teaspoon of a single plant hydrosol
4 tablespoons aloe vera gel
20–100 drops of essential oils and/or absolutes chosen from chapters 1 and 2

---

*Myrrh is an integral ingredient in the eye makeup khol, traditionally used for beautification and to protect against the sun and the evil eye.

In a six-cup (or larger) Pyrex measuring cup add base oils, butters, and wax. Fill a medium-sized pot halfway with water and bring to a simmer. Place the Pyrex measuring cup inside the pot. Stir frequently, keeping a close eye on it to not let it boil. Once melted, add the lecithin, mix well, and remove from heat. Place in a large bowl, surround it with ice, then add the arrowroot powder and mix well, then add the hydrosol, aloe vera gel, and all essential oils and absolutes, and continue to stir frequently for about five minutes. Place the bowl with cup in the freezer for about ten minutes, take out and stir well, place back in the freezer for about twenty more minutes. Remove, stir well, and scoop mixture into clean containers with lids. Keep out of direct sunlight and high heat. Shelf life is from two to six months depending on the environment you live in. Note that this body butter may take longer to set, so stick with the process until the desired texture is reached.

Soul Mates

Once upon a time, Baucis, an elderly woman, lived in Phrygia with her husband and true love, Philemon. Although poor in material goods, their lives were rich in love and their spirits rich with generosity. As the gods are wont to do, Jupiter and Mercury disguised themselves as beggars, which allowed them to get the true measure of anyone they encountered. Going door to door seeking shelter and a meal, door after door was closed to them and no hospitality offered. Finally, they knocked on Baucis and Philemon's door, and the couple warmly invited them in and offered the best of what they had. While trying to catch their beloved guardian goose to cook and serve them, the poor animal sought shelter in Jupiter's lap. The gods then reveled their true identities and invited the old couple to follow them to a mountaintop. From there they watched as the valley below flooded, and all but their home was swallowed beneath the water's surface. Then in an instant their humble home was transformed into a glorious temple. The gods asked them what they wanted as a reward for their kindness and generosity of heart. They only asked to serve at the temple, and when it was time to die, they would die at the same moment, so they would never have to live without each other. When the time came for them to shed their earthy bodies, Philemon transformed into an oak tree and Baucis a linden tree, their roots growing together and branches intertwined, as they continued to grow together for eternity.

❧ Soul Mate Blend

½ cup papaya seed oil (*spiritualizing love energies, working together as a team*)
½ cup poppy seed oil (*touching the Divine*)
1 cup fractionated coconut oil
1 cup mango butter
½ cup shea butter
6 tablespoons beeswax
3 tablespoons lecithin powder
1 tablespoon arrowroot powder
1 teaspoon rose hydrosol (*perfect love rooted in another*)
4 tablespoons aloe vera gel
6 drops white rose oil absolute (*devotion to the Divine*)
6 drops lavender (*gentleness*)
1 teaspoon linden blossom absolute (*perfection of the archetype of the wife*)
8 drops oak bark absolute (*perfection of the archetype of the husband*)
1 teaspoon lime essential oil (*detaching from the material as a measure of value*)

A Time for Work and a Time for Play

Once upon a time on a bright day in late autumn, a family of ants was bustling about in the warm sunshine, drying out the grain they had stored up during the summer, when a starving grasshopper, his fiddle under his arm, came up and humbly begged for a bite to eat. "What?" cried the ants in surprise, "you mean you haven't stored anything away for the winter? What in the world were you doing all last summer?"

"I didn't have time to store up any food," whined the grasshopper. "I was so busy making music that before I knew it the summer was gone."

The ants shrugged their shoulders in disapproval. "Making music, were you? You reap what you sow." And they turned their backs on the poor grasshopper and went on with their work.

ꙮ Procrastination Recipe

- ½ cup broccoli seed oil (*creating your to-do list from a place of joy and happiness that follows from imagining a job well done*)
- ½ cup corn oil (*finding happiness in work that leads to safety and comfort*)
- 1 cup fractionated coconut oil
- 1 cup olive butter (*invoking Athena, goddess of wisdom and handicrafts, to understand the practicality of a situation*)
- 1 cup kokum butter (*promotes new ways of thinking, helping counterproductive mindsets to fall away*)
- 2 tablespoons beeswax
- 2 tablespoons lecithin powder
- 1 tablespoon arrowroot powder
- 1 teaspoon cucumber hydrosol (*offsets exhaustion when you feel too tired to go on*)
- 4 tablespoons aloe vera gel
- 6 drops vetiver essential oil (*making a step-by-step plan and following through*)
- 6 drops black pepper essential oil (*opens your inner sun for the energy and mental power to finish a job*)
- 6 drops cinnamon leaf essential oil (*pulls you out of self-defeating attitudes that lead to ruin, such as "I cannot" or "I do not want to"*)
- 10 drops lemon essential oil (*versatility of thought, pulling from all that you are to accomplish something*)
- 1 drop Spanish broom absolute (*beginning and closing the day with meaningful work*)

Think Before You Speak

Once upon a time, a young man spread a false rumor about an old man who lived at the end of his street. Overcome with guilt, he worked up the courage to apologize. He humbly walked up to the old man's door, knocked, and when the old man answered the young man said he was sorry. The wise old man looked at him. He said that he would forgive him but first he must take a feather pillow to the top of a hill and pop it open so that all the feathers would spread in the wind. The young man thought it a strange request, but he did as the old man asked. Afterward, he went to report this to the old man and asked for forgiveness again. The old man said that when the young man collected all of the feathers, then he would be forgiven. Words, like feathers, get scattered everywhere. The next time you are tempted to pass gossip along, remember that once your words are spoken, they can never be taken back.

Words Are Like Feathers Recipe

- ½ cup cantaloupe seed oil (*working with the shadow*)
- ½ cup cranberry seed oil (*teaches restraint*)
- 1 cup fractionated coconut oil
- 1 cup macadamia butter (*kindness as an operating system, and making choices from this space*)
- 1 cup kokum butter (*understanding the ramifications of a single action*)
- 4 tablespoons beeswax
- 3 tablespoons lecithin powder
- 1 tablespoon arrowroot powder
- 1 teaspoon lavender hydrosol (*gentleness*)
- 4 tablespoons aloe vera gel
- 6 drops blue chamomile essential oil (*using words to create your environment in a thoughtful manner*)
- 6 drops benzoin absolute (*understanding why you do something*)
- 6 drops orris root absolute (*finding the first cause of a discordant behavior and undoing it*)
- 10 drops narcissus absolute (*using words in a garrulous manner*)

Necessity Is the Mother of Invention

Once upon a time, a clever crow happened upon a pitcher of water out in the wilderness. Relieved, the thirsty Crow believed his troubles were over. To the parched bird's dismay, however, there was so little water in the container that his tiny beak could not reach the life-saving liquid within. Ever industrious and thoughtful, the crow began to collect as many pebbles as he could carry and dropped them into the pitcher until the water had risen enough for him to bend down and drink.

❧ Creative Solutions Recipe

- ½ cup red cabbage seed oil (*try, try again until you succeed*)
- ½ cup sunflower seed oil (*helps you to be analytical*)
- 1 cup fractionated coconut oil
- 1 cup coconut butter (*the gumption to keep going*)
- 1 cup kokum butter (*each new experience brings clearer understanding*)
- 2 tablespoons beeswax
- 2 tablespoons lecithin powder
- 1 tablespoon arrowroot powder
- 1 teaspoon lavender hydrosol
- 4 tablespoons aloe vera gel
- 6 drops peppermint essential oil (*keeping a cool head; opens the door to achieving the seemingly impossible*)
- 6 drops cardamom essential oil (*opens up unexplored aspects of the psyche that bring new perspectives and understandings*)
- 6 drops labdanum absolute (*singleminded focus*)
- 10 drops lemon essential oil (*helps you reach goals and desires*)

Think Before You Act

Once upon a time there was a king named Midas who did a good deed for a satyr, a wise nature spirit with the body of a horse and a man. Dionysus, the god of wine, then granted the king a wish. For his wish, Midas asked that whatever he touched would turn to gold. Despite Dionysus's efforts to prevent it, Midas insisted this was a perfect wish, so it was granted. Eager to use his newly bestowed powers, Midas started touching all kinds of things, turning each item into pure gold. Soon, Midas became hungry, and as he picked up a piece of food, he found he couldn't eat it—it had turned to gold in his hand.

Realization set in, and Midas exclaimed "I'll starve! This is not an excellent wish after all!"

Seeing his dismay, Midas' beloved daughter threw her arms around him to comfort him, and she, too, turned to gold. "The golden touch is no blessing," Midas lamented.

༄ Consider the Consequences Recipe

- ½ cup macerated saffron oil (*energy of gold*)
- ½ cup macerated orchid oil (*energy of a satyr*)
- 1 cup fractionated coconut oil
- 1 cup macadamia butter (*love as a ruling principle*)
- 1 cup babassu butter (*accessing the softer traits within, including remorse*)
- 6 tablespoons beeswax
- 3 tablespoons lecithin powder
- 1 tablespoon arrowroot powder
- 1 teaspoon rose hydrosol (*love of daughter*)
- 4 tablespoons aloe vera gel
- 6 drops neroli essential oil (*finding value in the nonmaterial; riches from a life filled with true value*)
- 6 drops petitgrain essential oil (*discrimination*)
- 6 drops labdanum absolute (*internal gold that arises from wisdom*)
- 10 drops sandalwood essential oil (*a spiritualizing force helping one see all that glitters is not gold*)

The Prideful Rose

Once upon a time, a beautiful rose who was very full of herself would insult and tease her neighbor, the cactus, about his looks, without seeing who he truly was. The cactus, a sensible, self-contained fellow, remained quiet and knew his own worth. All the other plants nearby tried to make the rose see the truth, but she was too self-absorbed to even notice the things she and the cactus had in common (both being a prickly bunch), as well as the strengths that came from their differences.

As summer wore on, the earth became dry, and there was no water left for the rose to drink. She quickly began to wilt. Her soft petals dried up, losing their lush color. Looking to the cactus, she saw a sparrow dip his beak into the cactus to drink some water. Though ashamed, the rose begged the cactus if she could have some water. The kindly cactus agreed, helping her through the difficult summer.

❧ Calm the Ego Recipe

- ½ cup prickly pear seed oil (*allows you to stay centered in oneself and not be reactionary*)
- ½ cup tomato seed oil (*how to be in community*)
- 1 cup fractionated coconut oil
- 1 cup macadamia butter (*a sunny, serene disposition, counterbalancing the energy of being easily upset*)
- 1 cup babassu butter
- 6 tablespoons beeswax
- 3 tablespoons lecithin powder
- 1 tablespoon arrowroot powder
- 1 teaspoon rose hydrosol (*helps the more feminine, compassionate aspects of your personality to unfurl*)
- 4 tablespoons aloe vera gel
- 6 drops pink rose absolute (*truly seeing and caring for another, for what makes them unique, and celebrating that with them*)
- 6 drops white rose absolute (*learning through experience*)
- 6 drops frankincense essential oil (*how to read energy in the environment and respond from an evolved space*)
- 10 drops narcissus absolute (*heals egoic issues*)

Kindness Prevails

Once upon a time, two brothers lived at the forest's edge. The older brother was always unkind to his younger brother, eating the best food and taking the warmest clothes. The older brother daily ventured into the forest in search of firewood to sell in the market. As he walked through the forest, he chopped off the branches of every tree he passed until one day he came upon a magical tree.

The tree stopped him before he chopped its branches and said, "Oh, kind sir, please spare my branches. If you spare me, I will provide you with golden apples."

The older brother agreed, but since he was never satisfied, he was disappointed with how many apples the tree gave him. Consumed by greed, he threatened to cut the entire tree down to a stump if he didn't provide him with more apples. Instead of giving him more apples, the tree showered him with hundreds of tiny, sharp needles. The brother fell to the ground, crying in pain as the sun began to set.

When the older brother didn't return, the younger brother became worried and went to search for him. He looked and looked until he found him at the trunk of the tree, lying in pain with hundreds of needles in his body. He rushed to his aid and started to painstakingly remove each needle with great love. Once the needles were out, the older brother apologized for mistreating his younger brother. The magical tree saw the change in the older brother's heart and gifted them both with all the golden apples the brothers could need.

Kindness Recipe

- ½ cup apple seed oil (*supports accessing hidden layers of the self for improvement*)
- ½ cup apricot seed oil (*empowers one to take responsibility for one's actions; supports changing for the better*)
- 1 cup fractionated coconut oil
- 1 cup shea butter
- 1 cup kokum butter
- 3 tablespoons beeswax
- 2 tablespoons lecithin powder
- 1 tablespoon arrowroot powder
- 1 teaspoon cucumber hydrosol (*cooling to hot, unkind behaviors*)
- 4 tablespoons aloe vera gel
- 1 teaspoon Siberian fir absolute (*exploring the maze of why you do what you do and coming out the other side a better person*)
- 6 drops grapefruit essential oil (*balances power dynamics in relationships*)
- 6 drops lime essential oil (*detachment and freedom from limited mindsets*)
- 1 drop benzoin absolute (*helps to release selfish actions and attitudes*)

The Negligent Milkmaid

Once upon a time, a milkmaid filled her pails to the tippy-top with rich, delicious milk. Her job was to milk the cows and then carry the milk to the market to sell. She loved to think about what to spend her money on. As she walked along the road, she thought of buying some ribbon and a basket full of fresh strawberries.

A little further down the road, she spotted a chicken. She thought, "With the money I get from today, I'm going to buy my own chicken. That chicken will lay eggs; then I can sell milk and eggs and get more money! With more money, I can buy a dress that fans out as I twirl around." Out of excitement she started skipping, forgetting about the milk in the pails, which started sloshing to the ground as she continued daydreaming. When she arrived at the market and handed the merchant her pails, he exclaimed, "These are empty!"

"Oh, dear!" she lamented. "I was so busy dreaming about all the things I wanted to buy that I forgot about the pails!"

❧ Staying Present Bath Blend

This recipe expresses a youthful exuberance and balances the energies of daydreaming (the element of air pulling you forward) and being rooted in the present enough to make those dreams happen. Though this is a bath blend and not a body butter, the same blending principles apply, just in a different base. This is a great example of how you can take the general idea of what you want to blend and explore different mediums.

- 1 tablespoon virgin coconut oil (*supports completing tasks*)
- 1 tablespoon chia seed oil (*teaches the art of tenacity and keeping with one's goal even after setbacks*)
- 1 tablespoon strawberry seed oil (*tasting the sweetness in life*)
- 1 cup sheep's milk (*creating a safe and abundant life that allows all the frills and fun*)
- Optional: 1 tablespoon of artic cranberry fixed oil to 1 cup sheep's milk (*helps one take stock of life; what do you need to do to create an emotional and physical state of satisfaction? What goals or desires does this entail? This includes physical rewards and comforts that come from fulfillment of your wildest dreams. This is*

not the energy of instant gratification, rather, the life you have worked so hard to build, long sought-after security and well-being coming together.)

Milk Baths and Salt Scrubs

While the previous blends are on the more serious side, these recipes are all about simplicity and playfulness, as one of the best ways to grow is by dispelling difficulties through merriment.

Naming your blends is a delight! If your friends and family are anything like mine, they appreciate a little cheekiness. Naming also anchors in the intention behind the blend. One can infer what these blends do based on the name of the blend. For example, "Having Athena Set Your To-Do List" is great for procrastinators. "Looking into the Dalai Lama's Eyes" is a solid meditation blend to help someone get started if they don't know how to meditate. "You're Keepin' Me Down, Man" is great to gift for someone who is experiencing a lot of negativity in social settings.

Most of the following milks can be found in both fresh and powdered form. Use powdered milk if you want to make your recipe in bulk so you can gift it to others.

Having Athena Set Your To-Do List Salt Scrub

½ cup Cyprus flake salt (*spiritual guidance during times of change*)
½ cup olive oil (*Athena archetype*)

Looking into the Dalai Lama's Eyes Milk Bath

3 tablespoons dried yak's milk (*time traveling, shamanic journeying*)
1 teaspoon blueberry seed fixed oil (*star eyes to see in the dark*)
1 teaspoon borage fixed oil (*helps your newly emerging truth connect to your outer path*)
1 drop lemon essential oil (*bursts of spiritual insight*)
1 drop neroli blossom essential oil (*serenity and being in the moment*)
1 drop white lotus absolute (*deepens your meditation practice*)

꙳ It's True Love, Not Infatuation Milk Bath

- 1 cup sheep's milk (*heavily featured in Inanna's Sumerian hymns, in love songs to her human consort, with themes of watching over him and ensuring his safety*)
- 1 tablespoon guava seed fixed oil (*spiritualizes the energy of the heart*)
- 1 drop basil essential oil (*refined love, an elevated love*)
- 1 drop pink rose absolute (*creating a home that is a sanctuary*)

꙳ Pan's Consort Milk Bath

- 1 cup goat's milk (*wild abandon*)
- 1 tablespoon banana macerated oil (*culmination of pleasure*)
- 1 tablespoon orchid macerated oil (*naturalized sexuality, feeling juicy in your skin*)
- 1 drop vanilla essential oil (*helps heal emotional conflicts that keep you from giving yourself to another, the ecstasy of surrender*)

꙳ You're Keepin' Me Down, Man, Salt Scrub

- 1 cup Molokai red sea salt (*detoxifies emotions, dispelling heavy energy*)
- ¾ cup okra seed oil (*not being pressured to do something you don't want to*)
- ¼ cup milk thistle oil (*firm, safe boundaries set without guilt*)
- 6 drops kumquat essential oil (*not being ensnared in obligatory situations or relationships*)

꙳ Taking a Nap in Oz Milk Bath

- ¼ cup Kilauea onyx sea salt (*a portal to dreamtime*)
- ¼ cup powdered yak's milk (*allows you to travel to other dimensions of time and space*)
- 3 tablespoons poppy seed oil (*slipping into the holographic universe*)
- 1 drop frankincense essential oil (*day trip into the mystic*)

Song Blends

The following four blends reflect the essence of some of my favorite songs. A wonderful way to make and absorb these blends is to listen to the song as you make it and then apply it. Once you are comfortable with the technique, explore your own music library. We often listen to music to shape mood and atmosphere. Use your song blends the same way, anchoring your favorite music into both body and soul.

"This Is to Mother You," by Sinéad O'Connor

This is to mother you
To comfort you and get you through
Through when your nights are lonely
Through when your dreams are only blue
This is to mother you.

- 3 tablespoons oat oil (*the comfort of feeling safe and loved when your heart and soul ache*)
- 1 drop spinach absolute (*Universal mother energy*)

"Sisters Are Doin' It for Themselves," by The Eurythmics

Now this is a song to celebrate
The conscious liberation of the female state

- ¼ cup okra oil (*helps eliminate dominant/submissive dynamics, you are free*)
- 1 drop grapefruit essential oil (*helps you find a way out when you're trapped in authoritarian powers*)

"Draggin' the Line," by Tommy James and the Shondells

Makin' a livin' the old hard way
Takin' and givin' my day by day
I dig snow and rain and bright sunshine
Draggin' the line.

- 1 tablespoon broccoli oil (*helps you choose your tasks with freedom and joy*)
- 1 drop lemon essential oil (*gaiety that frees you from what shackles you, encouraging you to do what you dig*)

"Wuthering Heights," by Kate Bush

Out on the wily, windy moors
We'd roll and fall in green
You had a temper like my jealousy
Too hot, too greedy

- ¼ cup Epsom salt—for this body scrub blend
- 3 tablespoons Japanese shinkai deep sea salt (*healing the deep wounds of the soul that have resulted from faith betrayed, love dishonored, trust forsaken*)
- 1 drop spinach absolute (*rolling and falling into the green and jealousy*)
- 1 drop cinnamon leaf essential oil (*too hot, too greedy*)
- Fractionated coconut oil—enough to completely saturate the salt

Body Oils That Smell Like a Place

These blends offer a delightful scent holiday, inviting you to journey and explore the world—all from the comfort of your home. Allow yourself to be transported.

Smells are surer than sounds or sights
To make your heart-strings crack.
— RUDYARD KIPLING

🌿 South of Italy

This blend smells like a caprese salad, a sun-filled afternoon, and lunch on the patio. Your senses are refreshed with the wholesome fragrances of tomato ripening on the vine, lemon and basil, uplifting mind and spirit.

- 1 cup tomato seed fixed oil (*slightly sweet, with fresh soil notes and a green, vine-like dry out, hands in the garden*)
- 6 drops lemon essential oil (*bursting with brightness, tangy zest, and refreshing sharpness, accented by a clean, slightly acidic vibrancy*)
- 3 drops basil essential oil (*slightly sharp herbaceous notes with light peppery elements, warmth of midday*)

❧ Napa, California

This blend smells like luxury and indulgence—warm sunshine, lush vineyards, the air scented with grapes and orange blooms—inviting you to relax and savor every moment.

- 1 cup grapeseed oil (*sweet, juicy aroma with a hint of tartness and a fresh, fruity essence; depending on the variety, may also include subtle musky or floral notes*)
- 1 tablespoon avocado fixed oil (*buttery, rich, and indulgent*)
- 6 drops bergamot essential oil (*bright, sparkling aroma that captures the essence of liquid sunshine; this charmingly fresh blend of citrusy notes is accented with a subtle dash of spiciness, radiating warmth and vitality*)
- 4 drops neroli essential oil (*flower of the orange tree produces an oil with a bright white floral and green aroma, delicately layered with hints of honey and sweet orange*)

❧ Finnskogen Forest ("Forest of the Finns")

Finnskogen ("Forest of the Finns") Forest is an area in Sweden and Norway that was settled by immigrants from Finland in the 1600s. The Forest Finns, as they were known, understood nature from an eastern shamanistic tradition, and they are often associated with magic and mystery. Rituals, spells, and symbols were used as a practical tool in daily life that one could use to heal, protect, or safeguard against evil.

- ¾ cup cloudberry oil (*hints of peach and vanilla offer a white scent, like a first snow—fresh and new*)
- ¼ cup Artic cranberry oil (*tart, refreshing berry scent with a cool touch, reminiscent of fresh cranberries and subtle green or herbal notes*)
- 12 drops Siberian fir absolute (*fresh, piney aroma with hints of citrus and wood, crisp and green with a balsamic quality and a slightly camphorous undertone, reminiscent of a classic Christmas tree*)
- 3 drops peppermint essential oil (*strong, penetrating, fresh, cold, and sharp minty scent*)

❧ American Midwest Road Trip, Windows Down

The very essence of Ward and June Cleaver—comfort, safety, and the charm of suburban life—this blend evokes a sense of wholesomeness, warmth, and nurturing, where home and family are the heart of everything.

- ¾ cup oat oil (*comforting, warm aroma reminiscent of freshly baked oatmeal cookies, with a nutty hint of toasted grain*)

¼ cup wheat germ oil (*freshly baked bread*)
6 drops bergamot essential oil (*wholesomeness of sitting on the porch in the sun*)
4 drops lilac absolute (*sweet, floral, and powdery scent with notes of green, almond, and jasmine, reminiscent of an elegant, old-fashioned perfume your grandmother would wear*)
4 drops sweetgrass absolute (*the neighbor mowing his lawn*)
1 drop spinach absolute (*the fresh green of the hedgerow being trimmed*)

New York, New York

This scent takes you to the raw, eclectic atmosphere of CBGB—a dive bar on a worn street where a new musical scene emerged, shaping the careers of artists like Patti Smith, Blondie, and the Ramones. With hints of hot garbage on a summer night, vibrant cultures, exotic foods, and urban decay, it's balanced by a subtle floral sweetness, evoking a night that never ends until dawn.

½ cup dragon fruit oil (*mildly sweet, floral scent with hints of tropical fruit, blending honeyed sweetness with a subtle funk characteristic of exotic fruits*)
½ cup passion fruit oil (*a slightly sulfurous element to its aroma, with tropical sweetness and a hint of tangy brightness*)
1 tablespoon apple seed fixed oil (*fresh, crisp, and slightly sweet with a mouthwatering quality, reminiscent of biting into a fresh apple*)
6 drops blood orange essential oil (*sparkling, charismatic, bright orange scent*)
3 drops patchouli essential oil (*controversial fragrance that can smell earthy, musky, or offer hints of urban decay*)

New Orleans

This blend smells like getting your cards read at voodoo priestess Marie Laveau's old herb shop, having a black cat cross your path, getting lost in the Garden District, and feeling musical elements of syncopation, improvisation, and call-and-response feed your soul.

1 cup black currant oil (*primary note is a fresh, dark fruit aroma reminiscent of ripe blackberries with a touch of tartness*)
6 drops black currant absolute (*tart, juicy fruit; slightly green, leafy with "catty" undertones; often described as a fruity scent with an animalic quality*)

- 3 drops magnolia absolute (*the scent of a magnolia flower is often linked to hot summer nights in the South, its sweet and creamy fragrance hanging heavy during humid evenings*)
- 2 drops jasmine essential oil (*sweet, heady, and intoxicating with a thick, powdery scent that's a cross between heliotrope and honeysuckle*)

Namdroling Tibetan Monastery Golden Temple, Northern India

This blend smells like the essence of a puja in India. The word puja is derived from the Dravidian term pu, meaning "flower." In its simplest form, puja involves offering flowers, embodying devotion, humility, and the seeking of inner peace and contemplation.

- ½ cup borage seed oil (*fresh cucumber scent*)
- ½ cup goji berry oil (*a scent similar to cranberry with earthy and herbal hemp notes*)
- 14 drops sandalwood essential oil (*warm, creamy, earthy, rich, and comforting with subtle sweet, spicy, and musky undertones; smells like being uplifted and cloaked in reverence, holding the fragrance of a sacred puja*)
- 3 drops juhi absolute (*reminiscent of gardenia flowers with top notes of olibanum, tropical fruits, and a rich balsamic undertone; smells like devotion and prayer*)
- 1 drop gardenia absolute (*creamy scent with notes of coconut and peach skin, complemented by a heady indolic element of jasmine and the energy of wanting to connect to all that is*)
- 1 drop white lotus absolute (*a warm green floral aroma with earthy, sweet, and fruity-floral undertones, balanced by traces of indole and smells of stillness*)

My Grandmother's Kitchen (on my dad's side)

This blend smells like freshly baked treats, the warmth of a favorite sweater, a grandmother's love, and a bear hug.

- ½ cup fractionated coconut oil
- ¼ cup pumpkin seed oil (*warm, rich, and nutty*)
- 6 drops marjoram essential oil (*a mild, sweet scent with hints of mint and woody undertones and the energy of hygge—embracing simplicity, creating comfort, and taking time to connect with those you care about*)
- 6 drops common orange essential oil (*a warm citrus scent that exudes cheerfulness, with bright, uplifting notes and inclusive coziness*)

3 drops cinnamon leaf essential oil (*warm, sweet, slightly spicy, and woody; this is comforting and inviting aroma that smells like baked treats and cozy moments*)

My Grandmother's Kitchen (on my mom's side)

This blend smells like learning to cook at someone's knee, Sunday dinner with friends and family—filled with rich, hearty aromas and the warmth of togetherness.

½ cup corn oil (*cornfields have a sweet, honey-like scent, especially when ripe, with a hint of floral and the richness of damp earth, creating a warm, earthy aroma*)
¼ cup wheat bran oil (*freshly baked bread*)
3 tablespoons tomato seed oil (*sweet, slightly tangy scent with a touch of earthiness, often described as a "fresh summer" aroma, blending juicy fruit with a hint of green vine—happiness in your nose*)
3 drops lemon essential oil (*bright, zesty, tangy, citrusy, and refreshing with a sharp, slightly acidic quality that offers an invigorating and clean burst of freshness with a distinct "pop"*)
1 drop oregano essential oil (*a strong, pungent, camphoraceous odor, often associated with Mediterranean cooking, bringing mouthwatering herbal and warming notes*)

Off the Beach in Encinitas, California

This blend smells like ocean breezes, warm sand, and suntan oil; the tang of citrus and the faint aroma of driftwood carried by the waves; it's the scent of endless summer—sun-soaked relaxation and carefree days.

½ cup golden jojoba oil (*sun-warmed skin*)
3 tablespoons virgin coconut oil (*Hawaiian Tropic suntan oil—oh, come on, you know you like it!*)
3 tablespoons pineapple oil (*the second half of the Hawaiian Tropic suntan oil*)
3 drops grapefruit essential oil (*citrus, fresh, tart, and lively with a subtle hint of bitterness*)
3 drops kumquat essential oil (*a bright, citrusy scent similar to orange but fruitier and lighter; it carries a touch of richness with notes of coconut milk and pineapple; smells like sunny Southern California coast*)
3 drops pink pepper seed oil (*sharp, spicy scent with rosy overtones, often described as bright, cheerful, and accented with woody notes; this tree grows in abundance in this area*)

Appendix

Practices for Growth, Heart Opening, and Deep Purification

Mindfulness Bath to Support Growth

Authentic growth always entails a life-death-rebirth experience, as expressed in archetypal stories of the hero's journey and in the literature of almost every culture in the world. In the Bible we have the story of Jonah: "For as Jonah was three days and three nights in the whale's belly, so shall the Son of man be three days and three nights in the heart of the earth" (Matthew 12:40). And there is the account of the Resurrection, where Jesus literally died on the cross, was entombed in a cave for three days, and then ascended in his light body.

The Sumerian culture has a similar story, as does Egypt and Vedic India. It was for three days and three nights that the Sumerian moon goddess, Inanna, hung dead from a hook in the Great Below until, revived by the water and food of life, she ascended back into the Great Above. It was for three nights that the left eye of Horus was torn into pieces and thrown into outer darkness, when Thoth reassembled it, piecing it together until it was whole. In Vedic India, it is believed that those who die on the dark moon will reincarnate three nights later during the crescent moon phase, when they fall into the wombs of their new mothers as a rain of soma.

The promise of a new beginning as experienced through the cycle of death and rebirth can feel frightening if the change is uninvited. In the tarot, this concept is expressed as the Tower card, the idea that once a powerful citadel offering security becomes a limiting prison, the walls must come down to allow new life in. As we all know, when the wheel of life turns there is no stopping it. Anyone who has lost a relationship, a job, a friendship, or simply an aspect of oneself that needed to be shed can relate to this energy.

This Mindfulness Bath allows you to see where you're at in your personal cycle so you can move into growth consciously and with a perspective that allows you to see that a cycle of loss will lead to gain. In this way you can experience a metaphorical death and rebirth without fear, resentment, or anger, as you see the bigger truth found in the blessings of growth. We will be calling on the energies of plant allies and archetypes to help you see what it is you need to shed, plant, and harvest for your continuing evolution.

Certain divinities arose in our mythologies by virtue of their embodying certain archetypes arising from the collective unconscious. Understanding gods and goddesses as archetypes lends credibility to their sacredness and their power to invoke divine energy. These energies are represented in the Mindfulness Bath in the choice of essential oils, milks, and salt.

In Greek mythology, the Moirae—in English, the Fates—are beings of destiny, three wizened crones who spin and weave the threads of your life. Destiny is often confusing—as it is unfolding it can be hard to see the horizon. Take heart, for all growth requires a time of initiation.

Initiation is one of those concepts that seems exciting on paper but in reality can feel like a trial by fire. Call on the Moirae, the Fates, for clarity in your next steps, and they will assist you on your way. It is important to stay grounded (patchouli), to keep a clear head and nimble mind (lemon, black pepper), and to go with the flow and make decisions on a moment-to-moment basis to best craft your reality (red spikenard, frankincense). If you must experience a loss before you can achieve a gain, take the time to really experience your emotions and mourn (lavender). Working with the Fates will allow you to stay centered amid challenging situations so you can trust the future and the unfoldment of right action.

The Fates resonate with all the essential oils, so choose intuitively those that support the nexus of where fate is guiding you.

Let's take a look at a few of nature's allies that specifically allow you to work with the energy of growth in a graceful way.

Mindfulness Bath Blend

3 drops cyclamen absolute
3 tablespoons strawberry seed fixed oil
¼ cup camel's milk (optional)
½ cup Himalayan pink salt (optional)

Cyclamen absolute encourages you to see where you have calcified ideas about life, about situations, or about other people so you can perceive in a fresh, new perspective. This shift is powerfully freeing—in fact, it is transformative. Cyclamen can help you crystalize your new understandings so you can anchor them in the material realm to grow them. Strawberry seed fixed oil evokes the brilliant colors of a fauvist painting, encouraging you to express your wildness, to be adventurous and daring and willing to take a risk. As you trust the Divine to deliver what it is you truly need, you feel the excitement of venturing out of the known to experience the vast wonders of the world.

If you wish to find additional plant allies for this Mindfulness Bath, close your eyes, right hand on your heart, shake out your left hand, and hover it over essential oil bottles that you've preselected. You are feeling for the strongest sensation. Once that sensation, whatever it is, is revealed, open your eyes and read the energy signature of the essential oil chosen in chapter 1. Then, if you feel called to do so, add the following to this Mindfulness Bath:

- **Camel's milk** brings the energy of caretaking by the archetypal Mother and Father. This opens you to feeling unconditional love, trust, and hope and supports you to persevere through your cycle with patience and resourcefulness. If using dehydrated camel's milk powder in this bath blend, you can top off with any fresh milk you have on hand (cow, almond, coconut, and so forth) if you wish.

- **Himalayan pink salt** offers an ancient healing energy from the highest peaks in the world. The energy of this salt combines the power of three: primal waters that represent pure potentiality; the wisdom of intuition that recognizes the truth that shapes lives and destinies; and the power of logic to organize, process, and use the divine information being expressed so you can act on it.

Fill your bath with warm to hot water, add this bath blend to the running water, and stir in a figure 8 while asking your higher Self to reveal what it is you need to know at this time. Allow your mind to wander as you submerge yourself in the bath and see what knowledge is revealed.

Following the Mindfulness Bath, apply just a touch of cyclamen absolute and fixed strawberry oil to the center of your forehead using a soft, circular motion. Circle to the left if you want to let something go; circle to the right if you want to root something new in or keep growing what is already in motion. The subtle energy of this blend will support you as you consciously work through the cycle you are in. You can also dab on pulse points to be cloaked in this heavenly scent.

Heart Opening Practice

Wisdom traditions from all cultures remind us that the cosmic body and the human body are reflections of each other. The intelligence that organizes the activity of humankind also orchestrates the activity of the universe. Understanding this allows us to have a deeper relationship with nature and how to use her to navigate our own human nature. So, when you engage with any of the plant distillations in this book, see them as an extension of yourself, an aspect of you, and you in them. We are interconnected, made from the same raw materials, the same recycled earth, life force, mind, and spirit. The inner intelligence of our bodies is also the ultimate and supreme genius of nature and mirrors the wisdom of the universe.

The following blend uses plant distillations to focus on your sensual nature and a healthy, open heart. Note that this recipe calls for a tisane, which is a hot water herbal infusion—basically, an herbal tea.

White Lilac Tisane

1 cup water
3–4 tablespoons dried lilac flowers

Pour freshly boiled water into your cup or teapot, swirl, and then discard. Add the lilac flowers (the resulting flavor depends on how long you allow the flowers to steep in hot water). Two to three minutes of steeping achieves a subtle floral taste but not much aroma. Steeping four to five minutes develops a heady scent with a distinct tangy flavor. Lilac resets energy, creating a blank slate on which to inscribe a new story and a true new beginning, a fresh start, allowing you to remove energy blockages so you can lay down new patterns. After you make your tisane, consider the following:

- Do you simply want the energy of white lilac? If so, hold the affirmation in your heart, "I am forgiveness."
- If you want to cultivate more self-love in your life, add 1/2 teaspoon pink rose powder (see Resources) to 1 cup white lilac tisane, and hold the affirmation "I am love" in your heart.
- If you want more passionate love in your life, add 1/2 teaspoon beet powder (see Resources) to 1 cup white lilac tisane and hold the affirmation "I am sensual" in your heart.

The Gift of Beauty

Some orchids use nectar to entice their pollinators, although according to Oxford Academic (Oxford University's academic research platform),

46 percent of orchid varieties use some other sort of enticement, meaning they also employ color, shape, and fragrance, and they will even imitate the flowers of other plants to attract pollinators. Orchids offer beautiful and even uncanny forms that mimic other aspects of nature, such as a bee, a monkey, a flying duck, and a dove.

The orchid oil described in this book (see chapter 4) is the green-winged or green-veined variety and is a food-deceptive terrestrial orchid. This is simply a clinical way of saying that this flower is so visually appealing and its fragrance so enticing that its pollinators come and visit even without it being a food source. I like to think of this as a case of beauty for beauty's sake. Perhaps this is the same reason why we pause to look at sunsets, enjoy natural perfumes, and look at art. An endearing aspect of this plant is that its primary pollinators are bumblebees, especially bumblebee queens.

To devour orchid with your eyes and see what gifts are revealed to you, place the orchid plant of your choice in a place where you can sit comfortably while gazing at it. Have some macerated orchid oil at the ready. Place a drop or two of the oil on the center of your forehead and softly trace a circle. Put the tips of your fingers together forming an inverted V, tuck your thumbs into your palms, then place the outer edge of your pointer fingertips on your third eye. Take three deep breaths, asking that your mind become soft and receptive so that it has the ability to listen to the orchid and hear what is communicated. Then open your eyes and really look at the orchid and ask telepathically to be in relationship with this plant to see if it has any information just for you. Once the knowing comes, anoint your second chakra with this oil in a crescent moon shape, sealing that blessing in. If you are lucky, you and your new plant friend will live together a long time, as the life cycle of an orchid properly cared for is fifteen to twenty years.

Themes that arise in this practice can include: cultivating magnetism, sensuality, healthy sexuality, fertility, and supporting more romance in your life. This can help attract new love or revitalize an existing relationship that feels lackluster. It can also energetically prepare the body for conception.

Deep Purification Practices

The following purification practice uses white birch to heal the subtle layers of who we are: a field of energy, one that can be influenced by the vibrational and energetic qualities of nature. This practice gives you what you need to address the root cause of any imbalances and maximizes your ability to heal and come into balance.

Although all essential oils work on a subtle level to affect positive change, white birch is especially dynamic for deep purification anytime your energetic, emotional, or mental body feels gummed up. This tree and its oil have a long tradition of purifying both the subtle and the physical bodies. White birch essential oil is perfect for a monthly purification ceremony for a general reset. It is also recommended as a first step when undertaking any intense healing journey. To this end it is commonly used in Native American sweat lodge ceremonies for preparation, prayer, and purification.

This purification blend holds the elemental energy of water along with the seed of fire. Birch as an expression of the element of water holds the energy of the divine feminine in the form of the White Goddess and Brigid, the Lady of the Forest. It shines light in the darkness for deep purification, expands your appreciation of beauty as well as your own inner radiance, and offers emotional succor, protection, and a profound sense of calm. The essential oil of the birch tree has the same effect on the spirit as the living tree has in dreary winter landscapes, bringing a glowing, silvery-white radiance into the dark winter months.

The element of fire used in this practice is very dynamic:

- It initiates projects with passion, enthusiasm, and warmth.
- It transmutes any situation that does not serve one's higher Self.
- As the element in which form first comes into being, fire supports the birth of the ego and experiences centered in one's personal identity.
- It relates to the mental body and the ability to direct one's personal will and act on ideas in the physical world.

- Representing the divine masculine, it offers protection and the sensations of bliss, growth, change, increase, and evolution.

On the shadow side, too little fire results in:

- an inability to stand up for oneself or deal with confrontation
- passivity

Too much fire leads to:

- arrogance, feeling superior, and "my way or the highway" attitude
- a lack of self-control, volatility, instability, a devouring force
- "hot" qualities like anger, quarrelsomeness, and confrontational behavior.

These are not abstract characteristics but living dispositions embedded in behaviors that are produced by the element of fire. White birch, as a representative of water and the divine feminine, calms the energy of fire and as such is a resonate gateway that makes the energy of water accessible.

Fire Diffusion Ritual

This practice works with the elemental energies of water and fire. We'll be using a tea light diffuser to work with fire, while white birch brings the energy of water. A fascinating aspect of using plant oils with intent involves incorporating numerology. In this practice we will explore the numbers 6 and 11. The number 6 represents structured dynamism, the ability to spontaneously respond in the moment and allow any feedback you get to assist in restructuring yourself. The number 11 represents the dissolution of form, disconnecting from the collective, intuition, and releasing limitations to advance new potentials.

1. Place a tea light diffuser on a white cloth and fill the diffuser bowl with water.

2. Close your eyes and take three deep clearing and grounding breaths, inhaling through your nose and exhaling through your mouth. Then ask your deep self what energy, that of the number 6 or the number 11, will most support your life at this time? Wait for the answer to intuitively arise in your mind.
3. Add the number of birch essential oil drops you have been guided to use to the water in the diffuser bowl, and as you do so, reflect on the properties of the number in your mind. The number 6 indicates that you are leaning into creating something; 11 shows you are moving away from something. Light the tea candle and gaze softly at the flame until your mind is settled.
4. Meditate on the subtle properties of white birch (see chapter 2) as an expression of beauty and the divine feminine. It brings light into darkness and provides deep purification, emotional succor, protection, and a profound sense of calm. It expands your appreciation of beauty and your own inner radiance as a reflection of that archetype.
5. Invoke the energy of water (see chapter 5). Water opens a portal to the soul and reflects the divine feminine and the collective unconscious. Dreams are the primary way this element communicates to us. Water is the most creative element for birthing new ideas, projects, or environments.
6. Invoke the element of fire (see chapter 5). Fire holds the energy of awakening, of creativity, in which all the rich, fertile information within is mined and brought to the surface for the intellect to use. Fire is the catalyst in life. It is the great transformer that consumes in order to renew.
7. Assume a comfortable meditative posture with your head, neck, and spine aligned. Set the tea light diffuser two feet in front of you, with the flame positioned at eye level.
8. Begin with your eyes closed, surveying your body and watching your breath until it becomes calm, regular, and even.
9. Open your eyes and rest your gaze on the middle part of the flame, right above the tip of the wick. Keeping your eyelids slightly more

open than usual, maintain your gaze without blinking or blurring your vision for as long as possible.
10. Observe any thoughts that arise, watching them come and go without becoming engaged.
11. Close your eyes only when they begin to feel strained or start to water and you can no longer sustain the steady gaze. You can cup your palms and place them gently over the eyes to ease any strain, but do not rub your eyes because the tears you have shed are carrying away impurities. Wipe them gently with a tissue if you wish.
12. With your eyes still closed, find the afterimage of the flame in your mind's eye, resting your awareness at the ajna chakra (the third eye or eyebrow center). If the image moves up and down or from side to side, stabilize it by bringing it back to the center and continue to inwardly fix your gaze on it until the impression disappears.
13. Allow yourself to come back to the present and, when you are ready, open your eyes. Allow the flame to burn on, holding space. You are now primed for the next practice.

Gayatri Mantra Practice

The Gayatri mantra, found in the Rig Veda and first transcribed on birch bark, is used for purification of the body, mind, and spirit. My favorite description of this mantra comes from Deva Premal, a German singer known for her recordings of chants, including the Gayatri mantra: "The name 'Gayatri' can be translated as the 'Song of Liberation,'" she says. "It is said to be the most ancient of the mantras, an indigenous prayer to the sun asking for the enlightenment of all beings. It invokes the radiant source of life itself, purifying our thoughts, words and actions."[1]

This mantra

- purifies negative emotions and ways of being
- strengthens the mind and improves concentration
- helps slacken the bondage of karmas
- builds good intentions

- cultivates prosperity consciousness
- opens the mind to fulfill deep desires

For this practice you will need to have a sheet of birch bark paper and a pen with gold ink at the ready. Birch bark paper is readily available online from various sources (see Resources). Gold ink represents the power of fire, the sun, and the divine masculine; birch bark represents water, the moon, and the divine feminine. You can anoint your third eye with birch essential oil before beginning the practice.

The Gayatri mantra:

> *Om Bhur Bhuvah Svah*
> *Tat savitur varenyam*
> *Bhargo devasya dhimahi*
> *Dhiyo yo nah prachodayat*

The approximate English translation of the Sanskrit: "We meditate on that most adored Supreme Lord, the creator, whose effulgence (divine light) illumines all realms (physical, mental, and spiritual). May this divine light illumine our intellect."

To begin the Gayatri purification ritual, perform the following steps:

1. Place your right hand on your heart and your left hand on your stomach. Close your eyes, deeply breathing in the scent of the distilled white birch.
2. Begin chanting the mantra, allowing its sound and vibration, along with the energy of white birch, to wash over you to repattern you. If you feel more comfortable doing so, chant along with a recording, such as Deva Premal's version, which is available online. Repeat the mantra as many times as you feel guided. When you feel ready, open your eyes.
3. Now begin writing the sacred syllables of the Gayatri mantra (as shown above) on the birch bark paper with your golden pen: Imagine that the golden ink is the luminous sun as you inscribe the sacred syl-

lables of purification and awakening on the birch bark paper, allowing your divine nature to synchronize with nature's heartbeat.
4. When you feel you are complete, sink silently into space and time and visualize repurposing any disturbing energy that does not serve you.

Now that you have purified yourself with diffused white birch, fire, and mantra, it is time to make your Gayatri purification blend. This blend ushers in the anticipation of miracles, movement into the light, passing on blessings, and service given from a place of strength.

❧ Gayatri Purification Blend

¾ teaspoon safflower fixed oil (*knowledge, consciousness, synthesis, spiritual empowerment*)
6 or 11 drops white birch essential oil (*deep purification, emotional succor, protection, and a profound sense of calm*)

1. Start by placing a dab of safflower fixed oil in your palms and rub your hands together. Feel its viscosity. Do your hands slide easily? Does the oil warm up and create heat? Does the oil feel cool? Neutral? What scents do you detect? What descriptive words come to mind? Sunny? Bright? Masculine? Calm? Safe?
2. Add either 6 or 11 drops of white birch essential oil to a half-dram (about 1/16 of an ounce) amber glass bottle filled with safflower oil. Recap. Gently rolling the bottle in your hands back and forth, quietly invite white birch to come and work with you, until it feels enlivened.
3. Invoke the spirit of white birch by repeating the following: *Uttering your very name wraps me in protection from disturbances both internal and external. I appeal to you to expand my knowledge into wisdom in the context of working with my disturbed energies. Support my desire that my heart, mind, and actions always reflect this wisdom, and that I understand and become one with universal truth, purifying any aspects of myself that limit this.*
4. Hold the bottle to your heart and ask for any limiting aspects of

yourself to be released. Do a body scan, feeling deeply into the physical and the subtle bodies for any limiting aspects of self that come to mind or that you intuitively feel.
5. Take some time to mindfully and with respect anoint yourself with this blend anywhere on your body where you feel called to do so.

Resources

Absolute and Essential Oil Suppliers

AnimaMundiHerbals.com
Aromatics.com
DivineArchetypes.org
EdensGarden.com
FragrantEarth.com
HermitageOils.com
LgBotanicals.com
LibertyNatural.com
MountainRoseHerbs.com
Oshadhi.co.uk
PhibeeAromatics.com
Starwest-Botanicals.com
YorkshireFlowerEssences.com

Fixed Oil Suppliers

BulkApothecary.com
LibertyNatural.com
MountainRoseHerbs.com
Starwest-Botanicals.com

Sources for Hard-to-Find Milks

Camel's milk: DesertFarms.com
Water buffalo's milk: AmosMillerOrganicFarm.com
Yak's milk: Finding a local source through health food stores or farmers markets is best. Powdered milks can be ordered online, often internationally.

Plant Butter Suppliers

BulkApothecary.com
LibertyNatural.com
MountainRoseHerbs.com
Starwest-Botanicals.com

Salt Sources

Redmond.life
TheMeadow.com

Other Supply Sources for Recipes and Rituals

Beeswax: MountainRoseHerbs.com
Beet root powder: MountainRoseHerbs.com
Birch bark paper: Rudraksham.com or Etsy
Pink rose powder: AnimaMundiHerbals.com
PlantWave: PlantWave.com
White lilac tea: ReverieFarmLLC.com

Sources for All Types of Diffusers

LibertyNatural.com
MountainRoseHerbs.com
Starwest-Botanicals.com

Bottle and Container Suppliers

ContainerAndPackaging.com
SKS-bottle.com

Recommended Reading

Aromatherapy for Healing the Spirit: Restoring Emotional and Mental Balance with Essential Oils by Gabriel Mojay

Essential Oils and Aromatherapy Workbook by Marcel Lavabre

Essential Oils for Mindfulness and Meditation: Relax, Replenish, and Rejuvenate by Heather Dawn Godfrey, PGCE, BSc

Essential Oils for the Whole Body: The Dynamics of Topical Application and Absorption by Heather Dawn Godfrey, PGCE, BSc

Essential Oils in Spiritual Practice: Working with the Chakras, Divine Archetypes, and the Five Great Elements by Candice Covington

The Healing Intelligence of Essential Oils: The Science of Advanced Aromatherapy by Kurt Schnaubelt, Ph.D.

Healing with Essential Oils: The Antiviral, Restorative, and Life-Enhancing Properties of 58 Plants by Heather Dawn Godfrey

Hidden Meanings in Chinese Art by Terese Tse Bartholomew

The Meaning of Trees: Botany, History, Healing, Lore by Fred Hageneder

Meeting the Melissae: The Ancient Greek Bee Priestesses of Demeter by Elizabeth Ashley

The Tarot Apothecary: Shifting Personal Energies Using Tarot, Aromatherapy, and Simple Everyday Rituals by Ailynn Halvorson

Working with Unusual Essential Oils by Helen Nagle-Smith

Notes

INTRODUCTION: MEETING NATURE IN STORY

1. "*The Son of Man*, 1946 by Rene Magritte," Renemagritte.org, accessed February 7, 2025.
2. Chodron, *How to Free Your Mind*, 19.
3. Henry David Thoreau, "Wild Apples," available online at Project Gutenberg.

CHAPTER 1. ABSOLUTES

1. As quoted by Hillman, *A Blue Fire*, 115–16.
2. Wolkstein and Kramer, *Inanna*, 52.
3. Wolkstein and Kramer, *Inanna*, 58.
4. Wolkstein and Kramer, *Inanna*, 58.
5. Wolkstein and Kramer, *Inanna*, 60.
6. Wolkstein and Kramer, *Inanna*, 64.
7. Heilmeyer, *Language of Flowers*, 64.
8. Guttman and Johnson, *Mythic Astrology Applied*, 100.
9. Shore, "An Absurdist Pantomime," 158.
10. Ovid, *Metamorphoses*, 4.167.
11. Philostratus, *Life of Apollonius*, 1.31.
12. Calaprice, *New Quotable Einstein*, 316.
13. Pollan, *Botany of Desire*, xv.
14. Pollan, *Botany of Desire*, xv–xvi.
15. Covington, *Vibrational Nutrition*, 36.
16. Bailey, *Esoteric Psychology*, 152.
17. Tolkien, *Two Towers*, 98.
18. Bartholomew, *Hidden Meanings*, 46.
19. Jung, *Collected Works vol. 14*, paragraph 689.
20. Ovid, *Metamorphoses*, Book X.
21. Herrera, "Holy Smoke."

22. Ovid, *Metamorphoses*, Book III.
23. Ovid, *Metamorphoses*, Book III.
24. Ovid, *Metamorphoses*, Book III.
25. Prabhavananda and Isherwood, *Shankara's Crest-Jewel*, 54.
26. Ovid, *Metamorphoses*, Book III.
27. Ryan and Matthews, *Wildwood Tarot*, 60.
28. Ovid, *Metamorphoses*, Book III.
29. Ovid, *Metamorphoses*, Book III.
30. Ovid, *Metamorphoses*, Book III.
31. Hageneder, *Meaning of Trees*, 176.
32. Hageneder *Meaning of Trees*, 176.
33. Bolen, *Gods in Everyman*, 49.
34. Teilhard de Chardin, *Heart of the Matter*, 63, 65.
35. Covington, *Vibrational Nutrition*, 3.
36. Arden, *Bear and the Nightingale*, 22.
37. Frazer, *Golden Bough*, 381.
38. Frazer, *Golden Bough*, 363.
39. Verner-Bonds, *Color for Healing*, 28.
40. Covington, *Vibrational Nutrition*, 34–35.

CHAPTER 3. FIXED OILS

1. Zaa, Marcelo, An, Medina-Franco, and Velasco-Velázquez, "Anthocyanins."
2. Pearson, *Flower Essences*, 429.
3. Hunter and Jacobus, *Modern Art*, 103.
4. Covington, *Vibrational Nutrition*, 68.
5. Ovid, *Metamorphoses*, Book IV, 214–55, 256–73.
6. Bolen, *Gods in Everyman*, 135.
7. Guttman and Johnson, *Mythic Astrology Applied*, 163.
8. Guttman and Johnson, *Mythic Astrology Applied*, 234.

CHAPTER 4. OTHER TANTALIZING TIDBITS

1. Seyedinia et al., "Saffron and crocin."
2. Frawley, *Ayurveda and the Mind*, 31.
3. Wolkstein and Kramer, *Inanna*, 39.

CHAPTER 5.
OUR BODY AS EXPRESSED IN THE ELEMENTS

1. Dandine-Roulland, Laurent, Dall'Ara, Toupance, and Chaix, "Genomic Evidence."
2. McGee, *Nose Dive*, xvi.
3. Saraswati, *Tattwa Shuddhi*, 56.
4. "*The Son of Man*, 1946 by Rene Magritte," Renemagritte.org, accessed February 7, 2025.

CHAPTER 7. SYMBOLIC ANATOMY

1. Moore, *Care of the Soul*, 171–72.
2. Talbot, *Holographic Universe*, 54–55.
3. Jimbo et al., "Effect of Aromatherapy"; Pandur et al., "Linalool and Geraniol Defend Neurons."
4. Anderson, *Ugly One*, "John Lilly."
5. "Man Ray (Emmanuel Radnitzky)," MoMA.org, accessed February 14, 2025.
6. Andrews, *Amulets*, 83.
7. Jung, *Collected Works vol. 9*, 282.
8. Schweitzer, "Beginner's Guide."
9. Schweitzer, "Beginner's Guide."
10. Hillman quoted in Guttman and Johnson, *Mythic Astrology*, 108.
11. Webster, *Palm Reading*, 170.

CHAPTER 8. ALCHEMICAL CREATIONS

1. Jung, *Collected Works vol. 9*, 6.
2. Klimt, quoted in Kandel, *Age of Insight*, 103, 104.
3. "Mars and Venus United by Love," MetMuseum.org, accessed February 14, 2025.
4. "The Veteran in a New Field," MetMuseum.org, accessed February 25, 2025.
5. "Broken Eggs," MetMuseum.org, accessed February 26, 2025.
6. "The Strange Thing Little Kiosai Saw in the River, 1897," Arthur.io, accessed February 25, 2025.
7. "The Dream of the Shepherd (Der Traum des Hirten)," MetMuseum.org, accessed February 14, 2025.

8. "Diana and Actaeon (Diana Surprised in Her Bath)," MetMuseum.org, accessed February 25, 2025.
9. "Watson and the Shark," MetMuseum.org, accessed February 26, 2025.
10. Covington, *Vibrational Nutrition*, 58.

APPENDIX.
PRACTICES FOR GROWTH, HEART OPENING, AND DEEP PURIFICATION

1. "Deva Premal: Gayatri Mantra Meditation," DevaPremalMiten.com, accessed February 27, 2025.

Bibliography

Anderson, Laurie. *The Ugly One with the Jewels*. Warner Brothers UK, 2007.

Andrews, Carol. *Amulets of Ancient Egypt*. Austin: University of Texas Press, 1994.

Arden, Katherine. *The Bear and the Nightingale: A Novel*. New York: Del Rey, 2017.

Bailey, Alice. *Esoteric Psychology Vol. I: A Treatise on the Seven Rays*. New York: Lucis Publishing, 1979; available online at Internet Archive.

Barks, Coleman, trans., with John Moyne. *The Essential Rumi*. Edison, NJ: Castle Books, 1997.

Bartholomew, Terese Tse. *Hidden Meanings in Chinese*. San Francisco: Asian Art Museum, 2006.

Bolen, Jean Shinoda. *Gods in Everyman: Archetypes That Shape Men's Lives*. New York: HarperPerennial, 1989.

Calaprice, Alice, ed. *The New Quotable Einstein*. Princeton, NJ: Princeton University Press, 2005.

Cashford, Jules. *The Moon: Myth and Image*. New York: Four Walls Eight Windows, 2003.

Chodron, Thubten. *How to Free Your Mind: Tara the Liberator*. Ithaca, NY: Snow Lion Publications, 2005.

Chopra, Deepak, ed., trans., and Fereydoun Kia. *The Love Poems of Rumi*. New York: Harmony Books, 1998.

Covington, Candice. *Vibrational Nutrition: Understanding the Energetic Signatures of Food*. Rochester, VT: Healing Arts Press, 2021.

Dandine-Roulland, Claire, Romain Laurent, Irene Dall'Ara, Bruno Toupance, and Raphaëlle Chaix. "Genomic Evidence for MHC Disassortative Mating in Humans." *Proceedings of the Royal Society Biological Sciences* 286, no. 1899 (2019).

Dante (Dante Alighieri). *The Inferno*. Translated by John Ciardi. New York: Signet Classics, 2009.

Dougans, Inge. *The Complete Illustrated Guide to Reflexology: Therapeutic Foot Massage for Health and Well-Being*. Element Books, 1999.

Frawley, David. *Ayurveda and the Mind: The Healing of Consciousness*. Silver Lake, WI: Lotus Press, 1997.

Frazer, James G. *The Golden Bough: A Study in Magic and Religion*. New York: Macmillan, 1925.

Govinda, Lama Anagarika. *Creative Meditation and Multi-Dimensional Consciousness*. Wheaton, IL: Theosophical Publishing House, 1976.

Guttman, Ariel, and Kenneth Johnson. *Mythic Astrology Applied: Personal Healing through the Planets*. St. Paul, MN: Llewellyn Publications, 2004.

Hageneder, Fred. *The Meaning of Trees: Botany, History, Healing, Lore*. San Francisco: Chronicle Books, 2005.

Heilmeyer, Marina. *The Language of Flowers: Symbols and Myths*. Prestel Publishing, 2006.

Herrera, Matthew D. "Holy Smoke: The Use of Incense in the Catholic Church." *Adoremus* 17, no. 10 (2012).

Hillman, James. *A Blue Fire*. New York: HarperPerennial, 1991.

Hunter, Sam, and John M. Jacobus. *Modern Art*, 3rd edition. New York: Harry N. Abrams, 1992.

Jimbo, D., Y. Kimura, M. Taniguchi, M. Inoue, and K. Urakami. "Effect of Aromatherapy on Patients with Alzheimer's Disease." *Psychogeriatrics* 9, no. 4 (2009): 173–79.

Jung, C. G. *The Collected Works of C. G. Jung, Vol. 9 (Part I)*. Princeton, NJ: Princeton University Press, 1969.

Jung, C. G. *The Collected Works of C. G. Jung, Vol. 14 (Part I)*. Princeton, NJ: Princeton University Press, 1970.

Kandel, Eric R. *The Age of Insight: The Quest to Understand the Unconscious in Art, Mind, and Brain*. New York: Random House, 2012.

Kollerstrom, Nick. *Gardening and Planting by the Moon*. London: W. Foulsham Ltd., 2022.

Lao Tzu. *The Way and Its Power: Lao Tzu's Tao Te Ching and Its Place in Chinese Thought*. Translated by Arthur Waley. New York: Grove Press, 1958.

Ladinsky, Daniel. *Love Poems from God: Inspirations from Twelve Sacred Voices of the East and West*. London: Penguin, 2002.

Lavabre, Marcel. *Aromatherapy Workbook*. Rochester, VT: Healing Arts Press, 1996.

McGee, Harold. *Nose Dive: A Field Guide to the World's Smells*. New York: Penguin Press, 2020.

Moore, Thomas. *Care of the Soul: A Guide for Cultivating Depth and Sacredness in Everyday Life*. New York: HarperCollins, 1992.

Moyne, John, and Coleman Barks, *Open Secret: Versions of Rumi*. Boston: Shambhala, 1999.

Ovid. *The Metamorphoses*. Translated by A. S. Kline (2000). Available online at Poetry in Translation.

Pandur, E., B. Major, T. Rák, K. Sipos, A. Csutak, and G. Horváth. "Linalool and Geraniol Defend Neurons from Oxidative Stress, Inflammation, and Iron Accumulation in In Vitro Parkinson's Models." *Antioxidants* (Basel) 13, no. 8 (2024).

Pearson, Nicholas. *Flower Essences from the Witch's Garden*. Rochester, VT: Destiny Books, 2022.

Pollan, Michael. *The Botany of Desire: A Plant's-Eye View of the World*. New York: Random House, 2002.

Prabhavananda (Swami) and Christopher Isherwood, trans. *Bhagavad-Gita: The Song of God*. Vedanta Society of Southern California/Signet Classic, 2002.

Prabhavanada (Swami) and Christopher Isherwood, trans. *Shankara's Crest-Jewel of Discrimination: Timeless Teachings on Nonduality*. Vedanta Society of So. California, 1947, 1975.

Ryan, Mark, and John Matthews. *The Wildwood Tarot: Wherein Wisdom Resides*. New York: Sterling Ethos, 2011.

Saraswati, Satyasangananda (Swami). *Tattwa Shuddhi: The Tantric Practice of Inner Purification*. Munger, Bihar, India: Bihar School of Yoga, 1984.

Schweitzer, Sophia. "A Beginner's Guide to Craniosacral Therapy—Core Connection." The Cranial Therapy Centre website.

Seyedinia, Seyed Ali, Parnia Tarahomi, Davood Abbarin, Katayoun Sedaghat, Ali Rashidy-Pour, Habib Yaribeygi, Abbas Ali Vafaei, and Payman Raise-Abdullahi. "Saffron and Crocin Ameliorate Prenatal Valproic Acid-Induced Autistic-Like Behaviors and Brain Oxidative Stress in the Male Offspring Rats." *Metabolic Brain Disease* 38, no. 7 (2023): 2231–41.

Shore, Barbara. "An Absurdist Pantomime: The Collision of Violence, Innocence, and Pseudoinnocence," in *Psychology at the Threshold*, Dennis Patrick Slattery and Lionel Corbett, eds. Carpinteria, CA: Pacifica Graduate Institute Publications, 2010.

Star, Jonathan, trans. *Rumi: In the Arms of the Beloved*. New York: Tarcher/Putnam, 1997.

Talbot, Michael. *The Holographic Universe: The Revolutionary Theory of Reality*. New York: HarperCollins, 1996.

Teilhard de Chardin, Pierre, *The Heart of Matter*. New York: HarperOne, 2002.

Tolkien, J. R. R. *The Two Towers* (first edition, fifth printing). Boston: Houghton Mifflin Co., 1982.

Verner-Bonds, Lilian. *Colour For Healing: Harnessing the Therapeutic Powers of the Rainbow for Health and Well-Being*. Lorenz Books, 2014.

Whitmont, Edward C. *The Symbolic Quest: Basic Concepts of Analytical Psychology.* Princeton University Press, 1979.

Wolkstein, Diane, and Samuel Noah Kramer. *Inanna, Queen of Heaven and Earth: Her Stories and Hymns from Sumer.* New York: Harper and Row, 1983.

Zaa, César A., Álvaro J. Marcelo, Zhiqiang An, José L. Medina-Franco, and Marco A. Velasco-Velázquez. "Anthocyanins: Molecular Aspects on Their Neuroprotective Activity." *Biomolecules* 13, no. 11 (2023): 1598.

Index

absolutes. *See also specific absolutes*
  about, 8–9, 10
  blending, 10
  chakras and, 207–8, 210, 212–17
  dilution rate, 10
  solvent extraction, 9–10
abundance, 79, 160
aglaia (*Aglaia odorata*), 12–13
air element. *See also* elements
  about, 195–97
  invoking, 195
  physical gate, 197–98
  plant pairings, 199–200
  sacred shape, 198
  silence, 195
ajna (third eye), 216–17
akasha (ether), 45–47
allegory, 263
almond, sweet (*Prunus amygdalus* var. *dulcis*), 108
amygdala, 233
anahata (heart chakra), 213–15
anisotropy, 283
Annamaya kosha, 23, 24
apple seed (*Pyrus malus*), 108–9
apricot seed (*Prunus persica, Prunus armeniaca*), 109
archetypes, 229, 309
arms, 250–52
Aromatherapy Workbook (Lavabre), 262

art, blending, 281–93
ascent, 14–15
Athena, 5, 133, 227, 231, 328
avocado (*Persea gratissima*), 110

babassu butter (*Orbignya oleifera*), 163
Bailey, Alice, 45–46
balance, 67, 102, 109, 113, 127, 183
bamboo, 173–74
banana (*Musa paradisiaca*), 150–51, 223
basil, sweet (*Ocimum basilicum*), 86
beard, 237–41
beauty, 340–41
benzoin resin (*Styrax benzoin*), 13–20
bergamot (*Citrus bergamia*), 86–87
birch bark writing, 105
blackberry seed (*Rubus fruiticosus*), 110–11
black currant (*Ribes nigrum*), 20–23
black currant seed (*Ribes nigrum*), 111
black pepper (*Piper nigrum*), 87
blending
  art, 281–93
  exercises, 264–65, 300–301
  focus when creating, 309–10
  folk tales, 293–308
  poetry, 269–81
  principles, 263–64
blending tips
  aglaia, 13
  anisotropy, 283

benzoin resin, 20
black currant, 21–23
broom, 78
brown boronia, 27
carnation, 31
cyclamen, 33
damask rose, 36
elderflower, 38
fig seed oil, 125
frankincense, 40
gardenia, 45
goji berry seed, 126
grapefruit essential oil, 92
guava seed, 127–28
hyacinth, 47
jasmine essential oil, 93
jojoba, 128
juhi (jasmine), 49
kiwi seed, 129
labdanum, 52
lilac, 55
lily, 56
magnolia, 57
myrrh, 59
narcissus, 65
oak wood, 67
oat, 132
orris root, 72
peach kernel, 136
pineapple seed, 136
pistachio nut, 137
plum kernel, 137
prickly pear seed, 139
pumpkin seed oil, 140
Redmond Real salt, 176
safflower oil, 142
sel gris salt, 176
Siberian fir, 76
song, 329–31
spinach, 82
sunflower oil, 146
sweetgrass, 83
violet, 84
white rose, 73
blends
  air element, 199–200
  arms, 251–52
  beard, 239–41
  body butters, 320–28
  ear, 236–37
  ether element, 204
  fire element, 193–95
  galvanizing, 265
  hair, 224–25
  Handless Maiden, 301–2
  hands and fingers, 254–55
  heart opening, 340
  legs and feet, 257, 258–59
  library of sense memories, 267
  lip butter, 312–18
  milk bath, 156–57, 159, 160, 162, 328–29
  Mindfulness Bath, 338
  naming, 328
  neck and throat, 243–44
  painting-inspired, 285, 286–87
  place, 331–35
  poems to inspire, 273–81
  poetry, 271, 273
  purification, 342, 347
  Rapunzel-inspired, 307–8
  salt scrub, 328–29
  scent of childhood, 268–69
  skin, 227–28
  spine, 249
  water element, 189–90
blood orange (*Citrus sinensis*), 87–88
blue (color), 111–12

blueberry seed (*Vaccinium corymbosum*), 111–13
blue chamomile (*Matricaria chamomilla*), 88
body, the
　about, 219–20
　arms, 250–52
　beard, 237–41
　brain and head, 228–34
　ears, 234–37
　embodied self and, 23–27
　hair, 220–25
　hands and fingers, 252–55
　legs and feet, 255–59
　neck and throat, 241–44
　skin, 225–28
　spine, 245–49
body butters
　blends, 320–28
　morality stories, 318–28
　preparation guide, 318–19
Bolen, Jean Shinoda, 67, 145
borage (*Borago officinalis*), 113, 223
botanical extractions, 9–12
brain and head, 228–34
broccoli seed (*Brassica oleracea* var. *italica*), 113–14
Broken Eggs (Greuze), 288–89
brown boronia (*Boronia megastigma*), 23–27, 184, 227
buriti (*Mauritia flexuosa*), 114–15
butters
　body, 318–28
　lip, 310–18
　plant, 163–66

cabbage seed, red (*Brassica oleracea* var. *rubra*), 115
camel's milk, 156–57, 338–39
cantaloupe seed (*Cucumis melo*), 115–16
cardamom (*Elettaria cardamomum*), 88
carnation (*Dianthus caryophyllus*), 27–31
carrier oils. *See* fixed oils
cashew nut (*Anacardium occidentale*), 116
cedar (*Thuja occidentalis*), 89
chakras
　about, 205–7
　crown: sahasrara, 217–18
　depiction of, 207
　heart: anahata, 213–15
　opening, with plant allies, 207–8
　root: muladhara, 208–9
　sacral: svadhishthana, 209–11
　solar plexus: manipura, 211–13
　third eye: ajna, 216–17
　throat: vishuddha, 215–16, 242
cherry kernel (*Prunus avium*), 116–17, 227
chia seed (*Salvia hispanica*), 117
Chinese perfume tree, 12
cinnamon leaf (*Cinnamomum zeylanicum*), 89–90
circle, 198
citron, Buddha's hand (*Citrus medica*), 90
clary sage (*Salvia sclarea*), 90–91, 223
cloudberry seed (*Rubus chamaemorus*), 117–18
cocoa butter (*Theobroma cacao*), 164
coconut (*Cocos nucifera*) oil, 107–8, 118–19, 184–85, 223
coevolution, 41
cold expression, 11–12
collective unconscious, 22, 156, 187, 190, 194, 210–11
corn (*Zea mays*), 119
cosmic egg (oval), 203

cosmic library, 266–67
cow's milk, 157–58
cranberry seed (*Vaccinium macrocarpon*), 119–20
cranberry seed, arctic (*Oxycoccus palustris*), 120
craniosacral therapy, 246
crown chakra: sahasrara, 217–18
cube, 167
cucumber seed (*Cucumis sativus*), 120–22, 223
cyclamen (*Cyclamen europaeum*), 31–33
Cyprus flake salt, 169

daikon radish seed (*Raphanus sativus*), 123
daisy (*Bellis perennis*), 151
Dalai Lama, 8–9, 50
damask rose, pink (*Rosa damascena*), 33–36
Dante, 75
dark forest, 73–76
date (*Balanites aegyptiaca*), 123–24
de Chardin, Pierre Teilhard, 69
detachment, 95, 98, 112, 245
Diana and Actaeon (Corot), 291–92
divine feminine, 67, 104, 187, 203, 292, 342–44, 346
divine inspiration, 37, 128
divine masculine, 203, 343, 346
dragon fruit seed (*Hylocereus undatus*), 124
Dream of the Shepherd, The (Hodler), 290–91
dreams
  air and, 195–96, 198
  black currant bud and, 21–22
  fire and, 190–91

journeying to underworld and, 19–20
oceanic realm and, 211
portal to, 174
vision, 164
water and, 187, 190
writing down, 19

ears, 234–37
earth element. *See also* elements
  about, 180–81
  physical gate, 181–82
  plant pairings, 182–85
  sacred shape, 182
ego, 60–61, 63
Einstein, Albert, 40–41
elderflower (*Sambucus nigra* ssp. *caerulea*), 36–38
elements
  about, 178–80
  air, 195–200
  earth, 180–85
  ether, 201–4
  fire, 190–95
  water, 185–90
elemi (*Canarium luzonicum*), 91
embodiment, 23–27
emotions
  ether and, 46
  integrating, 90–91
  scent and, 5
  spiritualizing, 134
  water and, 61
empowerment, 131, 196, 347
endurance and perseverance, 118
enlightenment, 101, 102, 106, 154, 218, 290, 345
epiphany, 31, 33, 41, 198
Ereshkigal, 13, 16–17

essential oils
  about, 85–86
  aromatherapy with, 231
  basil, 86
  bergamot, 86–87
  black pepper, 87
  blood orange, 87–88
  cardamom, 88
  cedar, 89
  chakras and, 207, 208, 210, 212, 213, 215, 216, 217
  chamomile, 88
  cinnamon, 89–90
  citron, 90
  clary sage, 90–91
  current focus of, ix
  elemi, 91
  frankincense, 91–92
  grapefruit, 92
  heat sensitive, 11–12
  jasmine, 93
  kumquat, 93
  lavender, 94
  lemon, 94–95
  as lighter than water, 11
  lime, 95
  mandarin orange, 95
  marjoram, 96
  neroli, 97
  oakmoss, 97
  orange, 97
  patchouli, 98
  peppermint, 98–99
  petitgrain, 99
  pine, 100
  pink pepper seed, 100
  pomelo, 100–101
  rosemary, 102
  sandalwood, 102–3
  spikenard, 101
  steam distillation, 10–11
  tangerine, 103
  vanilla, 103
  vetiver, 103–4
  white birch, 104
  white lotus, 106
ether element. *See also* elements
  about, 46–47, 201
  emotions and, 46
  physical gate, 202–3
  plant pairings, 203–4
  sacred shape, 203
expeller-pressed oils, 12

fears, addressing, 95
feminine principle, 15, 55, 57, 67, 104, 163, 188, 201, 248
fig seed (*Ficus carica*), 124–25
fire element. *See also* elements
  about, 190–92
  physical gate, 192
  plant pairings, 193–95
  in purification practices, 342–45
  sacred shape, 192–93
fixed oils. *See also specific fixed oils*
  about, 107
  blending absolutes with, 10
  chakras and, 207, 208, 210, 212, 213, 215, 216, 217
  as expeller pressed, 12
  in macerated oil creation, 150
  in milk baths, 155
  in plant butters, 163–65
fleur de sel, 169–70
flow, staying in, 98
folk tales, blending, 293–308
food body, 27
forest, 73–76

fractionated coconut oil, 107–8, 140, 223
frankincense (*Boswellia carterii*), 91–92
frankincense (*Boswellia sacra*), 38–40, 92, 232
full moon, 57

gardenia (*Gardenia jasminoides*), 40–45
gardening, 30–31
gates (senses)
    about, 179
    sight, 192
    smell, 181–82
    sound, 202
    taste, 185–86
    touch, 197–98
Gayatri mantra practice, 345–48
ginkgo (*Ginkgo biloba*), 151–52
goat's milk, 158–59
goji berry seed (*Lycium barbarum*), 126
grapefruit (*Citrus paradisi*), 92
grapeseed (*Vitis vinifera*), 126–27
Great Below, 17–18
Great Salt Lake salt, 170
green (color), 78–80
grounding, 101, 103, 119, 128, 183, 185, 206–8, 255, 265
guava seed (*Psidium guajava*), 127–28

Hageneder, Fred, 66–67
hair, 220–25
Handless Maiden, The (Brothers Grimm), 293–302
hands and fingers, 252–55
harmonization, 94, 110, 206, 214
heart chakra: anahata, 80–81, 86, 213–15
heart healing, x, 100
heart opening, 136, 339–40

Heilmeyer, Marina, 28
hemp seed butter (*Cannabis sativa*), 164
Himalayan pink salt, 171, 339
hippocampus, 233
hyacinth (*Hyacinthus orientalis*), 45–47, 227
hydrosols, 310
hygge, 96
hypothalamus, 232–33

Icelandic birch-smoked sea salt, 171–72
Inanna, 13, 15–17, 18, 19
infused oils. *See* macerated oils
inherent self, 26
inner sun, 49–52
interconnectedness and wholeness, 89
irony, 263

Japanese Shinkai deep sea salt, 172–73
jasmine (*Jasminum grandiflorum*), 93
jojoba, golden (*Simmondsia chinensis*), 128
jugyeom bamboo salt, 173–74
juhi, jasmine (*Jasminum auriculatum*), 47–49
Jung, Carl, 56, 210–11, 281–82

Kilauea onyx sea salt, 174
Kindness Prevails, 325–26
kiwi seed (*Actinidia chinensis*), 128–29, 271
kokum butter, 164–65
kumquat (*Fortunella japonica*), 93

labdanum (*Cistus ladaniferus*), 49–52
Lao Tzu, 161
lavender (*Lavandula officinalis*), 94, 227, 232

lemon (*Citrus limon*), 94–95, 232
lilac (*Syringa vulgaris*), 52–55, 266, 340
lily (*Lilium candidum*), 55–56
lime (*Citrus aurantiifolia*), 95
liminal space, 22–23
lip butters
  blends, 312–18
  poetry, 310–18
  preparation guide, 311
love, 33, 34–36

macadamia butter, 165
macerated oils
  about, 150
  banana, 150–51
  daisy, 151
  ginkgo, 151–52
  making, 150
  orchid, 152–53
  saffron, 153, 154
magenta lilac, 54, 55
magnolia (*Magnolia champaca*), 57
mandarin orange (*Citrus reticulata*), 95
mango kernel (*Mangifera indica*), 129
mango seed butter, 165
manipura (solar plexus), 50, 51, 211–13
marjoram (*Origanum majorana*), 96
Mars, 13, 39, 66, 80, 282, 286–87
Mars and Venus United by Love (Veronese), 286–87
masculine principle, 15, 49–50, 55, 66–67, 175, 201, 212
meditation and prayer, 40, 83, 102
metaphor, 4, 264
microbiome, 203–4
milk baths
  about, 155–56
  blends, 328–29
  camel's milk, 156–57
  cow's milk, 157–58
  goat's milk, 158–59
  history of, 155
  sheep's milk, 159–61
  water buffalo's milk, 161–62
  yak's milk, 162
milk thistle (*Silybum marianum*), 129–31
Mindfulness Bath, 208, 336–39
mind-spirit connection, x, 91
mind support, 40, 80, 86, 90, 93, 113, 126, 151
Molokai red sea salt, 175
moon, the, 27, 29–31, 57, 186–87
morality stories, 318–28
muladhara (sacral chakra), 208–9
myrrh (*Commiphora myrrha*), 57–59, 227
myths and folklore, xi, 5, 60–65

nadis, 206. *See also* chakras
narcissus (*Narcissus poeticus*), 60–65
Narcissus myth, 60–65
nature
  awareness of, 6
  fauvism, 142–43
  as feminine principle, 55
  knowing, 40
  mutualism in, 125
  scent and, 5
  as storyteller, 4
Necessity Is the Mother of Invention, 322–23
neck and throat, 241–44
Negligent Milkmaid, The, 327
neroli (*Citrus aurantium*), 97, 186
nonlocal consciousness, 201, 203, 230
numerology, 343

oakmoss (*Evernia prunastri*), 97
oak wood (*Quercus robur*), 66–67
oat (*Avena sativa*), 131–32
okra seed (*Abelmoschus esculentus*), 132
olive (*Olea europaea*), 133–34, 166
onion (*Allium cepa*), 134
openness, cultivating, 37
oracles, 36–37
orange, common (*Citrus sinensis*), 97–98, 232
orchid (*Anacamptis morio*), 152–53, 340–41
orris root (*Iris pallida*, *Iris florentina*), 68–72
Ovid, 58, 60, 211

papaya seed (*Carica papaya*), 134–35
passion fruit seed (*Passiflora edulis*), 135
patchouli (*Pogostemon cablin*), 98
peach kernel (*Prunus persica*), 135–36, 188, 271
peppermint (*Mentha piperita*), 98–99
personal power, 51, 102, 143, 145, 212, 302
petitgrain (*Citrus aurantium*), 99, 223
pine (*Pinus sylvestris*), 100, 223
pineal gland, 233–34
pineapple seed (*Ananas comosus*), 136
pink pepper seed (*Schinus molle*), 100
pistachio nut (*Pistacia vera*), 136–37
place blends, 331–35
plant butters, 163–66
plant communication, 202–3
plant distillations, use of, 6, 9, 271
planting, 30, 43–44
plant resonances
    arms, 251–52
    beard, 239–41
    brain and head, 231–34
    ear, 236–37
    hair, 223
    hands and fingers, 254–55
    legs and feet, 256–59
    neck and throat, 243–44
    skin, 226–27
    spine, 248–49
plum kernel (*Prunus domestica*), 137
poetry
    blending and, 269–81
    blends, 271, 273
    to inspire blends, 273–81
    lip butters, 310–18
Pollan, Michael, 41–42
pomegranate seed (*Punica granatum*), 137–38
pomelo (*Citrus grandis*, *Citrus maxima*), 100–101
poppy seed (*Papaver somniferum*), 139
prakriti, 26, 48
pranayama, 214
prayer, 40, 83
prickly pear seed (*Opuntia ficus-indica*), 139
Prideful Rose, The, 324–25
psychoid space, 70
pumpkin seed (*Cucurbita pepo*), 140
purification practices, 342–48
pyramid, 167, 169, 171–72

quinoa (*Chenopodium quinoa*), 140–41

Ra (sun god), 57, 58
Rapunzel (Brothers Grimm), 302–8
raspberry seed (*Rubus idaeus*), 141
Redmond Real salt, 175–76
red spikenard (*Nardostachys jatamansi*), 101

reflexology, 256, 257–58
relationship, love, 33–36
resources, 349–50
root chakra: muladhara, 208–9
rosemary (*Rosmarinus officinalis*), 102, 232
rose otto, white (*Rosa alba*), 72–73

sacral chakra: svadhishthana, 209–11
sacred shapes
  about, 180
  circle, 198
  crescent moon, 186–87
  oval (cosmic egg), 203
  square, 182
  triangle, 192–93
safflower (*Carthamus tinctorius*), 141–42
saffron (*Crocus sativus*), 153, 154, 270
salts
  about, 166–68
  baths, 168
  crystal shapes of, 166–67
  Cyprus flake salt, 169
  fleur de sel, 169–70
  Great Salt Lake salt, 170
  Himalayan pink salt, 171
  Icelandic birch-smoked sea salt, 171–72
  Japanese Shinkai deep sea salt, 172–73
  jugyeom bamboo salt, 173–74
  Kilauea onyx sea salt, 174
  Molokai red sea salt, 175
  Redmond Real salt, 175–76
  sel gris salt, 176
salt scrubs, 328–29
sandalwood (*Santalum album*), 102–3
Satisfaction of Longing, The, 160–61

Saturn, 147–48, 284–85
Saturn Devouring His Son (Goya), 284
scent, 5, 39, 85, 181
scent of childhood, 267–69
self-containment, 98
self-knowledge, 62, 64–65, 211
self-love, 34, 60, 82, 137, 174
self-sufficiency, 117
sel gris salt, 176
senses. *See* gates
shea butter (*Vitellaria paradoxa*), 166
sheep's milk, 159–61
Siberian fir (*Abies sibirica*), 73–76, 183
sight, 192
silence, 195
simile, 264
skin, 225–28
smell, 181–82
solar plexus chakra: manipura, 211–13
solvent extraction, 9–10
song blends, 329–31
Son of Man, The (Magritte), 2–3
Soul Mates, 319–20
sound, 202
Spanish broom (*Spartium junceum*), 76–78
spinach (*Spinacia oleracea*), 78–82
spine, 245–49
spirituality
  exploring with your beloved, 35
  neroli and, 97
  red spikenard and, 101
  sensuality and, 154
square, 182
starflower. *See* borage (*Borago officinalis*)
steam distillation, 9–11
Strange Thing Little Kiosai Saw in the River, The (La Farge), 289–90

strawberry seed (*Fragaria ananassa*), 142–43
sun, 38, 39–40, 87, 144–45
sunflower seed (*Helianthus annuus*) oil, 143–46, 193
svadhishthana (sacral chakra), 209–11
sweetgrass (*Hierochloe odorata*), 82–83
symbolism, 47, 239, 253, 275, 289

tangerine (*Citrus tangerina*), 103
tanmatras, 188
taste, 185–86
Think Before You Act, 323–24
Think Before You Speak, 321–22
third eye: ajna, 216–17
thresholds, 20, 76–77
throat chakra: vishuddha, 215–16, 242
Time for Work and a Time for Play, A, 320–21
tomato seed (*Solanum lycopersicum*), 146
touch, 197–98
trapezoid, 167
trataka, 193
Tree of Life, 114, 179, 245, 246–48, 249
triangle, 192–93
twilight, 20, 21–23

underworld, 14, 16–17, 19, 138, 285
unrefined salts. *See* salts

vanilla (*Vanilla planifolia*), 103
Vedas, 25–26, 50–51, 187
Venus, 13, 39, 72, 80, 227, 282, 286–87

Veteran in a New Field (Homer), 287–88
vetiver (*Vetiveria zizanioides*), 103–4
vibrational fields, 26, 234
Vibrational Nutrition, 44, 81–82, 143, 302
violet leaf (*Viola odorata*), 83–84
violet lilac, 54
Virgin Mary, 28, 72
vishuddha (throat chakra), 242

water buffalo's milk, 161–62
water element
  about, 61, 185
  emotions and, 61
  energy of, 63–65, 187–88
  moon and, 186–87
  physical gate, 185–86
  plant pairings, 187–88
  sacred shape, 186–87
watermelon seed (*Citrullus vulgaris*), 146–47, 223
Watson and the Shark (Copley), 292–93
wheat germ (*Triticum aestivum*), 147, 227
white birch (*Betula lenta*), 104, 342, 343
white lilac, 54, 340
white lotus (*Nelumbo nucifera*), 106, 291
Wise Woman archetype, 76–78

yak's milk, 162

Zeus, 66–67, 137–38

About the Author

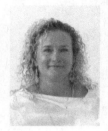

Candice Covington is a certified aromatherapist, massage therapist, healing arts master, and energy worker. A former instructor at Ashmead College and former aromatherapist for the Chopra Center, she is the founder of Divine Archetypes, an essential oil and flower essence company: **DivineArchetypes.org**.

Other Books by Candice Covington

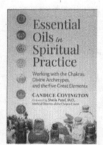

Essential Oils in Spiritual Practice
Candice Covington details how to use essential oils energetically to affect the *tattvas*, the elemental energies behind your unique personal characteristics. She provides energetic profiles of each tattva, chakra, and essential oil, explains their relationships to one another, and details how to craft your own ritual practice with essential oils.

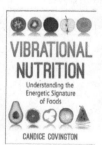

Vibrational Nutrition
In this hands-on guide, Candice Covington explores the vibrational signatures of the foods we eat and how they influence our behaviors and spirit. She details the energetic and spiritual qualities of more than 400 common foods, drinks, and seasonings. She also includes recipes with their energetic interpretations.